# *Outlines of*
# Meat Science and Technology

# *Outlines of* Meat Science and Technology

**Second Edition**

**BD Sharma** MVSc PhD
Ex–Principal-Scientist and Head
Division of Livestock Products Technology
Indian Veterinary Research Institute
Izatnagar, Uttar Pradesh, India

**Kinshuki Sharma** MSc MPhil PhD
Ex-Assistant Professor
IMS Engineering College
Ghaziabad, Uttar Pradesh, India

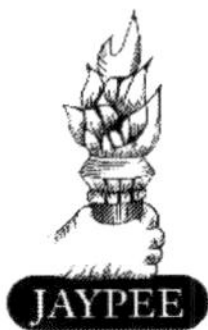


JAYPEE BROTHERS MEDICAL PUBLISHERS
*The Health Sciences Publisher*
New Delhi | London

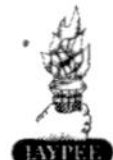

**Jaypee Brothers Medical Publishers (P) Ltd**

**Headquarters**
EMCA House
23/23-B, Ansari Road, Daryaganj
New Delhi - 110 002, India
Landline: +91-11-23272143, +91-11-23272703
+91-11-23282021, +91-11-23245672
E-mail: jaypee@jaypeebrothers.com

**Corporate Office**
4838/24, Ansari Road, Daryaganj
New Delhi 110 002, India
Phone: +91-11-43574357
Fax: +91-11-43574314
E-mail: jaypee@jaypeebrothers.com

**Overseas Office**
J.P. Medical Ltd
83 Victoria Street, London
SW1H 0HW (UK)
Phone: +44 20 3170 8910
E-mail: info@jpmedpub.com

**EU GPSR** Authorised Representative
Logos Europe, 9 rue Nicolas Poussin
17000, La Rochelle, France
Phone: +33 (0) 6 67 93 73 78
E-mail: contact@logoseurope.eu

Website: www.jaypeebrothers.com
Website: www.jaypeedigital.com



**Inquiries for bulk sales may be solicited at:** jaypee@jaypeebrothers.com

***Outlines of Meat Science and Technology***

First Edition: 2011
Second Edition: 2024
*Reprint:* **2026**

ISBN: 978-93-5696-298-9

*Printed in India*

**Dedicated to**

The young members of the profession

# Preface to the Second Edition

First edition of this book received a very good response from students and faculty members throughout the country. Meanwhile, syllabus has been revised at graduate and post graduate level. So, the earlier chapters required to be oriented and updated accordingly. Fresh chapters were needed to be added to incorporate new developments. The suggestions received from faculty and post graduate students for the betterment have also been taken care of in the second edition. Still, the book deals with the subject of meat science and technology in a systematic, concise, and yet comprehensive manner. Due weightage has been given to fresh meat technology, processed meat technology, poultry products technology, fish technology and quality control systems. Recent developments in packaging and sensory evaluation of muscle foods have also been incorporated.

I thank Dr SK Mendiratta (IVRI), Dr Manish Chatli (CIRG), Dr Nitin Mehta (Ludhiana), Dr SP Suman (Kentucky, USA), Dr Sunil Kumar (Jammu), Dr Vikas Pathak (Mathura), Dr UK Pal, Dr PK Mandal (Pondicherry), Dr AR Sen, Dr Prince (IVRI), Dr Girish Patil, Dr BM Naveena (Hyderabad), Dr Vinita Puranik (Allahabad), Dr Rajiv Ranjan (IVRI), Dr Bandu Mane (Palampur), Dr Anurag Pandey (Jaipur), Dr Arun Soni (Udaipur) and Dr M Irshad (Kerala) for their suggestions from time to time.

I hope second edition of the book will also receive a very good response from the students along with patronage of the faculty of Livestock Products Technology.

**BD Sharma**
**Kinshuki Sharma**

# Preface to the First Edition

My earlier books on the subject received an overwhelming response from the students and academicians. More than half of the veterinary students hail from vegetarian families and they have very little exposure to meat as such. The book deals with the science of meat and meat products in a systematic, concise, and yet comprehensive manner. The basic and emerging concepts in fresh meat technology, processed meat technology, and quality control systems have been incorporated in right earnest. Due importance has been given to the poultry and fish products technology in order to have an integrated approach in a single volume. The book is primarily designed as per new syllabus of Veterinary Council of India. The book will be useful to undergraduate students specializing in veterinary science, food science and technology, postgraduate students and research fellows in concerned specializations at the university level. This volume will serve as a handbook for meat plant managers, quality control supervisors and processing technicians at the industry level.

This book could not have been written but for the inspiration provided by Dr SPS Ahlawat, Director, Indian Veterinary Research Institute (IVRI), Izatnagar, Uttar Pradesh, India who constantly encourages his scientists to do their best in research, teaching and extension. We have been fortunate enough in having the benefit of the advice of leading meat professionals especially Dr N Sharma, Dr Sushil Kumar and Dr N Kondaiah. Besides, cooperation extended by Dr R Somvanshi, Dr JS Berwal, Dr VK Rao and Dr VV Kulkarni has been a big help. We take this opportunity to thankfully acknowledge the help rendered by Shri Ashish Kumar Saxena for giving special effects in figures and photographs.

We shall be satisfied if this book serves the intended purpose. There is no limit for the betterment and in that spirit, suggestions extended by senior professionals and colleagues for the improvement of the book will be highly appreciated.

**BD Sharma**
**Kinshuki Sharma**

# Contents

# 1 CHAPTER

# Indian Meat Industry

## LIVESTOCK RESOURCE

India has the largest livestock population in the world. There are 192.4 million cattle, 109.8 million buffaloes, 74.2 million sheep, 148.8 million goats and 9 million pigs and 851.8 million chickens in the country (Indian Livestock Census, 2019). Livestock sector is an important contributor to the income and employment of large number of rural people of India. This sector contributes 4.11% of the national GDP. Further, the share of livestock sector is as much as 25.6% of the total share of agricultural GDP, which is poised to increase further.

Our country shares about 55% of the buffaloes, nearly 18% of cattle and 14% goat population of the world. India ranks first in buffalo, second in goat and third in sheep population in the world. National sample survey has reported that in India livestock activities are carried out by over 90% of small cultivators and low wage earners to supplement their income. This is in contrast to the concept of large sized livestock farms in the developed countries. It is also noteworthy that 75% of our livestock population does not conform to the specific breed characteristics and has significantly reduced their production potential.

For a long time, meat industry has remained confined to a very small section of people in our country. These people had little knowledge of clean meat production and effective utilization of valued slaughterhouse byproducts. The scene is now changing. However, industry is still largely based on spent animals except for pig and farm poultry. Most animals are utilized for meat production after loosing their economic viability in the primary field. Cow (not bullock) slaughter is banned in India except in West Bengal and Kerala. The concept of meat type animals is yet to take roots in our country, although an awakening in this regard is discernible. Of late, particularly due to export potential, buffalo is emerging as a prospective meat animal and is being referred as 'Black Gold of India'. Buffalo meat is now being exported to more than 60 countries.

Meat industry provides direct and indirect employment to nearly 2.5 crore people at present. Presently, meat and meat products account for about 20% of the income from entire livestock sector.

## MEAT PRODUCTION

Meat is an important livestock product, which in its widest sense includes all those parts of the animals that are used as a food by man. Though meat has a very high biological value, its production and processing has always been the subject of social prejudice. This factor has adversely affected the growth of meat industry. In many cases, social resistance and ignorance have resulted in inordinate delay and deferment of abattoir modernization schemes. An important milestone in this area was the establishment of a modem abattoir at Bombay in 1973. Further, in the Fourth Five Year Plan, eight bacon factories were established with the foreign assistance. A few meat corporations were also formed to take up the development of slaughterhouses.

**Tables 1.1 and 1.4** show the population, slaughter rate and meat production figures of our traditional meat species annually yielding 8.6 million tonnes of meat. It may be noted that poultry with a population of 851 million contributes 4.3 million tonnes of meat (50% of total meat production). It has become possible because of an impressive rise in the share of poultry meat during the last decade **(Table 1.2 and Fig. 1.1)**. Nearly 22% meat production is contributed by sheep and goats whereas cattle and buffaloes contribute about 23%. An entire

**Table 1.1:** Livestock and poultry population in India.

| *Species* | *Population (million)* | *Share in the world (%)* | *Rank* | *Top ranks* |
|---|---|---|---|---|
| Cattle | 192.4 | 18 | I | India, Brazil, China |
| Buffalo | 109.8 | 55 | I | India, Pakistan, China |
| Sheep | 74.2 | 6 | III | China, Australia, India |
| Goat | 148.8 | 14 | II | China, India, Pakistan |
| Pig | 9.0 | 1.2 | — | China, USA, Brazil |
| Poultry | 851.8 | 3.2 | V | China, USA, Indonesia, Brazil, India |

*Source:* 20th Livestock Census, 2019 and FAO.

**Table 1.2:** Livestock and poultry population: 2012–2019—changing pattern in India.

| *Species* | *2012 (million)* | *2019 (million)* | *Change (%)* |
|---|---|---|---|
| Cattle | 190.90 | 192.49 | 0.8 |
| Buffalo | 168.70 | 109.85 | 1.0 |
| Sheep | 65.7 | 74.26 | 14.1 |
| Goat | 135.17 | 148.88 | 10.1 |
| Pig | 10.29 | 9.06 | -12.0 |
| Poultry | 692.6 | 851.8 | 16.8 |

*Source:* 19th Livestock Census (2012) and 20th Livestock Census (2019), Govt. of India.

**Table 1.3:** Production of major livestock and poultry products in India.

| *Products* | *Production 2019–20* | *Per capita availability* | *ICMR Recommendation* |
|---|---|---|---|
| Milk (million tonnes) | 198.4 | 395 g | 280 g/day |
| Meat (million tonnes) | 8.6 | — | 11 kg/year |
| Wool (million kg) | 36.7 | — | — |
| Eggs (million numbers) | 1,14,383 | 80 eggs/year | 182 eggs/year |

*Source:* DAHD, Annual Report 2020–21.

**Table 1.4:** Food animal population, slaughter and meat production (2019).

| *Species* | *Population (million)* | *Slaughter rate (%)* | *Meat production (million tonnes)* | *Share in meat production (%)* | *Average carcass weight (kg)* |
|---|---|---|---|---|---|
| Cattle | 192.4 | 1.5 | 0.34 | 4.0 | 103 |
| Buffalo | 109.8 | 10.8 | 1.64 | 19.1 | 138 |
| Sheep | 74.2 | 68.4 | 0.72 | 8.4 | 12 |
| Goat | 148.8 | 65.2 | 1.15 | 13.4 | 10 |
| Pig | 9.0 | 112.4 | 0.43 | 4.9 | 31 |
| Poultry | 851.8 | 330.2 | 4.32 | 50.2 | 0.45 |

*Source:* BAHS-2019, FAO-2019.

equivalent pig population is slaughtered annually contributing about 5% of the total meat production. **Table 1.3** depicts the production of major livestock and poultry products in India.

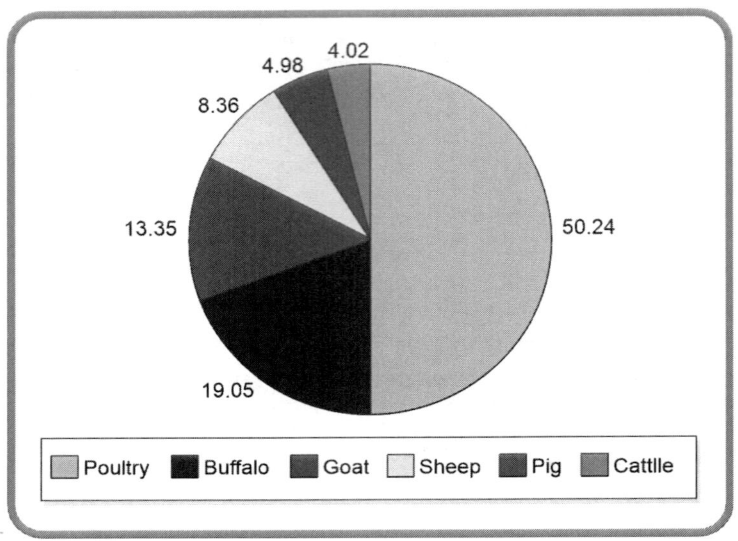


**Fig. 1.1:** Share of meat species in meat production in India.

The traditional form of meat industry is characterized by unorganized sector in the hands of butcher-workers with very little knowledge of personnel hygiene. At present, there are 3600 licensed slaughterhouses in the country. A large number of them are outdated and substandard according to the present production and processing technology specifications. These slaughterhouses operate as service abattoirs where butchers slaughter the animals for a fee and both edible and non-edible parts of the carcasses are delivered to the butchers. Most of them need modernization with facilities for lairage, slaughter hall, chilling room, rendering plant, etc. While it is imperative to have all these facilities in big cities, a semi-modern approach with mechanical hoist facility is the workable proposition for medium and small sized towns.

Eight new projects on modern mechanized abattoirs were initiated in 1990–91. In the next decade, five private sector export abattoirs became functional and ten modern abattoir complexes came up in public sector. Presently, there are as many as 77 APEDA approved integrated abattoirs-cum-meat processing plants and standalone abattoirs in the country. In the retail sector, more than 25,000 small scale retail meat shops are functional. The developmental activities are necessary to improve the image of the Indian meat sector.

## WORLD SCENE

Meat industry, although in a very developing stage in India is the top food industry in the world. An analysis of world meat scenario reveals that Europe leads in production followed by Asia. Developed continents (N. America, Europe and Oceania) contribute about 40% to total meat production but their share in meat exports is as high as 60%. Nearly 25% of all world meat exports are being shared by European countries alone. The share of Asia in world meat export is only 12% but it is on the rise.

India ranks 6th in the world in meat production **(Table 1.5)**. It is disheartening to note that India with a vast raw material base, contributes barely 2.5% to the world meat production. Our share in the export of meat is also of the same magnitude. The export of meat from India mainly comprises of fresh chilled meat, frozen meat and frozen meat products. A major chunk of meat exports amounting to ₹ 23,400 crores is contributed by buffalo meat (2020–21). Hong Kong, Vietnam, Malaysia, Egypt, Indonesia and UAE are the principal importers of buffalo meat from India (**Table 1.6** and extension). However, Indian exports of meat constitutes barely 3.2% of global export of this commodity. A great potential exists for exporting buffalo meat, beef and poultry in view of increased demand in gulf countries and higher cost of meat from developed countries. India has additional advantage of geographic proximity to gulf countries. There is a need to tap more of the world meat export market by hygienic meat production and quality maintenance in the entire chain.

**Table 1.5:** Top meat producers and their share in world.

| | *Production ('000 tonnes)* | | *Share in world* | |
|---|---|---|---|---|
| *Countries* | *2004* | *2020* | *2004* | *2020* |
| China | 74306 | 88156 | 28.5 | 29.6 |
| USA | 38891 | 63845 | 14.9 | 21.4 |
| Brazil | 19919 | 46341 | 7.6 | 15.5 |
| Russia | ** | 10629 | ** | 3.5 |
| Germany | 6798 | 8118 | 2.7 | 2.7 |
| India | 6032 | 7454 | 2.3 | 2.5 |
| Mexico | ** | 7051 | ** | 2.3 |
| Spain | ** | 7028 | ** | 2.3 |

Compiled from different sources ** Not among top ten

**Table 1.6:** Export of livestock and poultry products from India (2020–21).

| *Products* | *Quantity (tonnes)* | *Values (₹ in crores)* |
|---|---|---|
| Buffalo meat | 1085619 | 23400 |
| Sheep/Goat meat | 7050 | 330 |
| Poultry products | 255686 | 435 |
| Dairy products | 54693 | 1490 |
| Animal casings | 13887 | 416 |
| Processed meat | 774 | 12 |
| Other meats | 896 | 18 |

If the quality of Indian meat is strictly controlled, the country may boost its meat exports by selling to developing Asian, African and Latin American countries, that import about 25% of the world meat exports. These measures will also help in fetching better prices for our produce which is nearly 30% lower than the average world meat export price.

### Major Export Destinations

- *Buffalo meat:* Hong Kong, Vietnam, Malaysia, Egypt, Bangladesh, UAE, Indonesia, Saudi Arabia, Jordan, Oman
- *Sheep/Goat meat:* UAE, Qatar, Kuwait, Saudi Arabia, Oman, Bahrain, Maldives, UK
- *Processed meat:* Hong Kong, Qatar, Jordan, Russia, Oman, Seychelles, Bahrain, Singapore
- *Poultry products:* Oman, Maldives, Indonesia, Vietnam, Russia, Bangladesh, UAE, Saudi Arabia, Maldives, Japan, Philippines
- *Animal Casings:* Hong Kong, Vietnam, Malaysia, Myanmar, Italy, Spain

## PROCESSED MEAT INDUSTRY

Most of the meat produced in the country is sold by the retail butcher shops to the consumers as fresh hot meat (unchilled). This meat is then cooked in the households in many different ways depending on their taste and preferences. A very small proportion—less than 3% is sold as processed meat and nearly 8% as processed poultry products. The production of processed meat products in the organized sector got a fillip with the establishment of bacon factories in the Fourth Plan. These bacon factories stimulated the establishment of many processing units in those areas. There were 270 licensed manufacturers under MFPO (1973) producing about 30,000 tonnes of processed meat before it got merged in Food Safety and Standard Authority of India (2006). Our processing figures are far less than developed countries where 65 to 80% of the total meat produced is sold in the processed form. Lately, however, Indian dynamics is changing in favor of processed meat products especially in metropolis and big cities.

A look at the utilization pattern of meat in India will reveal that almost 90% of the meat is hot processed at home as per traditional methods. Nearly 8% of the production (mostly buffalo meat) is exported whereas only 2.2% is converted into value added meat products.

Several traditional meat products like meat kabab, chicken biryani, tandoori chicken, meat curry, etc., are popular in the non-vegetarian population for a long time. Some other foods products adopted in meat like meat samosa, meat tikka, meat kofta, meat pickle, etc., have been able to create an impact on the urban consumer. Various region-specific meat products like Nihari (Delhi), Goa sausage (Goa), Pork pickle (Himachal Pradesh), Yakini and Gustaba (Kashmir), Rapka (Arunachal Pradesh), etc., have good acceptability in their traditional consumers.

Western type meat products like cured ham, bacon, sausages, frankfurters, hot dog, meat patties, burgers, luncheon meat and loaves, liver paste, etc., have good demand in cities. Eight bacon factories, five meat corporations and a fairly good number of meat business operators in private sector have taken up the production of a wide range of these products. They are catering to the requirements of defence, restaurants and household consumers. Canned meat products are primarily being manufactured for defence supplies. These are now paving the way for retort pouched meat products in the domestic market. The prices of canned meats are comparatively high rendering them beyond the reach of common consumers, although their presence can be noticed in the departmental stores in the metropolitan cities. Retort pouched meat products are gaining popularity and have a shelf life of 3–6 months.

Animal protein consumption is lowest (11 g/capita/day) in India, lower than even the low income countries. This is mainly due to lower consumption of meat. ICMR has recommended per capita consumption of 11.0 kg meat and 183 eggs per year, whereas the present per capita consumption is only 5.0 kg meat and 80 eggs per annum **(Table 1.7)**. It points to the very high potential for growth of livestock and poultry sector in the country.

**Table 1.7:** Per capita consumption of livestock products (kg/year).

| *Country* | *Milk* | *Meat* | *Eggs* | *Fish* | *All* |
|---|---|---|---|---|---|
| India | 73.0 | 5.0 | 4.1 | 5.5 | 87.6 |
| Pakistan | 111.4 | 13.7 | 1.7 | 2.3 | 129.1 |
| Malaysia | 57.5 | 50.4 | 13.8 | 54.1 | 175.8 |
| USA | 254.9 | 120.0 | 13.3 | 21.7 | 408.3 |
| UK | 222.6 | 73.5 | 10.2 | 20.2 | 326.5 |
| Australia | 266.6 | 115.0 | 7.7 | 19.8 | 401.0 |
| Japan | 68.7 | 43.2 | 19.8 | 71.2 | 202.9 |
| Brazil | 109.8 | 58.6 | 7.6 | 5.9 | 181.9 |
| China | 7.4 | 38.6 | 12.9 | 18.3 | 77.2 |

Processed meat products are poised for continuous growth in the country. In big cities, there is an ever increasing demand for 'heat and serve' and 'ready to eat' convenience or fast foods. These are delicious, nutritious and if required, easy to carry home. The growth of fast food parlors and restaurants is attributed to the rapid urbanization, changing life styles and upwards in the number of women entering the outdoor work force. It may be pointed out that increase in consumption of value added processed meat products is closely linked with increase in disposable income and growth of urbanization. Thus convenience type meat products are going to have spectacular growth in the coming years. Due to nutritional awareness and liberal food habits of the newer generation, the adoption of western type products with indigenous flavor profiles is bound to take place at a rapid rate.

Processed convenience and value added meat and poultry products sector has a very good potential in the country due to:

- Increase in double income families
- Increase in disposable income
- Less time availability for cooking

At present India has a large population of over 300 million economically strong consumers having an adequate purchasing power for buying food, as a result of which the domestic demand for the livestock and poultry product is poised for rapid growth.

We must strive to export processed meat products rather than live animals and fresh meat. There is a need to study the consumption pattern of meat products in importing countries, so that we can tailor our products according to their requirements. A shift from primary products to value added products besides fetching more profits will decrease the transportation cost and generate more employment. It will also encourage more efficient utilization of meat byproducts.

## NATIONAL MEAT AND POULTRY PROCESSING BOARD (NMPPB)

Ministry of Food Processing Industries contemplated the establishment of National Meat and Poultry Processing Board for an integrated approach to the development of meat sector and drive the sector forward in a professional manner.

The NMPPB was formally launched in February, 2009, with the following objectives:

- Helping the meat industry to establish viable new/modern slaughterhouses, slaughterhouse byproducts plants.
- Set up quality control and analytical laboratories for meat and meat products.
- Promoting GMP (good manufacturing practices), HACCP (hazard analysis and critical control points) and ISO-9001 in meat production.
- Collaborating with others, like Ministries, Departments, NGOs and private sector for improving backward and forward linkages.
- Work as a Central! National hub to address all issues related to meat and poultry sector.

NMPPB functioned for about five years. Several activities were undertaken to achieve the desired objectives. About 100 training programs were organized for butures/meat plant workers covering all parts of the country and hygiene enhancing/safety kits were distributed to them. An extensive survey was conducted for bench marking of abattoirs. Some schemes were approved and work started to set up new abattoirs and modernization of existing abattoirs for various species, inclusive of committed liabilities in respect of 8 on-going projects of 11th plan. Thus NMPPB was to address issues related to production of hygienic, safe and wholesome meat and meat products. The board, which was to be an industry driven body, with provision of funding by the government for first three years, i.e., up to 2012–13, had to generate its own revenue. However, the board was unable to generate resources to continue its activities without government funding. It was, therefore, decided by the government to wind up the NMPPB.

2

CHAPTER

# Structure, Composition and Nutritive Value of Meat Tissues

Meat is predominantly composed of muscle tissue along with various types of connective tissue. The skeletal muscle is the principal muscle tissue in meat, although very little of smooth tissue is also present. The main connective tissue types are adipose tissue (fat), bone and connective tissue proper.

## STRUCTURE OF MUSCLE TISSUE

Animal musculature is mostly of mesodermal origin. There are more than 300 muscles in the animal body. These muscles constitute about 30–45% of the live weight or 35–60% of the carcass weight of meat animals. In addition to the skeletal muscle, which forms the bulk of meat, a little of smooth and cardiac muscles are also present in blood vessels and heart respectively. Smooth and cardiac muscles are involuntary in nature. Skeletal and cardiac muscles are sometimes referred as striated muscles due to their specific microscopic appearance.

### Skeletal Muscle and Associated Connective Tissue

In general, skeletal muscles are directly attached to the bones, although some attach indirectly via ligament, cartilage, fascia and skin. Each muscle is surrounded by a sheath of connective tissue known as epimysium **(Fig. 2.1)**. Inner surface of epimysium, a septa of connective tissue penetrates into muscle and surrounds the bundles of muscle fibers or fasciculi. This connective tissue is called perimysium. It contains major blood vessels and nerves. Muscle fibers or specialized muscle cells are the structural units of the skeletal muscle tissue. Each muscle fiber **(Fig. 2.2)** is surrounded by a connective tissue layer called endomysium, beneath which is delicate sarcolemma or

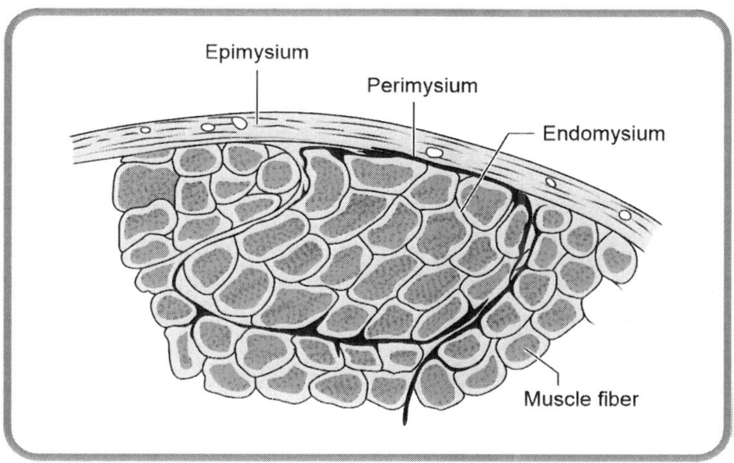


**Fig. 2.1:** Cross-section of a typical striated muscle depicting arrangement of connective tissue and muscle fiber.

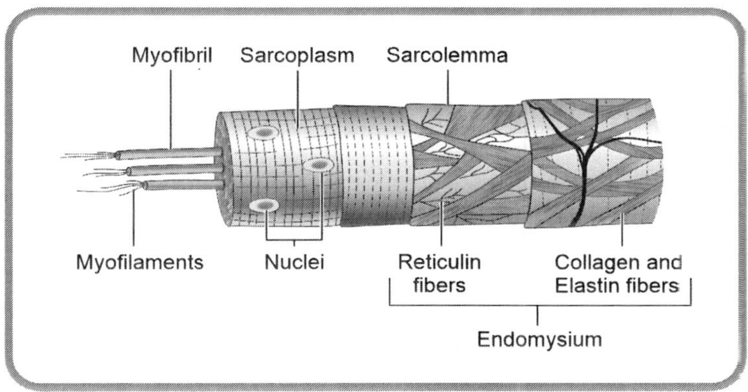


**Fig. 2.2:** Schematic diagram of a muscle fiber.

muscle cell membrane. It transmits nervous signals along the surface of muscle fiber.

*Skeletal muscle fibers* are long, narrow, almost tubular multinucleated cells which may extend from one end to the other end of the muscle **(Fig. 2.3)**. The nuclei are distributed peripherally close to the sarcolemma. Muscle fibers are usually 10–100 μ diameter with conical or tapering ends and their length ranges from 1–40 mm. The individual fiber may also be classified as red, intermediate and white. Most

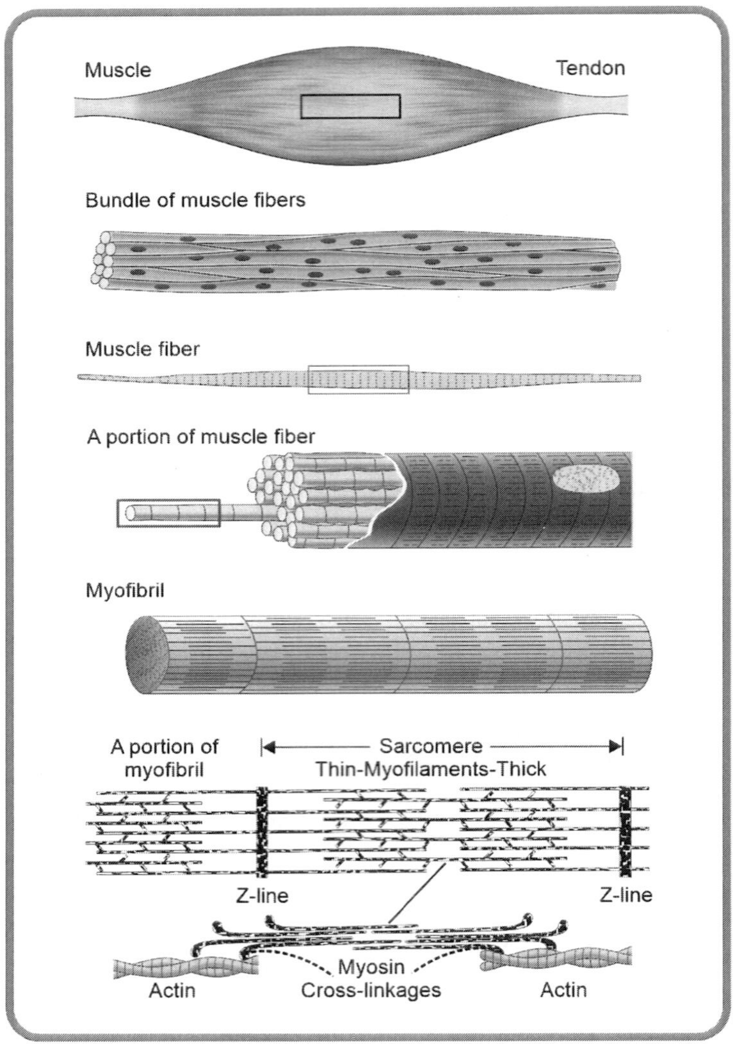


**Fig. 2.3:** Structure of a skeletal muscle (schematic).

animal muscles contain a mixture of these three types. Red muscle fibers have smaller diameter, lower glycolytic metabolism and ATPase activity but higher oxidative metabolism as compared to white muscle fibers.

*Myofibrils* have a number of elongated unbranched contractile muscle fibers that occupy almost 80% of its volume. They are responsible for the cross-striated appearance of the muscle fiber. Each myofibril is about 1 μ thickness and may run the length of muscle fiber. The cross-striated myofibrils remain embedded in the cytoplasm of the muscle fiber called sarcoplasm. The myofibrils are surrounded by a complex system of membrane tubules. The longitudinal tubules called sarcoplasmic reticulum run parallel to myofibrils. Another series of tubules run transversely as invaginations of the sarcolemma. The sarcoplasmic reticulum and T- tubules are arranged in a sequence and play an important role in generating Ca fluxes in the excitation-contraction mechanism. Sarcoplasm also contains glycogen particles, lipid droplets, etc.

At *low magnification (2000X)*, myofibrils, the intracellular contractile elements, show characteristics banded or striated pattern **(Fig. 2.4)**. This situation arises due to the orderly arrangement of dark or A-band and light or I-band. A clear area in the center of dark band

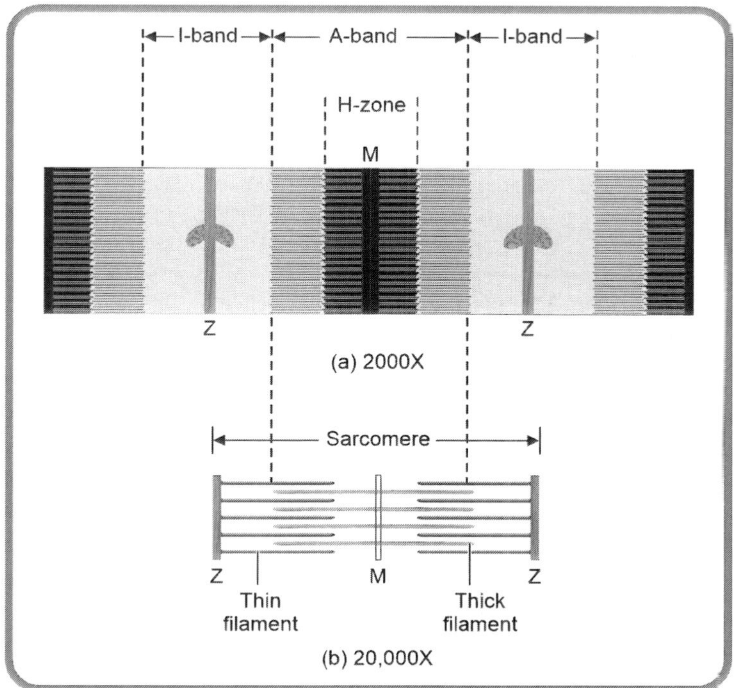


**Fig. 2.4:** Myofibril depicting (a) Typical dark A-band, light I-band, H-zone, M-line and Z-lines; (b) Thick and thin filaments.

called H-zone is bisected by a dark M-line. The light or I-band is also bisected by a dark Z-line. The distance between two adjacent Z-lines is called sarcomere. In fact, the sarcomere is the functional unit of myofibril.

At *20,000X magnification*, the myofibril itself is seen to be composed of a number of thick and thin filaments. Thick filaments traverse the entire width of A-band whereas thin filaments extend from Z-line to the edge of H-zone. Thus, only thick filaments are present in the H-zone. These thick and thin filaments consist of contractile proteins myosin **(Fig. 2.5)** and actin **(Fig. 2.6)** respectively.

*Connective tissue* serves as the major supportive element of the animal body. It envelops the muscle fibers (endomysium) and bundles (perimysium) and finally, the entire muscle (epimysium)

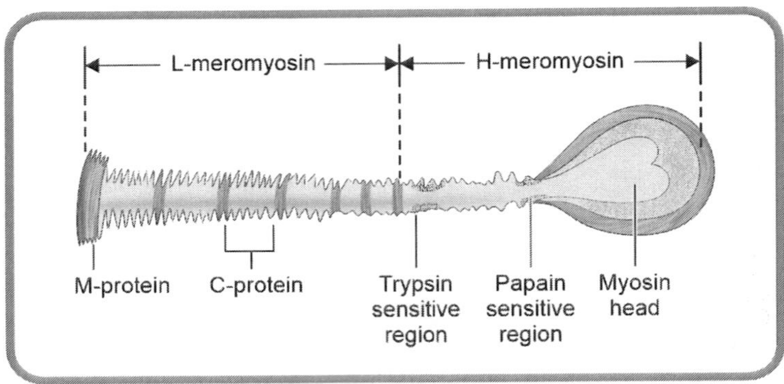


**Fig. 2.5:** Sketch showing one myosin molecule.

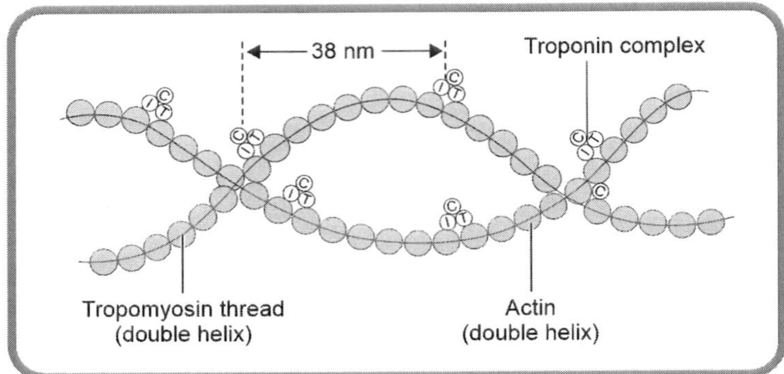


**Fig. 2.6:** Sketch showing arrangement of actin molecules.

connective tissue fibers form the bulk of tendons and ligaments. The tendons attach muscle with bone whereas ligaments connect two bones or support organs. Connective tissue consists chiefly of a mucopolysaccharide matrix in which fibers of collagen, elastin and reticulin are embedded. Collagen fibers predominate over those of reticulin and elastin. Adipose tissue is a specialized type of connective tissue which is primarily made up of cells storing fat droplets. It is seen around kidneys, omentum and in and around various muscles and organs.

### Smooth Muscles

Smooth muscle is found in the gastrointestinal tract, blood vessels, lymphatics and skin in close association with the connective tissue layers. It is involuntary in nature. Smooth muscle fibers are long, unevenly thickened in the center and tapering on both the sides. The myofibrils are homogenous and do not show alternating dark and light bands like those of skeletal muscle. There are no Z or M-lines. The sarcoplasmic reticulum is also not much developed.

### Cardiac Muscles

The cardiac muscles found in the heart are also involuntary. Their muscle fibers are rounded to irregular in shape and give off branches which get mixed up with those of nearby fibers. The nuclei are placed in the center of the fiber. Myofibrils depict striations similar to skeletal muscle. The sarcoplasm shows numerous and much more mitochondria than the skeletal or smooth muscles. The intercalated discs are present at the position of Z-lines.

## COMPOSITION OF MUSCLE TISSUE

Muscle tissue contains approximately 75 percent water and 25 percent solids of which 19 percent are proteins. Lipids constitute about 2.5 to 5 percent of muscle. Chemical composition of a fresh animal muscle is presented in **Table 2.1**. For simplification, meat can be taken as the postmortem aspect of a muscle.

**Table 2.1:** Chemical composition of a typical animal muscle.

| | *Component* | *Percent (wet basis)* |
|---|---|---|
| 1. | **Water** | 75 |
| 2. | **Protein** | 19 |
| | a. *Myofibrillar proteins* | 11.5 |
| | Myosin | |
| | Actin | |
| | Tropomyosin | |
| | Troponin C, I and T | |
| | Connectins | |
| | Desmin | |
| | b. *Sarcoplasmic proteins* | 5.5 |
| | Glycolytic enzymes | |
| | c. *Stroma or connective tissue proteins* | 2.0 |
| | Collagen | |
| | Elastin | |
| | Sarcolemma | |
| | Sarcoplasmic reticulum | |
| 3. | **Lipids** | 2.5 |
| | Neutral lipid | |
| | Phospholipid | |
| | Cerebrosides | |
| | Cholesterol | |
| 4. | **Carbohydrates** | 2.5 |
| | Glycogen | |
| | Glucose-6-phosphate | |
| | Glucose | |
| | Lactic acid | |
| 5. | **Miscellaneous soluble non-protein substances** | 2.3 |
| | a. *Nitrogenous substances* | |
| | Creatine | |
| | Inosine monophosphate (IMP) | |
| | Nucleotides | |
| | Carnosine, anserine | |

*Contd...*

*Contd...*

| | *Component* | *Percent (wet basis)* |
|---|---|---|
| | b. *Inorganic substances* | |
| | Total soluble phosphorus | |
| | K, Na, Mg, Ca, Zn and trace elements | |
| 6. | Vitamins | Minute quantities |
| | Fat-soluble vitamins | |
| | Water-soluble vitamins | |

*Source:* Lawrie (1975).

## Water

This is the largest component comprising two-third to three-fourth of the muscle tissue. Due to polar behavior, water molecules are attached with the electrically charged groups of muscle proteins. About 4.5% of the total water in muscle is so tightly bound that it is almost impossible to dislocate it. The attraction of molecules keeps on decreasing as the distance from the reactive groups increases, most of the water exists in immobilized and free forms. When pH of meat is more than isoelectric point, the enhanced negative charge increases the interfilamental space resulting in retention of excess water. It may be noted that almost 70% of water content in fresh meat is located within the myofibrils. Further, an increased water holding capacity is associated with juiciness and tenderness of cooked meat.

## Protein

Muscle proteins have been broadly classified into three categories:

1. Myofibrillar proteins—soluble in dilute salt solution
2. Sarcoplasmic proteins—soluble in water or very dilute salt solution
3. Stroma or connective—almost insoluble tissue proteins

### *Myofibrillar Proteins*

These proteins constitute contractile part of the muscle and make up about 60% of the total protein in the skeletal muscle. Thick filaments constitute the A-band of the sarcomere and consist of the protein myosin. There are 200–400 molecule of myosin in each thick filaments. Myosin is a long asymmetrical molecule containing a globular head and two identical polypeptide chains. It has a relatively high charge and shows a strong affinity for the divalent cations, calcium and magnesium. Tryptic digestion splits myosin into two large pieces heavy and light meromyosin. Heavy meromyosin head portion carries the ATPase activity and possesses actin binding ability. This ATPase activity of myosin is stimulated by $Ca^{++}$ ions and inhibited by $Mg^{++}$ ions.

The thin filament constitute I-band of the sarcomere and extent on either side of the Z-line beyond I-band also into the A-band between the thick myosin filaments. Actin is the main protein of the thin filament. Actin occurs in two different forms. Globular or G-actin is a monomer form, each molecule of which binds one molecule of ATP or ADP with high affinity. Further, each molecule of G-actin binds one $Ca^{++}$ ion very tightly. At high ionic strength and usually in the presence of ATP, G-actin is polymerized to a high molecular weight fibrous or F-actin. At low ionic strength, F-actin depolymerizes to yield G-actin usually with bound ADP.

Relatively small quantities of other proteins generally referred as regulatory proteins are associated with major myofibrillar proteins. Tropomyosin is a fibrous protein which occurs as a double helix. These helical strands are present in close association with in filaments, extending through the grooves of action helix. Troponin is another important regulatory protein which is present in association with thin filament cementing the long chain of tropomyosin thread into the grooves of actin at a regular interval. Troponin is composed of three sub-units:

**Troponin T**—Binds to tropomyosin and links it to F-actin filaments
**Troponin C**—Binds to calcium ions
**Troponin I**—Inhibits or prevents the interaction between actin and myosin in relaxed state. It allows their interaction only in the presence of calcium ions.

*Actinin* is a globular protein having similar amino acid composition as actin. It has two subunits. The alpha-actinin is a constituent of Z-line and has been shown to accelerate the polymerization of G-actin to F-actin. The beta-actinin regulates the length of thin filament (For the convenience of the students, the phenomena of muscle contraction and relaxation is given in **Flowcharts 2.1** and **2.2** which are self-explanatory).

*Myofibrillar* proteins are of special interest to the technologists because they contribute approximately 95% of the water holding capacity, 75% of the emulsifying capacity and to a large extent the tenderness of meat.

**Flowchart 2.1:** Mechanism of muscle contraction.

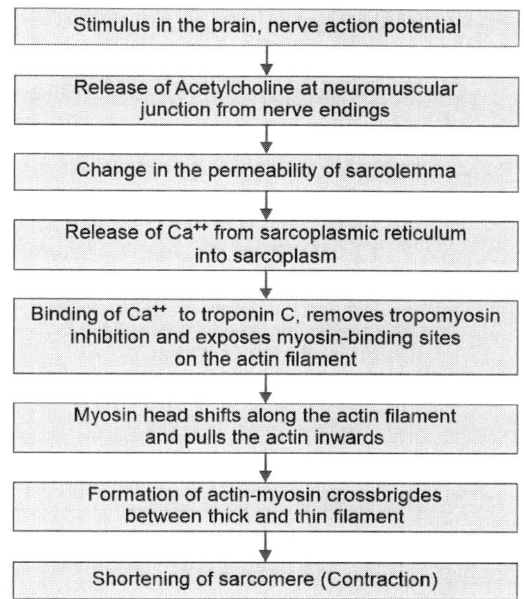


### *Sarcoplasmic Proteins*

These proteins make up about 30–35% of the total protein in the skeletal muscle. They contain hundred of enzymes for the normal functioning of muscle cell. Sarcoplasmic proteins have mostly glycolytic enzymes and associated proteins like creatine kinase, lactic dehydrogenase, myoglobin, aldolase, etc. In general, these proteins are very susceptible to heat.

*Myoglobin* is a conjugated protein consisting of a prosthetic heme moiety and a protein moiety (globin). It provides red color to the muscle and serves as a carrier of oxygen to the muscle fiber. It is the most important pigment of meat color. Cytochrome enzyme, flavin, etc., contribute very little to meat color. The amount of myoglobin present generally shows considerable variation.

In loin muscle of different species, the concentration of myoglobin (%) are:

Rabbit - 0.02
Pig - 0.06
Sheep - 0.25
Cattle - 0.50
Blue whale - 0.91

**Flowchart 2.2:** Mechanism of muscle relaxation.

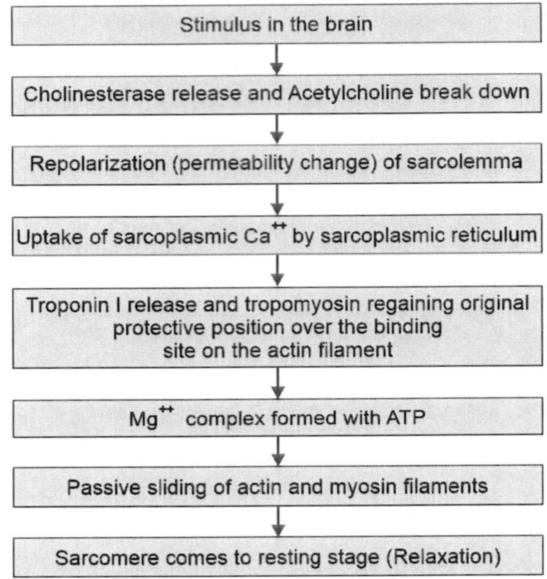


At a given time, meat color depends on the chemical state of myoglobin.

*Stroma or Connective Tissue Proteins*

The connective tissue is composed of an amorphous ground substance or matrix in which formed elements mostly fibers and a few cells are embedded. The ground substance is a viscous glycoprotein solution. The extracellular connective fibers are:

a. Collagen
b. Reticulin
c. Elastin

**Collagen** is the main fibrous protein the muscles and significantly influence the meat toughness. It makes up to 40–60 percent of the total stroma protein and 20–25 percent of the total protein in the body. A fine network of collagen fibers is present in almost all tissues and organs including skeletal muscles. It is the most common constituents of tendons. While colored collagen fibers are straight, inelastic and nonbranching, these fibers shrink or shorten at a temperature of 60°C but higher temperatures or boiling causes transformation to water soluble gelatin. Acid or alkali treatment results in the marked swelling of these fibers. Collagen is the only protein possessing a fair amount of hydroxyproline (approximately 14 percent) and low concentration of hydroxylysine. The smallest unit of collagen molecular structure is tropocollagen which aggregate to form more massive structures—the fibril, primitive fiber and mature fiber. High tensile strength and insoluble nature of mature collagen fibers is due to increased inter-molecular linkages.

**Reticulin** is composed of small fibers which resemble that of collagen except for its intimate association with a lipid containing myristic acid. Reticular fibers form a network around blood vessels, neural structures, epithelium, etc.

**Elastin** is common in ligaments and its yellow fibers can be easily stretched. Elastin fibers are branched and do not hydrolyze on boiling. Elastin contains two unique amino acids: desmosine and isodesmosine which contribute to its highly insoluble nature. The nutritive value of elastin is practically nil due to its resistance to digestive enzymes.

## Lipids

Lipid is a major component of the carcass of a meat animal. It is highly variable and is inversely proportional to the moisture content. Animal lipids are mainly neutral lipids and phospholipids. The neutral lipids are mostly glycerol esters of the straight chain carboxylic acids or triglycerides, with small amounts of mono- and diglycerides. Though animal lipids generally contain fatty acids of even carbon atoms (simple triglycerides), mutton and beef have odd number and branched chain fatty acids (mixed triglycerides). The saturated and monounsaturated fatty acids predominate in meat lipids. The principal saturated fatty acids are palmitic and stearic acids with little amount of other fatty acids, whereas most commonly occurring unsaturated fatty acids are oleic, linoleic and linolenic acids. The composition and distribution of meat lipids depend on the diet of meat animal.

*Phospholipids* are found in muscle tissue in small percentages (0.5–1%). These are principal structural and functional constituents of cell membranes and have a key role in the flavor and shelf stability of meat and meat products. Phospholipids are generally found in meat as phospholglycerides, the less common are phosphatidylcholine, phosphatidylethanolamine, phosphatidylserine and sphingomyelins. Meat phospholipids are more susceptible to oxidation than triglycerides. They may cause discoloration and off flavor in meat products when exposed to air and heat.

*Cholesterol* is a minor but important component of animal tissues. Most of it is in unesterified or free form. It has been noticed at high levels in patients with heart disease. A reduction in animal fat intake is usually advised as precaution, since cholesterol is formed in the body even without any dietary intake.

## Carbohydrates

Immediately after slaughter, muscle normally contains a very small amount (nearly 1%) of glycogen. It is a macromolecule of glucose residues which serves as a reserve polysaccharide of animal tissue. However, it gets worked up before the completion of rigor mortis and plays a key role in attaining the ultimate muscle pH. Both the rate and amount of glycolysis influence the color, tenderness and water holding capacity of meat. Insulin deficiency results in decreased tissue glycogen. Glucagon administration causes rapid degradation of liver glycogen to glucose. Besides, several mucopolysaccharides are widely distributed in animal body. Their quantity is less but many of them like heparin, hyaluronic acid, chondroitin sulphate, keratosulphate and glycoproteins are biologically important substances.

## Minerals

About 3.5% of the total body weight is inorganic matter. Most of the total body inorganic material is located in skeletal tissue primarily as salts of calcium and phosphorus and some other minerals especially magnesium. In living meat animal, essential minerals like calcium, phosphorus, sodium, potassium, sulfur, chlorine, magnesium, iron, etc., and trace elements like manganese, copper, iodine, zinc, cobalt, etc., serve a variety of important functions. These functions may be physical, chemical or biological depending on the chemical form and the location in body tissues and fluids.

In the conversion of muscle to meat, inorganic elements play an important role. Their main function relates to development of rigor mortis and alteration of fluid balance which causes a drop in pH and water holding capacity. Inorganic constituents also influence the meat color and tenderization. Several inorganic ions act as catalysts during oxidation of meat fat, enhancing the process of rancidity development.

### Vitamins

The vitamin content of meat is variable, depending on the species and age of the animal, the degree of fatness and type of feed received by the animal. Water soluble vitamins are localized in lean tissues, whereas fat-soluble vitamins in fatty tissues. Variety meats have substantial amounts of B-complex vitamins. Pork contains 5–10 times more thiamine content as compared to mutton. The exudates from cut meat surfaces and drip loss during thawing of frozen meat contain an appreciable amount of B-complex vitamins and amino acids. Most of the vitamins in meat are relatively stable during processing or cooking. However, thiamine or to some extent vitamin $B_6$ are susceptible to heat treatment.

## NUTRITIVE VALUE OF MEAT TISSUES

Meat is a very nutritious food. It is almost fully digestible. It is appealing to the eyes and pleasing to the sense of olfaction. The nutritive value of meat is attributed to its abundant high quality proteins, essential fatty acids, some important minerals and B-complex group of vitamins.

**Meat proteins:** Meat is a concentrated source of proteins which are far superior to the plant proteins due to very high biological value. Most lean meat cuts contain 16.5 to 20% protein **(Table 2.2)**. This protein is rich in essential amino acids. Essential, because there is no provision in the body for the synthesis of these amino acids and a deficient diet will lead to protein malnutrition. In fact, among meat proteins, myofibrillar and sarcoplasmic proteins are of very high quality because they contain enough of essential amino acids **(Table 2.3)**. Connective tissue proteins have lower levels of tryptophan and sulfur containing amino acids. Collagen is especially poor in lysine content.

**Table 2.2:** Proximate composition and caloric value of fresh meats.

| *Meat* | *Percentage* | | | | *Calorie (per 100 g)* |
|---|---|---|---|---|---|
| | *Moisture* | *Protein* | *Fat* | *Ash* | |
| Lamb, composite cuts of trimmed, good grade (lean 79%, fat 21%) | 62.5 | 16.8 | 19.4 | 1.3 | 247 |
| Lamb leg—separable lean, good grade | 73.8 | 19.9 | 4.7 | 1.6 | 127 |
| Pork ham, trimmed thin (lean 77%, fat 23%) | 59.2 | 16.7 | 23.2 | 0.8 | 281 |
| Pork ham, thin separable lean | 72.0 | 20.4 | 6.6 | 1.1 | 147 |
| Beef carcass—total edible, good grade (lean 66%, fat 34%) | 54.7 | 16.5 | 28.0 | 0.8 | 323 |

*Source:* USDA Handbook no. 8.

**Table 2.3:** Essential amino acids as percentage of crude protein in fresh meats.

| *Amino acid* | *Lamb* | *Pork* | *Beef* |
|---|---|---|---|
| Lysine | 7.6 | 7.8 | 8.4 |
| Methionine | 2.3 | 2.5 | 2.3 |
| Cystine | 1.3 | 1.3 | 1.4 |
| Tryptophan | 1.3 | 1.4 | 1.1 |
| Leucine | 7.4 | 7.5 | 8.4 |
| Isoleucine | 4.8 | 4.9 | 5.1 |
| Phenylalanine | 3.9 | 4.1 | 4.0 |
| Valine | 5.0 | 5.0 | 5.7 |

*Source:* Schweigert and Payne (1956).

**Meat fats:** Meat fats contain an ample amount of essential fatty acids and the nutritional demand of the body is easily met by intramuscular fat itself. The caloric value of fat in meat is attributed to fatty acids in triglycerides. The number of calories from lean meat is frequently less than those derived from equal weights of many other foods. In fact, the caloric value of a particular meat depends on the amount of fat in the meat cuts. The most abundant fatty acid in meat fat is oleic acid (an unsaturated FA) followed by palmitic and stearic acids

**Table 2.4:** Occurrence of fatty acids as percentage of total meat fat.

| *Fatty acid* | *Lamb* | *Pork* | *Beef* |
|---|---|---|---|
| Palmitic acid (C 16) | 25 | 28 | 29 |
| Stearic acid (C 18) | 25 | 13 | 20 |
| Palmitoleic acid (C 16:1) | - | 3 | 2 |
| Oleic acid (C 18:1) | 39 | 6 | 42 |
| Linoleic acid (C 18:2) | 4 | 10 | 2 |
| Linolenic acid (C 18:3) | 0.5 | 0.7 | 0.5 |
| Arachidonic acid (C 20:4) | 1.5 | 2 | 0.1 |

(saturated FA). The essential fatty acids in human diets are linoleic, linolenic and arachidonic acids **(Table 2.4)**. Pork and organ meats are relatively good sources of linoleic and linolenic acids. It may be noted that excess dietary linoleic acid is converted to arachidonic acid in human body to meet its demand.

The phospholipids are essential components of the cell wall as well as mitochondria and play a vital role in cellular metabolism. Meat fat always contain some quantity of cholesterol and blood cholesterol level increases after ingestion of cholesterol in food. However, it is now well known that our body is capable of synthesizing more cholesterol than is normally ingested. Organ meats have remarkably high cholesterol content as compared to skeletal meat.

**Minerals:** In general, meat is a good source of all minerals except calcium **(Table 2.5)**. The minerals are in close association with lean tissues in meat. Of these, quantitatively potassium is most abundant followed by phosphorus. Meat is a good source of iron which is required for the synthesis of hemoglobin, myoglobin and certain enzymes and thus plays a vital role in maintaining good health. Since human body has a very limited capacity to store iron, mainly in liver, it has to be a part of regular dietary intake. Meat provides this important mineral in a form that is easily absorbed in the system.

**Table 2.5:** Mineral and vitamin contents of raw meat (mg/100 g meat).

| *Mineral/Vitamin* | *Lamb* | *Pork* | *Beef* |
|---|---|---|---|
| Sodium | 75 | 70 | 65 |
| Potassium | 295 | 285 | 355 |
| Magnesium | 15 | 18 | 18 |

Contd...

*Contd...*

| *Mineral/Vitamin* | *Lamb* | *Pork* | *Beef* |
|---|---|---|---|
| Iron | 1.2 | 2.3 | 2.8 |
| Calcium | 10 | 9 | 11 |
| Phosphorus | 147 | 175 | 171 |
| Thiamine | 0.15 | 0.76 | 0.06 |
| Riboflavin | 0.20 | 0.18 | 0.13 |
| Niacin | 4.7 | 4.1 | 3.6 |

*Source:* Walt and Merrill (1963).

**Vitamins:** Lean meat is an excellent source of B-complex group of vitamins. It has only traces of fat soluble vitamins which are restricted to body fat. Vitamin C is almost absent in lean meat, although certain organs contain it in minor quantities. Among the B-complex group of vitamins thiamine, riboflavin and niacin concentrations are quite high. It may be noted that pork surpasses several meats as far as B-complex vitamins are concerned. In fact, lean pork has 5–10 times more thiamine than other meats. It has been noted that in monogastric animals like pig intake of vitamins in feed is directly reflected in their tissues.

Several organ meats have slightly less protein and fat than skeletal meats. However, these are quite often more economical sources of protein and vitamins than retail cuts of skeletal meat. Liver is a very rich source of iron, riboflavin, niacin and vitamin A. Nutritive value of skeletal and organ meats should be properly utilized to alleviate the malnutrition.

# 3 CHAPTER

# Conversion of Muscle to Meat

Slaughter of food animal is followed by a series of physical and chemical changes over a period of several hours or even days resulting in the conversion of muscle to meat. There is immediate loss of oxygen supply to the muscle due to exsanguination (bleeding). As the stored oxygen in myoglobin gets depleted, there is inhibition of aerobic pathway through citrate cycle as well as cytochrome system. The store of creatine phosphate (CP) used for rephosphorylation of ADP to ATP (creatine phosphate + ADP = ATP + creatine) gets soon exhausted. Energy metabolism is then shifted to anaerobic pathway resulting in the breakdown of glycogen to lactic acid. This process continues till all the glycogen stored in the muscle is exhausted. This resynthesis of ATP by anaerobic pathway is not enough to maintain the required ATP level and as it depletes, there is formation of actomyosin resulting in the onset of rigor mortis. The important changes that take place during postmortem period are as follows:

## LOSS OF HOMEOSTASIS

Homeostasis mechanism, a system for the physiologically balanced internal environment which helps the body to cope up with the stresses of oxygen deficiency, extreme variation in temperature, energy supply, etc., is lost. The homeostasis is controlled by nervous system which ceases within 4–6 minutes after bleeding. In the absence of blood supply, there is loss of body heat and temperature starts declining.

## POSTMORTEM GLYCOLYSIS AND PH DECLINE

In the absence of oxygen, anaerobic glycolysis leads to the formation of lactic acid from the glycogen reserves:

$$\text{Glycogen} \xrightarrow[\text{Conditions}]{\text{Anaerobic}} \text{Lactic acid} + 2\ \text{ATP}$$

The accumulation of lactic acid lowers down the muscle pH which is an important postmortem change during the conversion of muscle to meat. The rate and extent of pH decline are variable, being influenced by the species of food animal, various preslaughter factors, environmental temperature, etc. In most species, a gradual decline continues from approximately pH 7 in the living muscle during first few hours (5–6 hours) and then there is a little drop in the next 15–20 hours, giving an ultimate pH in the range of 5.5–5.7 **(Fig. 3.1)**. The rate of pH decline is enhanced at high environmental temperature. A low ultimate pH is desired to have a check on the proliferating microorganisms during storage.

A sharp decline in postmortem pH even before the dissipation of body heat through carcass chilling may cause denaturation of muscle proteins which cannot hold water. So, the muscles depict pale, soft and exudative (PSE) condition. This is usually seen in pork obtained from animal having severe short term stress. Such meat is not desirable for processed meat products. Contrary to this, muscles of those animals suffering severe prolonged stress maintain a consistently high pH during postmortem conversion to meat and depict a dark, firm and dry (DFD) condition. This is sometimes encountered in buffalo meat and makes the meat susceptible to bacterial spoilage. Both PSE and DFD conditions are undesirable.

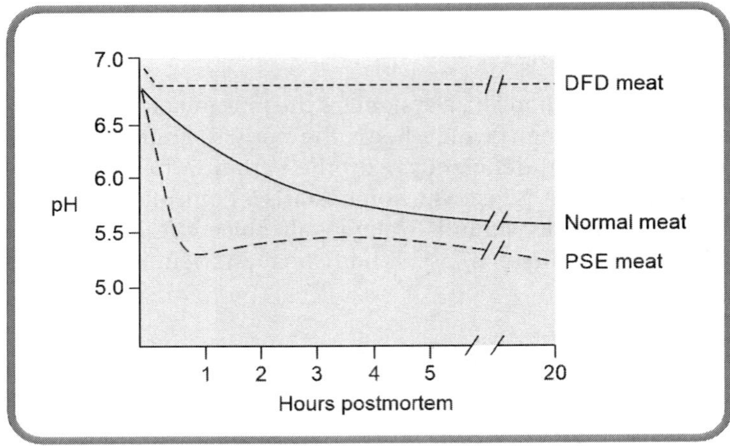


**Fig. 3.1:** Postmortem pH decline.

## RIGOR MORTIS

It refers to stiffening of muscles after death and is another important postmortem change in the process of conversion of muscle to meat. It is now very well known that a particular level or concentration of ATP complexed with $Mg^{++}$, is required for breaking the actomyosin bond and bringing the muscle to a relaxed state and as it drops, permanent actomyosin crossbridges begin to form and muscle gradually becomes less and less extensible under an externally applied force.

Rigor mortis occurs in three phases. During the period immediately following exsanguination, the actomyosin formation proceeds very slowly at first and the muscle is relatively extensible and elastic. This period is called the *delay phase* of rigor mortis. Then actomyosin formation picks up and the muscle begins to loose extensibility. This phase is called the *fast or onset phase* of rigor mortis. When all the creatine phosphate (CP) is depleted, ADP can no longer be phosphorylated to ATP, muscle becomes quite inextensible and stiff. This stage marks the *completion phase* of rigor mortis. When postmortem pH decline is very slow or very fast, the onset and completion of rigor mortis is rapid. The onset of rigor mortis is enhanced at ambient temperature above 20°C.

The phenomena of rigor mortis progresses from the muscles of face and neck which are the first to be affected and then rigidity spreads backward over the trunk and limbs. The relaxation of muscles also generally follows the same order.

The pattern of rigor mortis onset can be classified as acid rigor which is characterized in immobilized animals by a delay period and a short fast phase and in struggling animals by drastic curtailment of the delay period. At body temperature stiffening is accompanied by shortening. Alkaline rigor characterized by a rapid onset of stiffening and by marked shortening, even at room temperature. Intermediate type characterized in starved animals by a curtailment of the delay period but not of the rapid phase: there is some shortening.

The phenomenon of rigor mortis resembles that of muscle contraction in a living animal muscle, except that rigor mortis is irreversible under normal conditions. The resolution of rigor mortis takes place due to microbial degradation of muscle structure in due course of time.

Rigor mortis is very important in meat technology. The onset of rigor mortis and its resolution partially determines the tenderness of meat. If the post-slaughter meat is immediately chilled to 15°C, a phenomenon known as cold shortening occurs, where the muscle shrinks to a third of its original size. This will lead to the loss of water from the meat along with many of the vitamins, minerals, and water soluble proteins. The loss of water makes the meat hard and interferes with the manufacturing of several meat products like cutlet and sausage.

Pre-rigor meat is quite tender but its toughness keeps on increasing until rigor mortis is completed. It continues to be tough for some more time. However, with the resolution of rigor due to denaturation or degradation or ageing, meat again becomes tender. The onset of rigor mortis is also accompanied by a decrease in water holding capacity. This is true even when rigor mortis takes place at a high pH due to disappearance of ATP and consequent formation of actomyosin.

Electrical stimulation has been innovated to hasten the onset and resolution of rigor mortes. It helps in increasing the tenderness and improving the color of meat.

## LOSS OF PROTECTION FROM INVADING MICROORGANISMS

During postmortem period, body defense mechanism stops operating and membrane properties are altered. So, during conversion to meat, muscle is quite susceptible to invading microorganisms. Except for low pH, most of the other postmortem changes favor bacterial growth. Hence, utmost handling precautions are necessary to prevent contamination of meat.

## DEGRADATION DUE TO PROTEOLYTIC ENZYMES

Several autolytic lysosomal enzymes called cathepsins which remain inactive in a living muscle tissue, are activated as the muscle pH declines. These enzymes initiate the degradation of muscle protein structure. In fact, catheptic enzymes are capable of breaking down even collagenous connective tissue of the muscle and cause tenderization of meat during aging.

## LOSS OF STRUCTURAL INTEGRITY

Postmortem alteration of membrane properties initiates the degradation of muscular proteins. There is a progressive disruption of myofibrillar structure. The resolution of rigor mortis is known to occur due to disintegration of Z-line structure. A rapid decline in muscle pH also causes denaturation of collagenous connective tissue.

4

CHAPTER

# Some Meat Quality Parameters

Fresh meat can be referred as a product which has undergone imminent postmortem changes following slaughter but has not been subjected to any processing. However, fresh meat which has undergone freezing can be conveniently termed as raw meat. Some characteristics of fresh and raw meat need to be properly understood in order to achieve the best results in processing.

## MEAT COLOR

This is the total visual perception of meat. The hue (primary color), chroma (intensity) and the value (brightness) of meat color are based on the quantity of principal muscle pigment myoglobin and its chemical state. It is for this reason that meat color varies with species, sex, age and even among different muscles of the same species. Myoglobin content of more active species and muscles is higher than the passive ones. Typical color of meat from various species is:

| | | |
|---|---|---|
| Mutton or chevon | : | Light to dark red |
| Pork | : | Grayish pink |
| Poultry | : | Gray white to dull red |
| Buffalo meat and beef | : | Cherry red |

*Myoglobin* constitutes about 80-90% of the total meat pigments. The role of hemoglobin in meat color is negligible in a properly bled muscle. Catalase and cytochrome enzymes are of little consequence as far as meat color is concerned. Myoglobin molecule has a protein portion (globin) and a heme (iron containing) ring. It is one-fourth in size as compared to structurally similar hemoglobin molecule. In intact meat, iron in the heme ring of myoglobin exists in the reduced form. Upon cutting, grinding or exposure to air, myoglobin is oxygenated to form oxymyoglobin within 30–45 minutes. Oxymyoglobin has a bright red color (bloom) which is very much desired by the consumers. However, this pigment is comparatively unstable. In conditions of less oxygen, partial vacuum or semipermeable package, myoglobin as well as oxymyoglobin is oxidized to brown colored metmyoglobin. At the time of meat purchase, brown color is usually associated by the consumers with meat that has been stored for long, although it is not always true. In order to prevent the formation of brown color, fresh meat is often packed in films with very good gas (oxygen) transmission rate.

## WATER HOLDING CAPACITY

Water constitutes about 76% of fresh meat. It is a universal solvent and takes part in a large number of biological reactions. In muscles, water molecules carry positive and negative charges. The location of these molecules allows water to exist in three different forms—free water, immobilized water and bound water. The water molecules held by capillary forces on the surface make up free water which can be removed by application of even minor physical force. The middle layer of water molecules remain in contact with proteins and make up immobilized water, a large part of which can be removed by application of severe physical conditions. However, 4–5% of water molecules are so tightly bound to the charged hydrophilic groups on the muscle proteins that they do not allow this bound water to escape by application of any physical force. The capacity of meat to retain its water during the application of physical forces is known as water holding capacity (WHC). This property of meat has a special significance because it contributes to the juiciness of cooked meat besides influencing the texture and color. Fresh meat with a good WHC is less prone to shrinkage during storage. WHC of meat is very important in processing where meat is subjected to physical forces such as cutting, grinding, filling, pressing, heating, etc.

## MARBLING

It refers to the intramuscular fat which can be visibly detected when the muscle surface is cut. The solidification of this fat during chilling contributes to the firmness of meat. Marbling prominently figures in the USDA quality grades for meat because of its merchandising value. During handling of chilled meat, some special retail cuts like chops and steaks retain their uniform thickness and typical shape due to marbling. Besides, marbling also enables meat to bear the impact of comparatively high cooking temperature. During thermal processing, moderately marbled meat yields a juicy and flavorful product whereas too little marbling yields a dry and flavorless product. Excess marbling neither enhances the eating satisfaction nor desired in a fat conscious society.

## QUANTUM OF CONNECTIVE TISSUE

The amount of connective tissue in meat has a direct bearing on its textural characteristics. During animals life time, more active muscles tend to deposit more connective tissue to gain strength. This factor accounts for the coarse texture of biceps femoris and tenderness of loin eye muscle postmortem. The quantum of connective tissue per unit muscle does not increase with age and is not responsible for tough meat of older animals. In fact, it is the increase in muscle fiber diameter and consequent increase in muscle fiber bundles which account for the coarse texture of such meat.

Most meat cutting practices are based on separation of coarse textured meat from the tender meat, so as to facilitate the right kind of cooking procedure and derive maximum palatability pleasure.

## FIRMNESS

The firmness of meat is a good quality parameter which plays an important role in carcass setting, fabrication, ageing, processing, slicing and product display. During carcass chilling, the firmness increases due to loss of extensibility associated with the completion of rigor mortis. Fresh meat having a high water holding capacity shows good firmness and tight structure. It can be objectively measured by shear force apparatus or penetrometer. Meat with a good degree of firmness yields a comparatively better quality processed meat products.

## MEAT STORAGE CONDITIONS

### Cold Shortening

When prerigor meat is fast chilled below 15°C, there is shortening of muscles. This shortening or contraction is more at 0°C and still more at –2°C. However, it is minimum at 14–21°C. At 40% shortening, which is quite common, meat becomes very tough and large quantity of meat juices are exuded. However, in case cold shortening exceeds more than 40%, Z-lines are disrupted and meat becomes soft and tender. Otherwise also, cold shortening is a reversible phenomena and is resolved when glycogen content of muscle is exhausted. In the meat plant, cold shortening can be avoided by keeping the meat above 14°C for sufficient time to pass the rigor stage.

### Thaw Rigor

When prerigor meat is frozen, a severe type of rigor mortis ensues during thawing. The shortening so produced may be 60 to 80% of the original length of the unrestrained muscle. Although shortening is less in a muscle attached to skeleton, the condition results in a tough meat and heavy drip losses.

## ANTEMORTEM FACTORS AFFECTING MEAT QUALITY

Various stress factors such as extremes of environmental temperature, overcrowding, preslaughter transportation, struggle during immobilization and bleeding, etc. have ultimate bearing on the quality of meat. Exposure to low temperature may cause shivering which results in a reduction in muscle glycogen level. During any environmental stress, susceptible pigs, show Porcine stress syndrome which is characterized by muscle tremors, anxious behavior and reddening of skin. In such animals antemortem temperature rise, lactic acid build up and ATP depletion are the general features and postmortem changes are rapid. So conversion from muscle to meat is also fast due to a sharp fall in pH and muscle denaturation. Ultimately, meat becomes pale in color, soft in texture and exudative or moist during chilling itself. Stress resistant animals are able to withstand exercise, fasting, fatigue, fight, etc., but at the expense of their glycogen reserves. Slow and limited glycolysis often results in high ultimate pH and excellent water binding capacity. So meat appears dark, firm and dry.

Preslaughter handling such as long distance transportation and overcrowding in trucks is also stressful to the animals. This treatment causes shrinkage of muscular tissue and comparatively low dressing percentage. So holding of such animals for resting and feeding can be helpful in restoring their depleted glycogen level. However, basic principle of feed withdrawal and adequate water supply for 24 hours before slaughter has to be followed for ease of evisceration and to reduce microbial contamination of carcass from intestinal contents.

Like other livestock products, meat is also quite prone to the absorption of off odors from the surrounding environment. Hence, meat should not be stored in the presence of other strong smelling substances.

# 5 CHAPTER

# Meat Cutting Practices

Meat cutting refers to the skill of separation of carcass into wholesale primal cuts in order to facilitate requirements of meat trade, cater to the consumer preference and convenient handling by the butchers. It is a specialized work which requires expert butcher to have a fair understanding of animal conformation, a good knowledge of carcass components and break-up, consumer preference and on-the-job experience. Different cutting methods are followed in various countries. Hence, terms like British cutting method, American cutting method, French cutting method, etc., are common. Besides, regional variations within a country are also not uncommon. The primal cuts are divided into subprimals which are further made into retail cuts. Any technical bulletin on specialized meat cutting can give further details.

Whatever system is adopted, the underlying principles remain the same. In many developing countries, a centralized meat cutting room is attached to the slaughterhouse where primal cuts are prepared as in line operation and packed. Basic requisites in meat cutting are:

1. The carcass has to be essentially chilled for proper meat cutting and trimming job.
2. Meat cutting room should be maintained at a temperature of 15 to 20°C and relative humidity of 80 percent. This environment is wholesome for meat and convenient to workers.
3. All meat cutting equipment and machinery such as meat cutting tables, various types of knives, manual as well as electrically operated saws should be made up of stainless steel and be sufficiently sharp.
4. Meat cutting operation has to be done by adequately trained and experienced butchers. It is important to maintain uniformity in cuts and economy of merchandising.

5. Approved meat cutting method should be followed step by step as per standard specifications.
6. Thumb rules for meat cutting techniques are:
   - More valued primal cuts are separated from the less valued cuts.
   - The muscular portion is cut with a sharp knife.
   - The bony structure is severed with a manual/mechanized saw.
   - A limited force is applied while disjointing whenever joints are involved.
7. In line operations in a meat cutting room should be fully synchronized. Different cuts, fat, trimmings, etc. should be transferred to their natural destinations.

## WHOLESALE CUTS OF LAMB CARCASS

USDA and many other international standards specify the division of lamb carcass into foresaddle and hindsaddle by cutting between the last two ribs **(Fig. 5.1)**. The right and left sides are not separated. However, BIS specify the division of carcass into right and left sides.

### Foresaddle (53%)

1. Neck — Cut at last cervical vertebrae where it blends with shoulder
2. Shoulder — Cut between 5th and 6th ribs
3. Rack — Portion from 6th to 12th rib
4. Breast — Cut forward from midway of the last rib to ½" above elbow joint
5. Foreshank — Cut containing foreshank bones

### Hindsaddle (47%)

1. Loin — Cut hindquarter by sawing in front of hip bone in between last two lumber vertebrae
2. Leg — Remaining portion of hindquarter
3. Flank — Thin meat without bone from the natural seam starting from breast
4. Suet and kidney

In India, people generally go for six cuts only—neck, shoulder, rack, foreshank and breast, loin and leg **(Fig. 5.2)**.

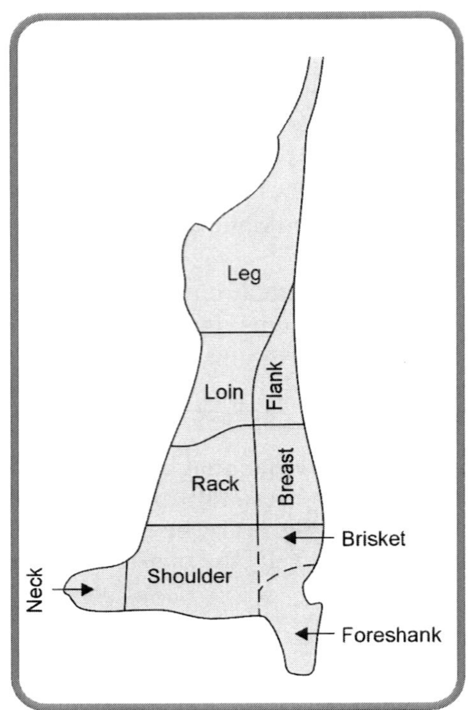


**Fig. 5.1:** Goat and lamb carcass—primal cuts (USDA).

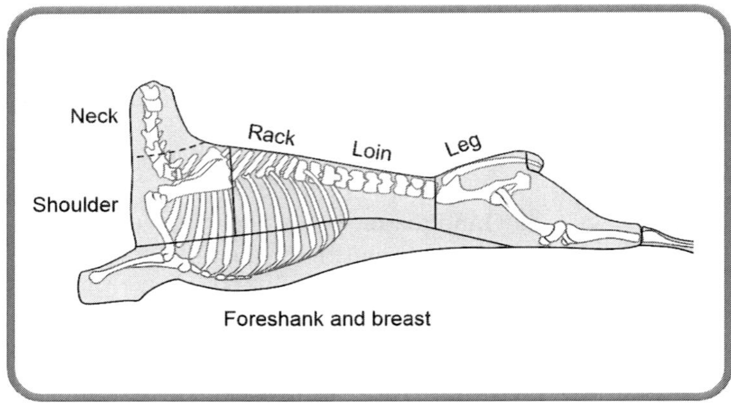


**Fig. 5.2:** Goat and lamb carcass—primal cuts (Indian method).

## WHOLESALE CUTS OF PORK CARCASS

Pork carcass is divided into right and left sides. Then front feet are removed 1" above knee and hind feet at the lower edge of the hock and each side is subjected to six cuts **(Fig. 5.3)**.

Anterior part called rough shoulder is separated from the posterior by cutting between 2nd and 3rd ribs. This is made into three wholesale cuts—jowl, butt and picnic.

1. Jowl — Cut close to the neck line
2. Boston butt — Upper 1/3rd of the skinned shoulder
3. Picnic shoulder — Lower 2/3rd of the shoulder
4. Ham — Cut between 2nd and 3rd sacral vertebrae at right angle to the line of leg
5. Loin — Upper middle portion
6. Belly — Lower middle portion between picnic shoulder and ham.

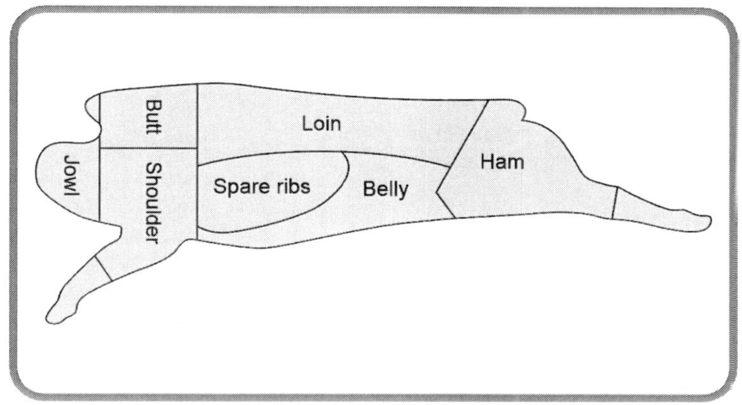


**Fig. 5.3:** Pork carcass—primal cuts.

## WHOLESALE CUTS OF BUFFALO OR BEEF CARCASS

1. Carcass sides are separated. The right side is called closed (kidney close) side whereas left side is called open (kidney free) side.
2. Each side is now subjected to quartering or ribbing. The forequarter and hindquarter are separated by making a cut between 12th and 13th ribs.

3. Forequarter is cut between 5th and 6th ribs to have shank, brisket and chuck in the anterior part and rib and plate in the posterior part **(Fig. 5.4)**.
   - *Rib and plate:* From the posterior part separate the upper rib from the lower plate by a straight and parallel cut to the backbone.
   - *Shank and brisket:* Place the anterior part on the table with rib side down. The shank is removed by cutting parallel to the underline and just dorsal to the lower extremity of the humerus. The brisket is removed by continuing the same cut through the breast bone and lower ends.
   - *Chuck:* This is the remaining large square cut with ribs.

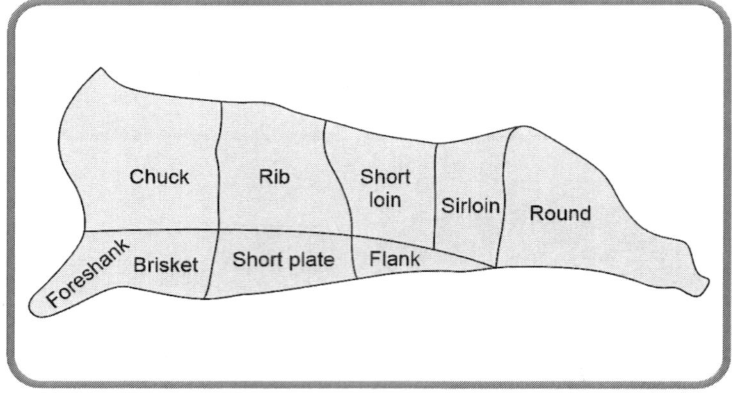


**Fig. 5.4:** Buffalo or beef carcass—primal cuts

4. From the hind quarter first remove kidney knob, i.e., kidneys along with the adjoining fat.
   - *Flank:* Cut below the aitchbone following the natural seam up to thick muscle of the flank and then extending straight upward cut up to 4 cm below the eye muscle.
   - *Round:* Start with a cut 4 cm anterior to the pelvic bone and go parallel to the rib and loin.
   - *Loin:* Leftover cut which can be further sectioned into anterior short loin and posterior sirloin by making a cut between lumber and sacral vertebrae.

## GRADING

There is lot of variation in the carcass conformation, size, and meat quality depending on the breed, age group, body conformation and health status of meat animals. Meat grading refers to the sorting or grouping of meat carcasses and cuts on the basis of their conformation, finish, and overall quality. Although this concept is yet to develop in our country, it is beneficial to the animal raiser at the farm, processor at the packing plant, purchaser at the retail outlet and above all to, the quality conscious consumers. Carcass conformation, trimming, meat to bone ratio, color, etc. play an important role in grading. Carcasses of buffalo, goat, sheep or calf may be graded for meat quality as prime, choice, good or poor. Pork carcasses are generally graded on the basis of yield in most of the developed countries.

Grading of meat carcasses and wholesale cuts is still confined in India at the export points, that too as per the agreement between the exporter and importer. Directorate of Marketing and Inspection, Government of India has already evolved its grades but the same are still to be implemented.

# 6
CHAPTER

# Aging of Dressed Carcasses

As the slaughter process completes, the animal carcasses have a temperature of 30 to 39°C which makes them highly perishable. This carcass heat has to be removed rapidly to check decomposition and weight loss due to evaporation. It is a general practice in meat industry to chill meat carcasses before wholesale distribution and even before freezing.

## CHILLING OF DRESSED CARCASSES

Chilling is a process of prolonging the shelf-life of meat with the help of low temperature. It retards the microbial growth in meat and slows down the enzymatic and chemical reactions which may contribute to deterioration and spoilage. As soon as the postmortem inspection is completed, the carcasses are passed on to chilling room on the overhead rails in the suspended state itself. Chilling room is maintained at a temperature of –1 to +3°C. For effective chilling an air speed of 0.5 to 0.75 meter/second is generally used. Besides, relative humidity of chilling room is kept at about 90% so that moisture loss or shrinkage is minimum. Warm carcasses will inevitably increase the temperature of chilling room, so care should be taken not to overload it.

The rate of carcass chilling depends on several factors—the temperature of chilling room, the size and fat covering over the carcass and the speed of air circulation in the chilling room. In general chevon, lamb, pork and veal carcasses require 24 to 36 hours to attain an internal temperature of 5°C or below whereas large animal carcasses require 48 hours or more to attain the same temperature. The chilling time can be reduced by 25% if high velocity air is passed through the carcasses. Two chilling rooms are sometimes used for heavy buffalo or beef carcasses. It should be noted that rapid chilling of hot carcasses may result in undesirable toughness of muscles. This phenomenon is called cold shortening. The initial chilling room, which receives warm carcass sides or quarters, is maintained at about 7°C whereas the latter is maintained at a temperature between –1°C and 2°C, air speed being 0.75 meters/second in both of them.

Due attention is needed to keep the moisture loss or shrinkage during chilling to minimum in order to retain quantity as well as quality. Excessive moisture loss can affect the color and appeal of meat surface making it dark, dry and shriveled. A relative humidity of 88 to 92% has been found to be ideal because higher relative humidity may encourage slime and mold growth. Even with these precautions, shrinkage loss of 1.5 to 2% is inevitable.

## Guidelines for Proper Chilling of Dressed Carcasses

- Chilling room temperature should be maintained between –1 to 3°C and it should be monitored on a regular basis.
- Relative humidity of the chilling room should invariably be kept at 88 to 92%.
- Hot carcasses should be hung separately from cold carcasses in the chilling room.
- Carcasses should not be allowed to come in direct contact with each other.
- Chilling room should not be overloaded with carcasses.
- Chilling room door should have a self-closing device so that it remains closed as much as possible.
- Temperature of chilling room should always remain above –1.4°C, since meat freezes at this temperature.
- Chilling room equipment has to be safeguarded against excessive condensation.

## Chilling of Dressed Poultry

As soon as the poultry carcasses are eviscerated, they are subjected to chilling. The purpose is to lower the temperature of carcasses from about 37°C to below 7°C. It retards the growth of microorganisms and increases the shelf life of meat. Due to increase in intramuscular osmotic pressure, water-holding capacity of meat is enhanced. Besides, there is increase in tenderness of meat due to rupture of chemical bonds and associated changes.

Chilling of poultry carcasses is accomplished with the help of chilling water or chilled air. Care is taken to avoid extremely rapid cooling so as to rule out cold shortening of muscles and the resultant toughness of meat. Due to this reason, slush ice (water and ice mixture, 50:50) has been widely accepted as an ideal medium of chilling. Immersion chilling may be either still water chilling or mechanically agitated water chilling. Cross contamination of carcasses through chilling process can be checked by adding chlorine in the chilling water to the extent of 25 ppm. It is also very important to control the uptake of water by the carcasses to the satisfaction of regulatory authorities and the consumers in general.

## AGING OF DRESSED CARCASSES

In the absence of microbial spoilage, the holding of unprocessed meat above freezing point is known as aging. It is also frequently referred as conditioning and sometimes ripening. During this period of holding at 0 to 3°C, i.e., above freezing point several changes occur in meat at a subtle rate. Atmospheric oxidation proceeds very slowly in the dark. Bacterial action is retarded to a large extent. Proteolytic enzymes (proteases) within muscle fibers remain active and fragment myofibrils in natural course. Cathepsins or autolytic enzymes also play their role. Maillard reaction also proceeds to a varying degree. A combination of these alterations bring about desirable changes in the sensory attributes of meat system especially increase in tenderness, flavor and to some extent in the juiciness. Increase in tenderness is relatively rapid during first 3 to 7 days postmortem and tenderization rate diminishes after that.

Two types of postmortem aging procedures are commercially practiced—dry and wet aging. Dry aging is the traditional procedure in which entire carcass or wholesale cuts, without any packaging, are hung in the chilling room at 0 to 1°C for 3 to 4 weeks at relative humidity of 86% and air velocity of 0.5 meter/sec. These conditions can vary widely at commercial level. Wet aging is the predominant commercial practice these days wherein wholesale or primal cuts are put in vacuum bags and held at 0 to 1°C for 7 to 10 days. In such a situation, humidity and air velocity provisions become superfluous.

Some of the significant changes in the meat system during aging are:

- **Protein denaturation:** Denaturation refers to physical rearrangement of chemical bonds in the amino acids of protein polypeptide chains without involving any hydrolysis. During postmortem aging myofibrillar and sarcoplasmic proteins denature to a varying degree. There is detachment of actin filaments at Z-lines resulting in the fragmentation of myofibrils. It enhances tenderness, although muscle proteins manifest some loss of water holding capacity. However, connective tissue proteins-collagen and elastin do not undergo denaturation.

- **Proteolysis:** Denatured proteins are particularly susceptible to the action of proteolytic enzymes. So myofibrillar proteins are very prone to these enzymes. During aging, sarcoplasmic reticulum looses the capacity to retain $Ca^{++}$ ions and their release initiate a water-soluble enzyme called calcium-activated sarcoplasmic factor (CASF). This factor degrades desmin (a Z-line protein), connectin (gap filaments), troponin T (above pH 6), tropomyosin and M-line proteins causing tenderization of meat.
  *Cathepsins* or lysosomal enzymes become active at low ultimate pH or comparatively high temperature and bring about degradation of myosin and actin to fragments. Besides, they also degrade crosslinks of non-helical telopeptides of collagen and mucopolysaccharides of ground substance. Some lysosomal enzymes operate during postmortem aging to cause hydrolysis of sarcoplasmic proteins to peptides and amino acids. Proteolysis, thus, brings about some improvement in water holding capacity of meat.
  Some collagen fibers appear to swell during aging suggesting partial damage to crosslinks in perimyseal and endomyseal collagen and solubilization to a limited extent.
- **Flavor enhancement:** During postmortem aging, ATP is broken down to mononucleotides-AMP and IMP which produce inosinic acid and hypoxanthine, enhancing flavor of meat. Besides, there is production of some flavor compounds such as hydrogen sulfide, ammonia, acetaldehyde, acetone and diacetyl, etc., by microbes, most particularly by yeast and in long-term aging by molds.

Due to break down of protein and accumulation of free amino acids and presences of traces of soluble carbohydrates contributing carbonyl groups, Maillard reaction can also take place during later part of aging. This non-enzymatic reaction can form brown compounds, which may cause some discoloration and may impart some bitter taste to meat.

7

CHAPTER

# Fraudulent Substitution of Meat and its Recognition

Adulteration of meat involves substitution of costly or superior quality with cheaper, undesirable or inferior quality meat. It is a fraudulent practice that is objectionable on the grounds of health, religion and economics. It is punishable under Prevention of Food Adulteration Act, 1955.

The substitutions generally practiced are mutton for goat meat (chevon), beef for buffalo meat, rabbit meat for chicken, etc. The instances of dog or cat meat or even veal as goat meat have also come to light. In United Kingdom, substitution of beef with horse flesh is the most likely one to be encountered whereas in Australia the possibility of substitution of beef with Kangaroo meat cannot be ruled out.

## RECOGNITION OF FRAUDULENT SUBSTITUTION OR ADULTERATION

It is necessary to assure the wholesomeness of meat to the public, which besides other measures, may necessitate the authentic identification of species of meats. The following methods can be used for meat differentiation:

1. **Physical methods:**
   - *General appearance:* Color, consistency, odor
   - *General characteristics of the body fat:* Color, consistency, quality, etc.
2. **Anatomical methods:**
   - Dentition
   - Bone percentage of carcasses
   - Rib numbers and their degree of curvature
   - Characteristics of long bones
3. **Histological methods:**
   - Muscle fiber length
   - Muscle fiber diameter

## Physical Methods

| S. No. | Meat | General Appearance | | | Characteristics of body fat | | |
|---|---|---|---|---|---|---|---|
| | | Color | Consistency | Odor | Color | Consistency | Quality |
| 1. | Chevon | Light red | Very firm | Goaty | Pure white | - | Practically no inter-muscular fat |
| 2. | Mutton | Light to dark | Firm and dense | Ammoniacal | White | Hard and firm | Abundant inter-muscular fat |
| 3. | Buffalo meat | Dark red | Firm | - | Pure white | - | - |
| 4. | Beef | Red | Fairly firm | - | Yellowish white | Firm | Intramuscular fat |
| 5. | Bullock | Light to dark red | Firm | - | White to yellow | Firm to loose as per age | - |
| 6. | Pork | Light red | Very soft | Urine like | White | Soft | Subcutaneous fat deposition |
| 7. | Vial | Pale to white | Firm | - | White | Firm | No intramuscular fat |
| 8. | Horse flesh | Dark red | Soft | - | Yellow | Soft and greasy | No intramuscular fat |
| 9. | Dog meat | Dark red | - | - | White | - | Slight intramuscular fat |
| 10. | Poultry meat | White | Firm | - | Yellow | Loose | Mostly subcutaneous |
| 11. | Camel meat | Red | Fairly firm | - | - | - | - |

4. **Chemical methods:**
   - Composition of meat
   - Myoglobin content
   - Glycogen content
   - Composition of body fat
5. **Immunological/Serological methods:**
   - Precipitation test
   - Double immunodiffusion test
   - Single radial immunodiffusion test
6. **Electrophoretic methods:**
   - Polyacrylamide disc electrophoresis
   - Polyacrylamide gel electrophoresis
   - Sodium dodecyl sulphate-polyacrylamide gel electrophoresis (SDS-PAGE)
7. **Isoelectric focusing**
8. **Enzyme-linked immunosorbent assay (ELISA)**
9. **PCR**

## Anatomical Methods

*Dentition*

| *S. No.* | *Species* | *Permanent dentition* |
|---|---|---|
| 1. | Cattle and buffalo | $2\dfrac{(0033)}{(4033)} = 32$ |
| 2. | Sheep and goat | $2\dfrac{(0033)}{(4033)} = 32$ |
| 3. | Pig | $2\dfrac{(3143)}{(3143)} = 44$ |
| 4. | Horse | $2\dfrac{(3133)}{(3133)} = 40$ |

*Bone Percentage of Carcass*

Proportion of bones in dressed carcasses can give indication of animal species:

| S. No. | Species | Percentage of bone |
|---|---|---|
| 1. | Mutton | 25 |
| 2. | Bobby calves | 50 |
| 3. | Veal calves | 25 |
| 4. | Pork | 12–20 |
| 5. | Bull | 15 |

*Ribs on the Thorax*

Paired ribs vary in number in different species of animals:

| S. No. | Species | Ribs in pairs | Sternal ribs |
|---|---|---|---|
| 1. | Ox | 13 | 8 |
| 2. | Pig | 14–15 | 7 |
| 3. | Sheep and goat | 13 | 8 |
| 4. | Horse | 18 | 8 |
| 5. | Dog | 13 | 9 |

*Characteristics of Long Bones*

| Bone | Species | Characteristics |
|---|---|---|
| Scapula | • Sheep<br>• Goat | • Short and broad, superior spine thickness and bent back<br>• Possesses distinct neck spine, straight and narrow |
| Radius | • Sheep<br>• Goat | • 1.25 times length of metacarpus<br>• Twice the length of metacarpus |
| Ulna | • Horse<br>• Ox | • Extends only 1/2nd the length of radius<br>• Extends and articulates with carpus |
| Femur | • Horse<br>• Ox | • There is no third trochanter. Fibula is only a small point projection<br>• Possess third trochanter. Fibula extends 2/3rd the length of tibia |

## Histological Methods

The diameter and number of muscle fibers, determined by a fiberoptic microscope, can also lead to species identification. Diameter of muscle fibers of buffalo is more than ox, whereas muscle fibers of buffalo are smaller in size and polygonal in cross-section as compared to large and irregular muscle fibers of ox. As far as other species are concerned, the size of muscle fibers decrease in the following order: pig, buffalo, sheep, goat, poultry.

## Chemical Methods

- **Composition of meat:** Muscular fat content varies according to the meat species. The intramuscular fat in mutton is higher (13.3 percent) as compared to beef (2.6 percent), buffalo meat (0.9 percent), chevon (3.6 percent) and pork (4.4 percent). Vitamin A is present in beef and mutton but absent in buffalo meat, chevon or pork.
- **Myoglobin content:** Horse flesh contains maximum myoglobin content (0.71 percent), much higher than the musculature of other animals.
- **Glycogen content:** Horse flesh is richer in glycogen as compared to most food animals.

*Composition of Body Fats*

- **Refractive index:** Horse fat has higher refractive index (53.5) than ox (less than 40) and pig (less than 50) fat.
- **Iodine number:** Iodine number of horse fat (70–85) is higher than even lard (50–70), whereas iodine number of ox and sheep fat is 35–46.
- **Carotene content:** Buffalo fat is white due to absence of carotene whereas cow fat is cream to yellow in color due to carotene content.
- **Fatty acid analysis:** Horse fat contains 1–2 percent linoleic acid whereas other fats contain less than 0.1 percent linoleic acid.

## Immunological/Serological Methods

These tests are based on the principle that a reaction between soluble antigen and its corresponding specific antibody in appropriate proportion yields a visible precipitate at the point of their interaction.

- **Precipitation test or ring test:** In this test, an antigen is overlayered on to antiserum contained in a test tube. This test has now become obsolete because precipitate often diffuses in a short period of time.
- **Double immunodiffusion (DID) test:** This test initially developed by Ouchterlony (1948) has been further improved and extensively used for the detection of meat species. The test is performed in wells punched in agarose. The buffalo anti cattle monospecific (BACM) serum and rabbit anti cattle monospecific (RACM) serum have

been found to be most suitable from the point of view of simplicity and reliability. Antiserum should be checked for sensitivity before use. It should have a sensitivity of 10 percent.

The precipitation lines produced by the interaction of homologous antigen and antiserum in this test remain distinct for quite sometime and can be preserved for future use. It is easy and cheap test for identification of raw or heated meat at 80°C for less than 10 minutes. Besides, it can detect adulteration up to 5 percent. However, it is time consuming and ineffective for the detection of thoroughly cooked meats.

- **Single radial immunodiffusion (SRID) test:** In this test, serum albumen content in meat extract is estimated on the ground that only this protein formed an immune precipitate in antiserum. Immunological species specificity of albumen is regarded as far superior than the globulin fraction.

## Electrophoretic Methods

Electrophoretic methods have been found to achieve the separation of proteins by their differential migration through a supporting medium under the influence of an electric field. The protein bands thus resolved are visualized for characteristic pattern by direct observation or densitometric scanning.

- **Polyacrylamide disc electrophoresis:** In this method, mitochondrial preparation of goat, sheep, cattle and buffalo meat has been used for the identification of the particular species of fresh meat. The species are identified according to the band pattern.
- **Polyacrylamide gel electrophoresis:** Initially, introduced as starch gel electrophoresis, it was improved with Polyacrylamide gel. Here buffer consisting of 0.5M NaCI and 0.034M EDTA is used at pH 5.4. After electrophoresis and staining, band pattern is observed for identification. It is applicable to meat cooked at less than 80°C for 10 minutes. However, every time we have to run the standard along with the sample.
- **Sodium dodecyl sulphate polyacrylamide gel electrophoresis (SDS-PAGE):** When electrophoresis of different meat samples is performed in a Polyacrylamide gel along with sodium dodecyl sulfate, proteins run according to their molecular weights. The resultant band patterns can be observed for species specificity. SDS-PAGE electrophoresis yields not only excellent results for globular proteins in native state but also for the highly helical rod

shaped molecules like myosin. This method is useful for cooked meat and meat products. However, complexity of bands in high molecular weight region hinder the identification especially in closely related species.

### Isoelectric Focusing

This method utilizes differences in the isoelectric point of fresh meat proteins for meat differentiation. Tissue sections are placed directly on the surface of agarose gels and the proteins are eluted electrophoretically. This is a speedy method with high resolving power.

### Enzyme-linked Immunosorbent Assay (ELISA)

ELISA is an important qualitative immunological tool which is not monitored by precipitation. In this test, antigen-antibody interaction occurs in a monomolecular layer immobilized on an inert surface and is followed by means of an enzyme chemically bonded to one of the immuno-reagents. This is a rapid test and the results are obtained in 2–3 hours. The test is very sensitive also because even 2 percent adulteration can be recognized by this test.

### Polymerase Chain Reaction Assay

PCR assay is a genetic method of meat species identification. This technique has several variants. Species-specific PCR is highly beneficial due to its simplicity, reliability and ability to detect and differentiate target nuclear or mitochondrial DNA. The mitochondrial D-loop based species-specific PCR can detect species in raw, cooked and adulterated meat samples with a limit of detection of 0.1%. The technique involves DNA extraction or isolation from raw or cooked sample, designing of PCR primers for specific amplification of species mitochondrial D-loop region and then PCR assay.

PCR technique has several variants. Multiplex PCR assay can amplify and identify several targets in a single PCR reaction but it requires skillful primer designing and validation. RT-PCR is highly sensitive but it requires costly reagent and equipment. Therefore, species-specific PCR would prove advantageous than other DNA-based methods.

It should be noted that no single test is good enough to differentiate all types of meats. Physical, chemical and anatomical methods are more suitable for raw meat whereas comminuted meat products require sophisticated techniques such as Ouchterlony method, SDS-PAGE, Isoelectric focusing, ELISA, etc. However, Ouchterlony method cannot distinguish between closely related species such as sheep and goat, cattle and buffalo, etc. The effectiveness of ELISA and SDS-PAGE is hampered by the cumbersome process of isolating species-specific serum. A new method called "Random Amplified Polymorphism DNA (RAPD) Fingerprint Technique" generates specific DNA fingerprint pattern for differentiation of red meats in a short time. Besides, some developed countries have patented field identification test kits. Such a kit is very much required in our field conditions also.

# 8

CHAPTER

# Principles of Various Preservation Techniques

Meat is a highly perishable commodity due to nearly neutral pH (low acid food), high moisture content and rich nutrients. Contamination with spoilage organisms is almost unavoidable which makes the preservation of meat more difficult than most other foods. Unless proper preservation methods are adopted, deteriorative microbial activity, enzymatic and chemical reactions along with physical changes are bound to occur. Efforts should be made to attain asepsis by avoiding contamination as much as possible. However, once meat is contaminated with microorganisms, their removal is difficult. Hence, preservation of meat is usually accomplished by the use of low temperature, high temperature, moisture control, direct microbial inhibition, etc. Various methods employed to prolong the shelf life of meat are:

1. Chilling/Refrigeration
2. Freezing
3. Curing
4. Smoking
5. Thermal processing
6. Canning
7. Dehydration
8. Irradiation

## CHILLING/REFRIGERATION

This is the most widely used method of preservation for short-term storage of meat because chilling or refrigeration slows down the microbial growth and enzymatic as well as chemical reactions. Storage of fresh meat is done at a refrigeration temperature of 2 to 5°C. Refrigeration of meat begins with the chilling of animal carcasses and continues through the entire channel of holding, cutting, transit, retail display and even in the consumer household before ultimate use. The relative humidity is generally kept 90% in order to check excessive shrinkage due to loss of moisture. Carcasses are first held in chill coolers (15°C) to remove their body heat and then passed on to holding coolers (5°C). It is important to maintain proper spacing between carcasses so as to allow thorough air circulation.

The refrigerated storage life of meat is influenced by species of origin, initial microbial load, packaging and temperature as well as humidity conditions during storage. Pork and poultry start with a comparatively high microbial load. Irrespective of species of origin, utmost care should be taken during handling of meat in order to check further microbial contamination. Since convenience of meat plant workers is also important, the temperature in cutting and packing halls generally exceeds 5°C. As such, operations should be accomplished by specialized hands within the minimum possible time. Refrigerated temperatures favor the growth of psychrophilic organisms causing spoilage of meat in due course of time.

Generally, fresh meat is maintained in good condition for a period of 5–7 days at a refrigerated temperature of 4±1°C. Processed meat products are also stored under refrigeration till these are finally consumed. These meat products are less perishable as compared to fresh meat. The refrigerated shelf life of these products depends on the processing steps followed in each case.

## FREEZING

Freezing is a method of choice for the long-term preservation of meat. It stops the microbial growth and retards the action of enzymes. It has the advantage of retaining most of the nutritive value of meat during storage, although a very little loss of nutrients does occur in the drip during thawing process. Since drip is not possible in cooked meat products, proper freezing conditions result in retention of most of the nutritional and sensory properties.

It is utmost important to wrap fresh meat in suitable packaging film before freezing, otherwise meat undergoes freezer burn. This abnormal condition occurs due to progressive surface dehydration resulting in the concentration of meat pigments on the surface. This discoloration in frozen meat due to sublimation of ice crystals is irreversible condition. On cooking, freezer burn meat is quite tough and lacks juiciness.

The quality of frozen meat is also influenced by freezing rate. In slow freezing, extracellular water freezes more quickly due to low solute concentration as compared to intracellular water. Thus, there is formation of large extracellular ice crystals which may cause mechanical damage to the muscular tissue, giving it a distorted appearance in the frozen state. Contrary to this, in fast freezing numerous small ice crystals are formed uniformly throughout the meat tissue. Thus, problem of muscle fiber shrinkage and distorted appearance is not there. Besides, drip losses during thawing are considerably low as intracellular water freezes within the muscle fiber itself. Numerous small ice crystals on the surface of fast frozen meat also impart it a desired lighter color as compared to slow frozen meat.

Various types of freezers are employed to freeze meat and meat products. In plate type freezers, meat is placed in trays which remain in direct contact with metal freezer plates. A temperature of –10°C or so is achieved. Blast type freezers are used in large meat plants. Such freezers render fast freezing of meat products due to rapid air movement. A temperature range of –10°C to –30°C is generally achieved.

The quality of meat and meat products can be preserved for months together during frozen storage at –10°C. However, a storage temperature of –18°C is recommended because at this level almost all water in meat is frozen and minor temperature fluctuations can be taken care of. At –18°C, storage life of buffalo meat, beef, mutton and chevon is approximately 6 months, while that of pork and poultry is less (4 months) because of associated unsaturated fat, prone to rancidity development. Storage life of cured and salted meat products is still limited (2 months) as salt is a pro-oxidant. However at –10°C, storage life of these meats is reduced to half or even less. Thawing of meat should be done within the package itself preferably in a refrigerator so as to minimize the drip losses. However, if thawing is to be accomplished at a short notice, warm air or lukewarm water may be used. Refreezing a thawed meat is not suggested in tropical countries and repeated freezing should not be practised.

At times, freezing and thawing of young chicken may pose the problem of bone darkening due to leaching of hemoglobin from the marrow of porous bones to the adjoining muscle tissue. This tissue appears gray or black after cooking, although other sensory attributes are not affected.

## CURING

Preservation of meat by heavy salting is an age old practice. It was applied as a thumb rule because refrigeration facilities were not available. Later, curing by common salt and sodium nitrite resulted in comparatively improved products. These days mild curing of meat products is practised mainly for specific flavor and color development and preservative effects of curing ingredients is an added advantage. Sodium chloride, sodium nitrite, sodium nitrate and sugar are the main curing ingredients.

**Sodium chloride** (common salt) exerts its preservative action as follows:

- It acts by dehydration and alteration of osmotic pressure that inhibits the growth of spoilage bacteria.
- Chloride ions in the salt directly act on the microorganisms.
- It slows down the action of proteolytic enzymes in meat.

Besides, sodium chloride interacts with fatty acids to enhance the flavor of the cured products. It also contributes to the tenderness of the product.

**Sodium nitrate and nitrite** serve to stabilize the attractive cured meat color and impart characteristics cured meat flavor. Color reactions of cured meats can be summarized as follows:

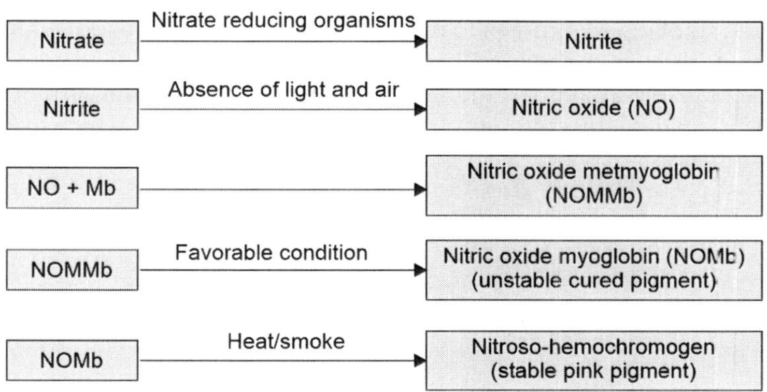


Nitrates and nitrites at permitted levels of 500 ppm and 200 ppm respectively act as preservatives by inhibiting the growth of a number of bacteria especially *Clostridium botulinum*. These chemicals also retard the development of rancidity. Cured flavor develops due to reaction between fatty acids and sodium nitrite resulting in the formation of benzonitrile and phenylacetonitrile. However, nitrite has been found to be involved in the formation of nitrosamine which is supposed to be carcinogenic. Sugar counteracts the harsh hardening effect of salt, adds to the flavor development and also serves as an energy source for nitrate reducing bacteria in the curing solution or pickle. Sucrose or dextrose is mainly used for this purpose. Traditionally, curing of meat is limited to pork (esp. ham and belly) and beef (esp. brisket and leg muscles).

There are several methods of curing:

- **Dry cure:** Dry ingredients are rubbed to meat, e.g., curing of bacon.
- **Pickle cure:** Meat cuts are immersed in ingredient solution (pickle), e.g., curing of pork shoulder.
- **Injection cure:** Concentrated solution of the ingredients is pumped into the meat through artery or injected by needles in the muscular pork, e.g., curing of pork ham **(Fig. 8.1)**.
- **Direct addition method:** Curing agents are added directly to finely ground meat, e.g., luncheon meat.

The temperature of curing room is maintained at 3±1°C and curing process is allowed for 3 to 4 days depending on the strength of curing pickle.

## SMOKING

Meat smoking was known to man as an aid in preservation for a long time, although its chemical basis was a mystery. It is now well known that smoke contains a large number of wood degradation products such as aldehydes, ketones, organic acids, phenols, etc., which exert

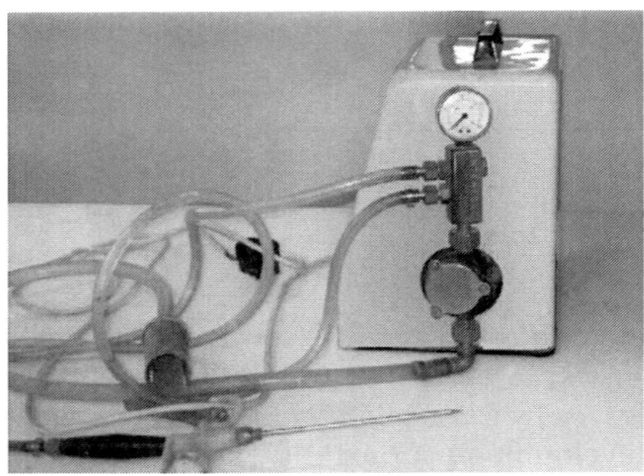

**Fig. 8.1 :** Cure injector.

bacteriostatic effect besides imparting characteristic smoky flavor. Preservation of smoked meat is also due to surface dehydration, lowering of surface pH and antioxidant property of smoke constituents. Curing and smoking of meat are closely inter-related and these days, curing is usually followed by smoking. Besides, smoking and cooking operations are accomplished simultaneously.

Smoke is produced in the specially constructed 'smoke house' where saw dust or hard wood and sometimes both are subjected to combustion at a temperature of about 300°C **(Fig. 8.2)**. High temperature is desirable to minimize the production of carcinogenic compounds. Smoke generation is accompanied by formation of numerous organic compounds and their condensation products. Aldehydes and phenols condense to form resins, which constitute 50% of the smoke components and contribute most of the color of smoked meat products. Phenols act mainly as bacteriostatic and formaldehyde as the chief bactericidal compound.

These days many liquid smoke preparations are commercially available in the developed countries. Liquid smoke is generally prepared from hardwood, wherein polycyclic hydrocarbons are removed by filtration. Application of liquid smoke on the product surface before cooking imparts it a smoky flavor which is very much liked by the consumers.

## THERMAL PROCESSING

Unlike refrigeration of meat that slows or stops microbial growth, thermal processing as a preservative method is employed to kill

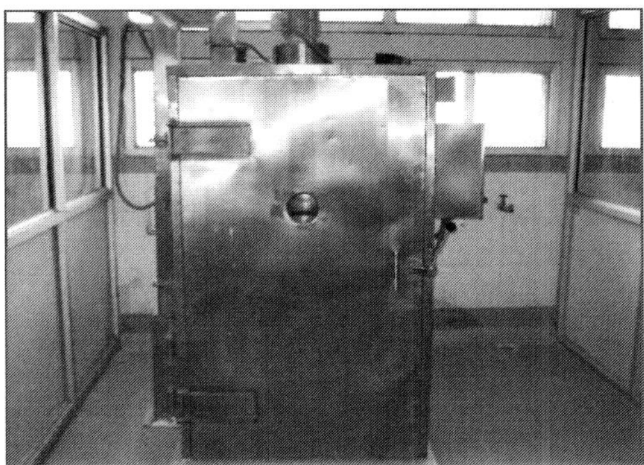

**Fig. 8.2:** Smoke generator.

the spoilage microorganisms. Two temperature regimes, that of pasteurization and sterilization are generally used. Pasteurization refers to moderate heating in the temperature range of 58°C to 75°C whereby most of the microorganisms present including Trichinae occasionally found in pork are killed. Incidentally, this is also the cooking temperature range of most processed meats. This heat treatment significantly extends the shelf life of meat, although such products also need to be stored under refrigeration. Sterilization refers to severe heating at temperatures above 100°C whereby all spoilage microorganisms in meat are killed or their microbial cells are damaged beyond repair. This heat treatment renders the meat products commercially sterile because some bacterial spores may still survive. Such meat products have a recommended shelf life of two years in cans and one year in retort pouches at ambient temperature in tropics. However, exposure of meat to high temperatures imparts sulfhydryl flavor in cans and modifies texture also.

Various meat products differ in water content, amount of fat and consistency. These factors have a definite bearing on the thermal processing schedule. For example, moist heat is much more effective in killing microorganisms and spores as compared to dry heat, so a meat product with higher moisture content will require comparatively less heat for sterilization.

## CANNING

It is a process of preservation achieved by thermal sterilization of a product held in hermetically sealed containers. Canning preserves the sensory attributes such as appearance, flavor and texture of the meat products to a large extent. Besides, canned meat products have a shelf life of at least 2 years at ambient temperature. Conventional canning is done in the following steps:

- **Preparation of meat and gravy:** Carcass is deboned and 4 cm meat chunks are prepared. Meat gravy is prepared using condiments, tomatoes, dry spices and salt, etc.
- **Precooking:** Meat and gravy, both are precooked at 70°C for 15 minutes. It causes the inevitable shrinkage of meat chunks and reduces the initial microbial load.
- **Filling:** Filling in cans may be done manually or mechanically leaving proper headspace as per BIS specifications. Half of the gravy

is filled first followed by meat chunks and finally the rest of the gravy. Special care is taken to avoid trapping of air during this operation.

- **Exhausting:** It refers to the removal of air from the container before it is closed. It is necessary to minimize the strain on the can seams due to expansion of air during heat processing. Mechanical exhausting may vacuum seal the cans.
- **Seaming:** This is usually done by a double seamer machine.
- **Retorting or thermal processing:** The product is subjected to high temperature under pressure for sufficient duration to achieve commercial sterility.
- **Cooling:** Retorting is followed by very fast cooling up to 30–40°C to give a shock to the thermophilic bacteria.
- **Storage:** Cans should be stored in a cool and dry place preferably at a temperature of about 20°C.

## DEHYDRATION

Removal of water from meat concentrates the water soluble nutrients making them unavailable to the microorganisms. The extent of availability of water to microbial cell is expressed as water activity ($a_w$). Dehydration lowers the water activity considerably to prevent the growth of spoilage organisms. Sun drying of meat chunks as a means of preservation was practised even in ancient days but rehydration of such meat chunks used to be limited. Mechanical drying process involves the passage of hot air with controlled humidity but here also there is difficulty in rehydration.

Freeze drying of meat is a satisfactory process of dehydration preservation due to better reconstitution properties, nutritive quality and acceptability. Freeze drying involves the removal of water from a food by sublimation from the frozen state to vapor state by keeping it under vacuum and giving a low heat treatment. Freeze drying of meat is carried out in three stages:

1. Prefreezing
2. Primary drying
3. Secondary drying

Meat is first frozen at –40°C. Then it is dried under vacuum for 9–12 hours at low temperature in plate heat exchangers at 1 to 1.5 mm pressure of mercury. Ice crystals get sublimated to water vapor and there is no rise of temperature. In the first phase of drying, free and immobilized water of meat which is freezable and constitutes about

90–95% of total moisture, is removed. Secondary drying is done at high temperature to remaining 4–8% bound water. Freeze dried products are packaged under vacuum and have very good storage stability. The process has been largely used for the preparation of dehydrated meat soup mixes.

## IRRADIATION

Radiation is the emission and propagation of energy in the material medium. Electromagnetic radiations are in the form of continuous waves. These are capable of ionizing molecules in their path. These radiations can destroy the microorganisms by fragmenting their DNA molecules and causing ionization of inherent water within microoganisms. Since microbial destruction of foods takes place without significantly raising the temperature, food irradiation is many times referred as cold sterilization.

Among radiations, alpha and beta-rays are charged particles and have limited use in food irradiation. However, lambda rays are electronic waves of short wave length and not the charged particles. These are easily obtained from isotopes like $^{60}Co$ and $^{137}Cs$ and have excellent penetration power. Gamma radiations produce desired effect only during food irradiation and have no effect after removal of source. These are widely used in food preservation. In foods, the radiation dose is expressed as Gray (Gy) which is equivalent to 100 rad of older unit. One kGy is equal to 1000 Gy. Radiation dose for food can be classified as:

1. *Radurization* (radiation pasteurization) refers to low dose treatment (generally <1 kGy) with the intent to eliminate parasites and extend the food product shelf life.
2. *Radicidation* refers to medium dose (generally 1–10 kGy) radiation pasteurization with the intent to eliminate spoilage and non-spore forming pathogens.
3. *Radappertization* (radiation pasteurization) refers to high dose radiation treatment (generally >10 kGy) with the intent to make the food product sterile and shelf stable.

A dose of 0.3–1 kGy can inactivate the tapeworm and trichinae in raw pork while a dose of 1–7 kGy can markedly reduce the spoilage and pathogenic bacteria and extend the shelf life of raw and fresh fish, refrigerated and frozen meat as well as poultry products. A dose of 20–70 kGy can sterilize pork, poultry and fish. Among the non-ionizing radiations, ultraviolet radiations of 2650 A° are most bactericidal in nature, but due to poor penetration power, these are used only for surface sterilization of meats. It may be mentioned that certain chemicals like ascorbates have been found to increase the sensitivity of the microorganisms to radiation.

In addition to the above mentioned preservation techniques, there are many chemicals which prevent microbial growth in foods and act as preservatives. Several organic acids have been generally recognized as safe (GRAS) for use as chemical preservatives. Citric acid, propionic acid, benzoic acid, sorbic acid and their salts are effective mold inhibitors. Acetic acid and lactic acid prevent bacterial growth, whereas sorbate and acetate are capable of arresting the growth of yeast in foods. It may be noted that modern meat food processors do not rely on any single preservative factor or technique. They employ a combination of preservative factor (hurdles) in a balanced manner to derive maximum benefit. Technologists have exploited the hurdle concept in the development and keeping quality enhancement of intermediate moisture and shelf stable food products.

# 9 CHAPTER

# Processing of Meat and Meat Products

Basic meat plant operations such as cutting, trimming, deboning and grinding do not constitute meat processing. In fact, processing refers to any treatment including salting which brings about a substantial chemical and physical change in the natural state of meat. Processing invariably imparts considerable shelf stability to meat. As a matter of fact, many processing techniques were evolved in the pursuit of preservation.

## BASIC PROCESSING PROCEDURES

### Comminution

All processed meats can be classified as either non-comminuted or comminuted products. Non-comminuted products are generally processed from intact cuts. These products are usually cured, smoked and cooked, e.g., ham and bacon. Comminution refers to subdivision or reduction of raw meat into meat pieces or particles. The degree of comminution or particle size varies with the processing characteristics of products. Such meat particle size reduction helps in the uniform distribution of seasonings and eliminates the toughness associated with meat of old animals and lowers the fuel cost for cooking (Padda *et al.*, 1987). Comminution is done with the help of meat mincer for coarse ground products whereas bowl chopper is also employed for making fine meat emulsion.

### Emulsification

A mixture of two immiscible liquids where one liquid is dispersed as droplets in another liquid is called emulsion. An emulsion has two phases, a continuous phase and a dispersed or discontinuous phase. These phases remain immiscible due to the existence of an interfacial tension between them. The emulsion remains unstable if interfacial tension is very high. The emulsion can be stabilized by reducing the interfacial tension with the help of emulsifying agents or emulsifiers. Homogenized milk is a good example of true emulsion in which fat droplets are dispersed in an aqueous continuous phase. The size or diameter of dispersed fat droplets in a true emulsion ranges from 1 to 5 micrometer (1 µm).

Meat emulsion comprises of a dispersed phase of solid or liquid fat droplets and a continuous phase of water containing salt and proteins. Here, continuous phase can also be referred as a matrix in which fat droplets are dispersed. Due to the presence of matrix, many people call meat emulsion as a multiphase system **(Fig. 9.1)**. For practical purposes, meat emulsion is an oil-in-water emulsion where solubilized meat proteins act as emulsifiers. The fat droplets are usually larger than 50 µm in size and remain coated with a soluble protein—either myofibrillar or sarcoplasmic. The amount of fat that can be incorporated in a stable emulsion depends on fat particle size, meat pH, temperature during emulsification and the amount and type of soluble proteins. It is very important to maintain low temperature during emulsion formation in order to avoid melting of fat particles, denaturation of soluble proteins and lowering of viscosity. This is done by adding ice flakes instead of chilled water during chopping.

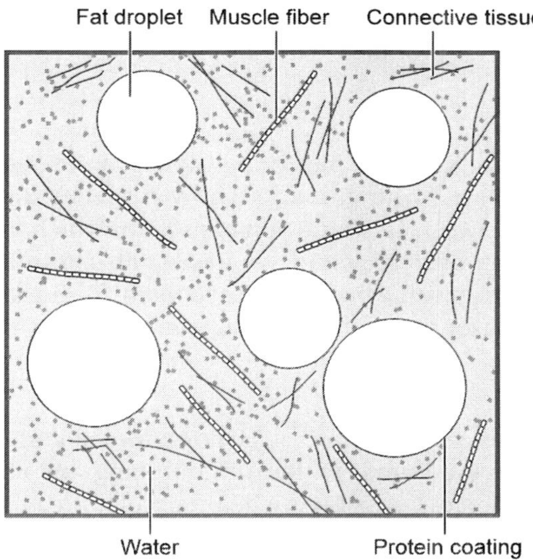


**Fig. 9.1:** Meat emulsion (Ultra view).

For the preparation of a good meat emulsion, lean meat is first chopped with salt to extract salt soluble proteins and then fat and other ingredients are added. Salt, soluble proteins have a relatively high emulsifying capacity. Once a good meat emulsion is formed, it has to be protected during cooking or heat treatment. The emulsion breakdown can occur due to sudden exposure to high temperature because of coalescence of finely dispersed fat particles into larger ones (fat pockets). The encased or moulded emulsion is first exposed to heat at 55°C so as to coagulate the coating proteins and stabilize the emulsion.

## Meat Extension

A lot of non-meat food items can be incorporated in meat products. These are generally termed as extenders, although these may be specifically referred as fillers, binders, emulsifiers or stabilizers depending on the purpose of their incorporation in the basic meat formulation. In developing countries soy products, potato starch and flours of wheat, rice, pea, corn, etc., are used as fillers to reduce the cost of formulations. Several milk products such as skim milk powder, dried whey, sodium caseinate, etc., are frequently used as binders. Some gums like sodium alginate, carrageenan, gum acacia, etc., may be used to stabilize fragile meat emulsions. Due to high cost, extension of meat should be taken up on a large scale in order to ensure the availability of meat products to the masses.

## Preblending

It refers to the mixing of a part or all the curing ingredients (salt, nitrite, nitrate, etc.) with ground meat in a specified proportion. This process allows better extraction of proteins which in turn helps in the formation of stable emulsion. It permits control of product composition by adjusting the desired fat content. Besides, processors get enough time for the analysis of meat samples.

## Hot Processing

It refers to the processing of carcass as soon as possible after slaughter (certainly with 1–2 hours) without undergoing any chilling. The term prerigor processing is used when muscular meat is processed in a prerigor condition. Though hot processing of meat has been a common practice in India, it is rather a new development in western countries. This technique has many advantages. It accelerates the processing steps and entire processing time is reduced to a great extent. There is improvement in the cooking yield and sensory quality of the product. In addition, there are financial benefits due to reduced chiller space and labor requirement. Thus, lot of energy is saved if hot processing is adopted at a pilot scale.

## Cooking

Meat and meat products are cooked by anyone or a combination of three methods—dry heat, moist heat and microwave cooking. Dry heat cooking is an accepted method for relatively tender cuts of meat such as pork chops, leg and chops of lamb, ground and comminuted meats, etc. The product yield is relatively high due to comparatively less shrinkage. Dry heat cooking involves either broiling, roasting or frying. In broiling, meat held on a wire grill, is exposed to heat from above as in electric and gas oven or below as in charcoal broiler. Meat is required to be turned for uniform and sufficient cooking on all sides. Roasting is also practised on tender cuts of meats such as pork shoulder and loin; shoulder, rack and loin of lamb and cured ham, etc. The roast piece, at least 8 cm thick, is adjusted in open roasting pan with fat side up and placed in hot-air oven at 115–150°C. Cooking temperature and time varies according to the cut. Roasting generally gives good browning and improves the flavor of the product. Frying—deep fat or shallow pan is also classified under dry heat cooking. This method is especially suitable for thin cuts of meat such as sliced steaks, mutton chops, chicken meat pieces, etc.

***Moist heat cooking*** is recommended for relatively tough cuts of meat. In this method, hot water or steam is continuously kept in contact with meat for cooking, so that moisture loss does not take place beyond a particular stage. Pressure cooking, stewing, simmering, etc., are popular moisture cooking procedures. Higher cooking temperatures can be achieved in pressure cooking facilitating the tenderization of tough cuts of meat. In stewing, tough meat pieces are first browned in small amount of fat and then covered with water along with curry stuff and allowed to cook at simmering temperature in covered container. The final product becomes tender along with a curry. Simmering involves cooking in hot water at a temperature of 70°C for considerable time. Braising utilizes both dry heat as well as moist heat for proper processing of meat products. Several meat cuts like pork chops and steaks, mutton breast and shanks, etc., are first fried in a frying pan and then put in a covered container along with water and seasoning for cooking at 80–90°C.

***Microwave cooking*** is relatively a recent development. Microwaves are high frequency, non-ionizing electromagnetic waves which are generated by magnetron vacuum tube within the oven. These waves are channelized into the oven cavity through a wave guide. A stirrer fan distributes the microwaves evenly. The microwaves penetrate the food from all directions simultaneously up to a depth of 2–4 cm causing water, fat and sugar molecules to vibrate at a very high speed. The vibrations cause tremendous friction which produces heat for cooking the food. The spread of heat throughout the three dimensional space in the food itself is called volume heating. Contrary to conventional heating, food is first to be heated in the microwave cooking which then transmits heat to container and oven environment. It saves a lot of time, taking only 25% time as compared to conventional thermal oven. Microwaves can pass through glass, pottery, wood and paper but reflected by metal. So, metallic utensils cannot be used in the microwave oven. There are some other disadvantages also. Food has to be frequently turned to ensure proper heating and browning of food does not take place in this cooking.

## PROCESSING OF MEAT PRODUCTS

Processing of meat products is divided into the following groups for further discussion:

- Cured and smoked meats
- Sausages
- Intermediate moisture and shelf stable meat products
- Restructured meat products
- Other popular meat products, e.g., meat samosa **(Fig. 9.15)**

### Cured and Smoked Meats

All meat products belonging to this class are cured, whereas only some of them are smoked. The primal cuts of pork especially ham and bacon have been subjected to curing and smoking for a long time. These days, it is a general practice to accomplish cooking also during smoking except for country ham, which is smoked without cooking.

*Hams*

These are classified in several ways:

- According to weight : Light, medium and heavy
- According to trimming : Rough, regular, skinned and skinless
- According to presence of bone : Bone-in, semi-boneless and boneless

**Commercial processing of ham**

Irrespective of classification, most hams are processed in three steps—curing, smoking and cooking. Most commercial hams are pickle cured. A typical curing solution consists of:

| *Ingredients* | *Quantity* |
|---|---|
| Table salt | 850 g |
| Phosphate | 225 g |
| Sucrose | 175 g |
| Sodium erythrobate | 15 g |
| Sodium nitrite | 8 g |
| Water | 40 liters |

Curing is usually done by artery pumping or stitch pumping to 10% of the green weight. However, best results with respect to color and flavor are obtained by keeping the hams in a cover pickle at 4°C for 5 days. The hams are now shifted to smoke chamber which is maintained at 75–85°C temperature and 30–40% relative humidity for 5–6 hours. Smoke generated from hardwood is preferred for good results.

The processing of some variety hams is given hereunder:

**Cooked ham:** These hams are deboned and cured in the pickle but smoking is not done. Instead, these hams are stuffed tightly into metal moulds and cooked in a water tank at 75–85°C for 2–3 hours depending on the weight of the ham. During cooking, the core temperature must reach 65–70°C. After cooking, the mould-in hams are chilled in a tank maintained at 0°C for 12 hours. These hams are then sliced and packed.

**Country ham:** These uncooked hams are manufactured in USA by dry curing method. The curing mixture usually contains 8 kg salt, 1 kg sugar and 100 g sodium nitrite. It is rubbed thoroughly at the rate of 30 g per kg of ham on 1st, 5th and 10th day. The entire production schedule is divided into three phases—(a) Curing is allowed to take place under refrigeration at a relative humidity of 70–90% for 30–40 days during which hams are overhauled at least three times, (b) Smoking is done at low temperature for 2–3 days till the hams become amber colored and (c) Aging is done for 6–9 months at a temperature of 20–30°C and relative humidity of 50–60%. During this period, country hams become progressively harder and develop a unique flavor. Country hams have a final salt level of 4–5% and a moisture content of 50–60%. The shrinkage loss during processing amounts to 18–20%.

**Prosciutto:** These hams are manufactured in Italy from certified trichinae free hams and traditionally consumed without being cooked. These are dry cured like country hams. Curing continues for 45 days at 40°C, followed by smoking for 2 days at 55°C and finally aging for 30 days at 20°C at a relative humidity of 65–75%. There is shrinkage of 3–5% in weight during the entire processing schedule.

#### *Bacon*

Pork bellies are generally processed as cured and smoked bacon. There are no fixed criteria for the classification of bacon. However, many processors grade them on the basis of weights of green bellies.

**Commercial processing of bacon**

Green bellies are first cleared of rind and stitch pumped with a curing pickle. These are now transferred to smoke chamber maintained at a temperature of 60–65°C and a relative humidity of 30–0% for smoking as well as cooking. The cooking time depends on the size of bellies although an internal temperature of 55°C must be achieved. Cooking also helps to stabilize the cured color. After smoking and cooking, bacon is chilled to 0°C to allow it to retain proper shape and facilitate slicing. These bacon slabs are processed in a forming machine to give uniform width and thickness. Bacon blocks are now sliced to 5–7 mm thickness with the help of slicer **(Fig. 9.2)**. The slices may be packed in a modified atmosphere if long-term storage is desired.

Some variations in the processing of bacon in different countries are inevitable. Canadian bacon is not manufactured from bellies but from larger muscles of pork loin and sirloin. In Europe and UK, Wiltshire bacon is produced from pork sides where shoulder, loin, ham and belly are processed as a single large piece.

### Sausages

Sausage term was derived in the ancient times from the Latin word 'salsus' meaning salt. It was literally coined to refer to ground meat

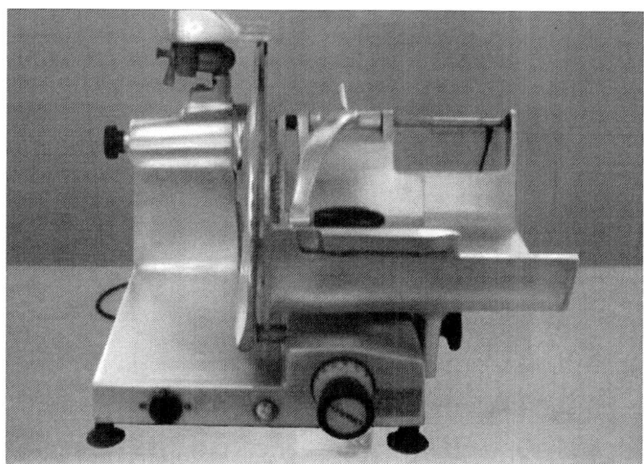

**Fig. 9.2:** Meat slicer.

which was salted and stuffed in animal casings. Presently, sausage may be defined as a meat product which is prepared from minced and seasoned MEAT and formed into cylindrical shape by natural or synthetic casings. Though sausages originated in the western world, these products acquired universal popularity due to variety and convenience to the consumers. Sausages are economical also because these are generally prepared from cheaper cuts of meat and byproducts of industry.

*Classification*

Sausages are such a large number of varying kinds of products that it is not possible to cover them in any classification system. Some overlapping is always there. Some of the popular classification systems are:

1. Based on degree of chopping
   a. Coarse ground sausage
   b. Emulsion type sausage
2. Based on moisture content
   a. Fresh sausage
   b. Smoked uncooked sausage
   c. Cooked sausage
   d. Dry and semi-dry sausage
3. Based on fermentation
   a. Fermented sausage
   b. Non-fermented sausage

*Processing Steps*

1. **Grinding or mincing:** Lean meat and fat are minced separately in a meat mincer **(Fig. 9.3)**. The choice of mincer plate or sieve depends on the type of meat.

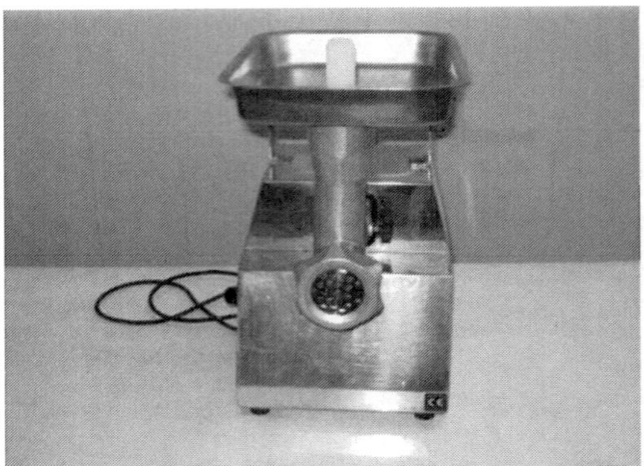

**Fig. 9.3:** Meat mincer.

2. **Mixing:** Meat and fat to be used for the preparation of coarse ground sausage are mixed uniformly in a mixer. Extender, condiments and spices should also be run in the mixer for even distribution.
3. **Chopping and emulsifying:** For emulsion preparation, lean meat is first chopped for few minutes in a bowl chopper **(Fig. 9.4)** with salt to extract myofibrillar proteins. This is followed by addition of fat and running for a few minutes again to get desired emulsion consistency. Now, all other ingredients are added and chopper is run for sometime for uniform distribution. The entire operation is conducted at low temperature by addition of ice flakes in place of chilled water.

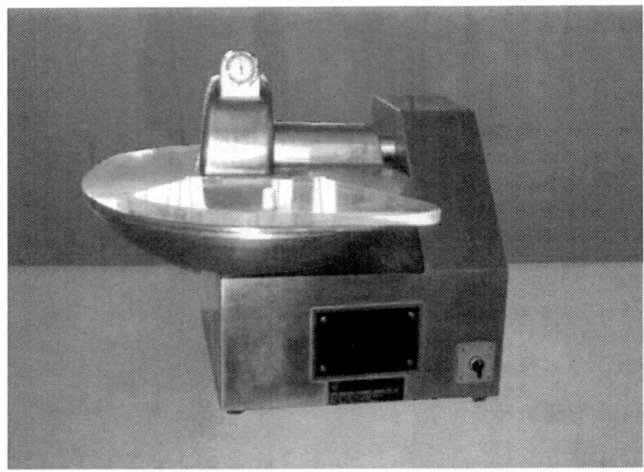

**Fig. 9.4:** Bowl chopper.

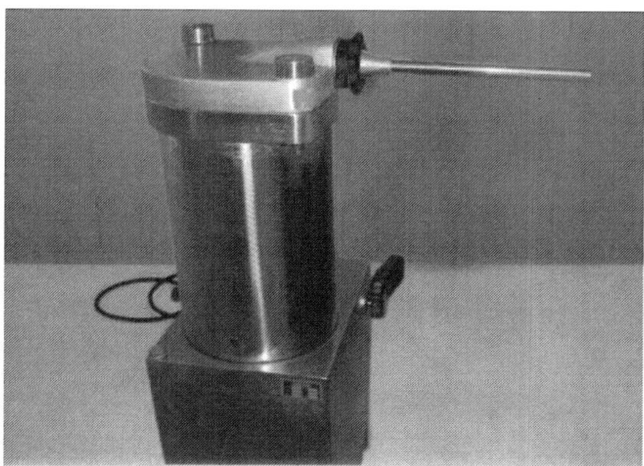

**Fig. 9.5:** Sausage filler.

4. **Stuffing:** Sausage emulsion or batter is taken to stuffer for extrusion into casings. The casings are first collected on the stuffing horn or nozzle and released to coincide with the extrusion **(Fig. 9.5)**.
5. **Linking and tying:** In small sausages, the encased mass is twisted to produce links either manually or mechanically whereas in large sausages, the encased mass is tied with thread at regular intervals.
6. **Smoking and cooking:** Sausage links are hung on the smokehouse trolley and transferred to smokehouse. The temperature of smokehouse is usually maintained at 68–70°C which is enough for coagulation of sausage emulsion, cooking and requisite drying of sausages.
7. **Chilling:** The cooked product is showered with chilled water to an internal temperature of about 4°C.
8. **Peeling and packaging:** While artificial or synthetic casings are peeled off before the product is packed, small sized natural casings need not be removed. The product is generally unit packed for retail outlets.

Formulations of some sausages with special features:

**Fresh pork sausages (Coarse ground type)**

| *Ingredients* | *Quantity* |
|---|---|
| Lean pork trimmings | 35 kg |
| Backfat | 15 kg |
| Table salt | 1 kg |
| White pepper | 125 g |
| Sugar | 75 g |
| Ginger powder | 15 g |

**Frankfurters (Cured, emulsion type meat sausages)**

| *Ingredients* | *Quantity* |
|---|---|
| Beef trimmings | 30 kg |
| Pork trimmings (50/50) | 20 kg |
| Ice flakes | 15 kg |
| Table salt | 1.2 kg |
| White pepper | 110 g |
| Nutmeg | 25 g |
| Cardamom | 25 g |
| Ginger powder | 25 g |
| Monosodium glutamate (MSG) | 25 g |
| Sodium erythrobate | 20 g |
| Sodium nitrite | 7.5 g |

**Salami (Fresh, emulsion type sausages)**

| *Ingredients* | *Quantity* |
|---|---|
| Pork trimmings (50/50) | 20 kg |
| Pork cheek meat | 10 kg |
| Pork hearts | 10 kg |
| Pork stomachs | 5 kg |
| Ice flakes | 5 kg |
| Table salt | 1.2 kg |
| Black pepper | 115 g |
| Sodium erythrobate | 25 g |
| Garlic powder | 25 g |
| Sodium nitrite | 5 g |

Batter is stuffed in broader casings, usually dried cattle esophagus and hanged for 2 days at 4°C. It is smoked and cooked simultaneously in India.

**Chicken sausages (Emulsion type)**

| *Ingredients* | *Quantity* |
|---|---|
| Chicken meat | 30 kg |
| Vegetable oil | 7.5 kg |
| Ice flakes | 5 kg |

*Contd...*

*Contd...*

| Ingredients | Quantity |
|---|---|
| Condiments | 3 kg |
| Bread powder | 3 kg |
| Table salt | 1.2 kg |
| Whole egg liquid | 1 kg |
| Spices mix | 800 g |
| Sodium nitrite | 5 g |

**Thuringer summer sausages (coarse ground, fermented, semi-dry type)**

| Ingredients | Quantity |
|---|---|
| Pork trimmings (75/25) | 25 kg |
| Beef trimmings | 20 kg |
| Table salt | 1.2 kg |
| Dextrose | 400 g |
| Black pepper | 115 g |
| Starter culture | 60 g |
| Coriander | 30 g |
| Sodium nitrite | 5 g |

The pH of sausage mix comes down to about 5 due to bacterial fermentation. Dextrose serves as a substrate for fermentation. Sausage mix prepared at 4°C is stuffed into casings and held in green or ripening room maintained at 25°C and 85–90% relative humidity until fermentation is complete (2–3 days). These are smoked and cooked at 60–65°C. The moisture content of finished product is nearly 50%.

**Dry sausages (coarse ground, fermented sausages, e.g., pepperoni)**

| Ingredients | Quantity |
|---|---|
| Pork trimmings (50/50) | 20 kg |
| Beef trimmings | 15 kg |
| Pork hearts | 5 kg |
| Pork cheeks | 5 kg |
| Table salt | 1.5 kg |
| Dextrose | 500 g |
| Black pepper | 175 g |
| Fennel seeds | 10 g |
| Sodium nitrite | 7.0 g |

Sausage mix is stuffed into 40–44 mm animal casings and held for 9–11 days at 4°C. It is transferred to green room for 2 days to be maintained at 20°C and 70% relative humidity and then smoked for 3 days at 35°C and 80% relative humidity. The product is not cooked but held for 21 days in the drying room at 35°C and 70% relative humidity during which it will have a shrinkage. The final product has only 30–35% moisture content **(Fig. 9.11)**.

**Bologna:** It is an emulsion type sausage prepared from the meat of old animals.

**Hot dog:** It is a fairly spicy sausage in broader casings, usually weasand in India.

**Mortadella:** It is a dry sausage prepared in cattle bladder or artificial broader casings.

## Intermediate Moisture and Shelf Stable Meat Products

Sun drying of meat was one of the earliest preservative techniques used by man. Such meat had meagre rehydration capacity resulting in poor juiciness and texture. Later studies revealed that meat products with 20–50% moisture had moderate juiciness and texture on rehydration. Such products were resistant to bacteriological spoilage and could be held without refrigeration. These products were referred as intermediate moisture meats (IMM). The basic reason for the stability of these products lay in the reduced availability of water to the microorganisms, since water activity generally remains in the range of 0.6 to 0.85. These semi-moist meats are of special significance to the developing countries where refrigeration facilities are not always available. Such products can be easily carried in defence expeditions and stress situations like floods, famines, etc., for air drop.

### *Humectants*

Various additives employed for lowering the water activity of foods are known as humectants. Some of the most commonly used humectants are:

- Glycerol
- Propylene glycol
- Sodium chloride
- Polyhydric alcohols (e.g., sorbitol)
- Sugars (e.g., sucrose, dextrose, corn syrup, etc.)

The humectants are generally low molecular weight compounds which are easily soluble in water. These are chemically inert and do not modify the normal sensory qualities of the product. Besides, these compounds are edible in large quantities without any adverse effect.

In addition to humectants, use of antimycotic agents like potassium sorbate, sodium benzoate, propylene glycol, etc., is a must in the semi-moist meats because 0.6 to 0.85 water activity range specifically permits the growth of molds.

*Basic Processing Techniques*

a. **Moist infusion or desorption:** It involves soaking and/or cooking of meat chunks or cubes to yield a final product having desired water activity level, e.g., sweet and sour pork, Hungarian goulash, etc.
b. **Dry infusion or adsorption:** It involves initial dehydration of meat chunks or cubes followed by soaking in an infusion solution containing desired osmotic agents, e.g., ready-to-eat cubes of roast pork, chicken a la king, etc.
c. **Component blending:** In this process, dry and wet ingredients or components are blended, cooked and extruded or otherwise mixed to give a final product of desired water activity.

Whatever process is adopted, the thumb rules for the preparation of IMM are: (a) reduction of water activity by addition of humectants, (b) retardation of microbial growth by addition of antimicrobial especially antimycotic agents and (c) improvement of sensory properties such as flavor and texture through physical and chemical treatments.

Composition of infusion solution developed by Brockmann (1970) for the preparation of sweet and sour pork ($a_w = 0.85$) is given below to give an idea about the balancing of various additives:

| *Ingredients* | *Percentage* |
|---|---|
| Glycerol | 25.00 |
| Catsup | 23.55 |
| Water | 15.00 |
| Vinegar | 13.50 |
| Sucrose | 11.84 |
| Starch hydrolysate | 14.50 |
| Salt | 2.59 |
| Corn starch | 2.30 |
| Monosodium glutamate | 1.15 |
| Potassium sorbate | 0.30 |

*Contd..*

*Contd...*

| *Ingredients* | *Percentage* |
|---|---|
| Mustard powder | 0.24 |
| Onion powder | 0.02 |
| Garlic powder | 0.01 |

#### *Stability of Intermediate Moisture Meats*

IMF products are fairly stable at ambient temperature for several weeks or even months. However, prolonged storage may result in some quality deterioration due to the following reasons:

a. Limited breakdown of both myofibrillar and sarcoplasmic proteins. Collagen being more susceptible to degeneration results in more hydroxyproline formation.
b. Degradation of hemoprotein (myoglobin and hemoglobin) causing loss of color.
c. Development of rancidity.
d. Non-enzymatic browning resulting in loss of color, consumer appeal, nutritive value and possibly off-flavor.
e. Formation of lipid-protein crosslinks causing decreased water binding capacity and net protein utilization of meat products.

#### *Hurdle Technology*

Intermediate moisture meat products mostly depend on lower moisture content and consequent decrease in water activity for their shelf stability. Use of high concentration of humectants including salt and sugar for desorption usually produces a disagreeable taste. This is true for Indian palate also. Leistner and Rodel (1976) coined the term hurdles for the parameters like chilling, heating, pH reduction, low water activity, enhanced Eh, use of preservatives and competitive microflora. Use of these hurdles or combination preservation technique in a balanced and judicious manner was named as hurdle concept and later the hurdle technology. It does not allow a single parameter to affect the product characteristics drastically. Thus, hurdle technology is the use of two or more factors, none of which is independently capable of sufficiently inhibiting the spoilage or pathogenic microorganisms to extend the shelf life of food products. Hurdle technology based meat products provide a desirable taste, juiciness, texture and safety.

### Restructured Meat Products

It has now become possible to utilize less desired or secondary carcass cuts into the production of highly preferred meat products such as steaks, roasts, chops, cutlets, etc. The less desired carcass cuts are carefully trimmed to remove sinews, excess fat and other connective tissue. Anyone of the following three basic procedures can be adopted depending on the appearance and texture targeted in the finished product:

1. Chunking and forming
2. Flaking and forming
3. Tearing and forming

**Chunking and forming:** The trimmed meat is put through a dicing machine and reduced to small chunks. One percent common salt and 0.25% phosphate are added at this stage and meat is put in a tumbler run at medium speed **(Fig. 9.6)**. During tumbling process, impact energy is utilized for the extraction of salt soluble proteins. The extracted proteins serve as cementing material when this meat is restructured by stuffing and pressing into suitable moulds. Restructured meat is frozen and then sliced to obtain uniform slices of desired thickness.

**Flaking and forming:** The trimmed meat is passed through a flaking machine to get flakes which are then mixed with 1% common salt and 0.25% phosphate. The material is run in a massager **(Fig. 9.7)**. During massaging process, frictional energy is utilized for the better extraction of salt soluble proteins. The meat mass is stuffed and pressed or formed into desired shapes—steaks, cutlets or chops. The restructured product is frozen and thawed just before cooking. The products have relatively good tenderness and uniform texture.

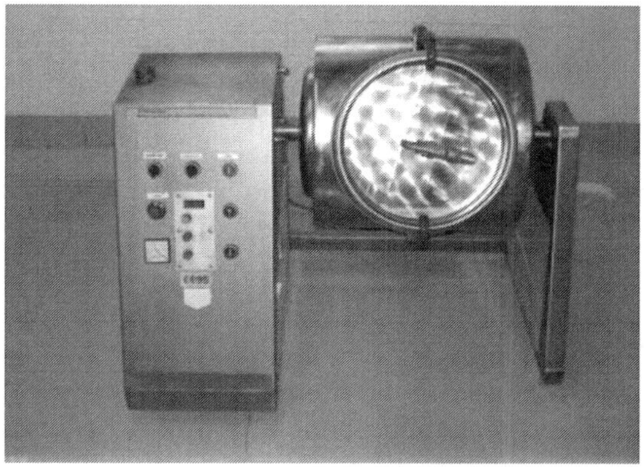

**Fig. 9.6:** Tumbling machine.

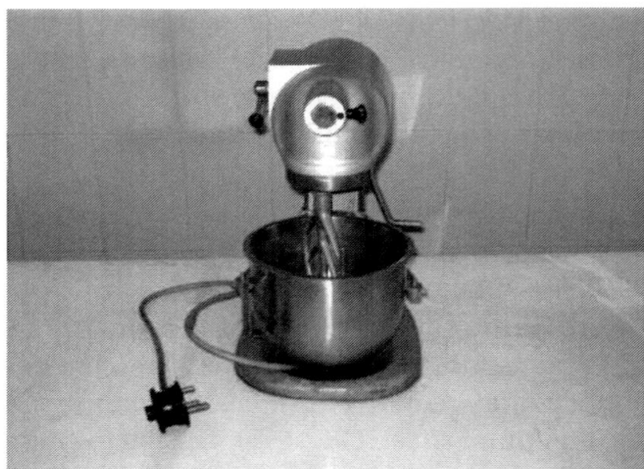

**Fig. 9.7:** Table top mixer.

**Tearing and forming:** In this procedure, meat fibres are torn apart. So there is less damage to the membrane resulting in less chances of autoxidation. Further, the structural integrity of meat tissue is maintained, though it becomes tender. Efforts are on to mechanize the process.

The advantages of restructured meat products are as follows:

- Production of quality meat products from lower value cuts and trimmings
- Convenience in preparation (RTC, RTE)
- Improved products characteristics such as texture, bind strength, and shape
- Low in fat content
- Can be formed as a block and then cut in various shapes and sizes such as slices, nuggets, steaks, cubes, etc., as per consumer demand
- Various new products can be developed for different markets
- Product with consistent quality and uniform nutritive value
- Better suited for nutrient fortification
- Comparatively economical to produce
- Less equipment required

## Other Popular Meat Products

**Luncheon meat:** It is a canned product usually prepared from pork along with some cereal component. The product contains not less than 80% pork including pork fat which should not exceed 30% in the final product. Besides, added water is limited to 3% and the cereal ingredients should not exceed 7% of the total formulation. Lean pork and pork fat are ground through 5 mm and 3 mm plate of the meat mincer, respectively. These are initially chopped along with chilled water or ice flakes, common salt and nitrite followed by other ingredients such as refined wheat flour, condiments and dry spices. A simple formulation of luncheon meat is being reproduced:

| *Ingredients* | *Percentage* |
|---|---|
| Lean pork | 67 |
| Pork backfat | 15 |
| Ice flakes | 3 |
| Table salt | 2.5 |
| Dextrose | 1.5 |
| Refined wheat flour | 5 |
| Condiments | 4.75 |
| Dry spices | 1.5 |
| Sodium nitrite | 150 ppm |

The batter or meat mix, maintained at 4°C, is filled compactly in cans which are sealed under vacuum. Commercial sterilization is done in retorts at 121°C for 75 minutes. Cans are then cooled with cold water shower until the contents reach 38°C. Canned luncheon meat is stable at ambient temperature for a period of two years.

**Meat patties:** Meat patty is one of the most popular products among the ground meat items and is generally used as filling for burger roll or sandwich **(Fig. 9.8)**. Some people prefer to consume it separately with tomato sauce or chutney. This product has a very good demand in big towns and cities in India. Patties are partially or completely emulsion based product, contain less than 30% fat and are moulded manually or mechanically. An optimum formulation is presented below:

| *Ingredients* | *Percentage* |
|---|---|
| Lean meat | 65 |
| Fat | 15 |
| Table salt | 2 |
| Texturized soy protein | 10 |
| Condiments | 6.5 |
| Dry spices | 1.5 |

Lean meat is minced twice through 6 mm plate and fat through 4 mm plate of a meat grinder. These are mixed thoroughly with all other ingredients in an electrically operated mixer or prepared into an emulsion. The batter weighing 80–100 g is moulded into 70–80 mm diameter and 15–20 mm thick patties. Raw patties may be frozen for future use or broiled in a preheated oven at 190°C for 20 minutes. The internal temperature must reach 72°C. These are deep fat fried in many commercial establishments. The patties are cooled and consumer packed.

**Meat loaves:** This important ready-to-eat comminuted meat product is prepared from coarse ground meat or meat emulsion or a combination of both **(Fig. 9.9)**. The formulation of a family loaf is given below:

| *Ingredients* | *Percentage* |
|---|---|
| Lean pork | 65 |
| Pork backfat | 15 |
| Ice flakes | 5 |
| Table salt | 2 |
| Refined wheat flour | 7.5 |
| Skim milk powder | 4 |
| Dry spices | 1.5 |
| Sodium nitrite | 150 ppm |

The meat mix or batter is tightly filled in aluminum or steel loaf pans which may be rectangular, cubical or cylindrical in shape depending on the requirement of slices for making the sandwiches. The pan-in mix is cooked in hot water maintained at 80°C or steam without pressure or broiled in hot air oven at 165°C for 2.5 to 3 hours. The internal temperature of 70°C must be achieved. It is then given a cold shower **(Fig. 9.14)** and chilled at 4°C. The chilled loaves are either packed as such or cut into slices of desired thickness and packed **(Fig. 9.12)**.

**Meatballs:** Indian consumers are familiar with this food item by the name of meat kofta **(Fig. 9.10)**. The product, stored raw or cooked offers a great convenience to restaurants, hotels and housewives who can just put few balls in the gravy and serve the food within 10 minutes. The product is prepared from ground meat which is mixed with fat, bread powder, salt, condiments and spices in an electrically operated mixer.

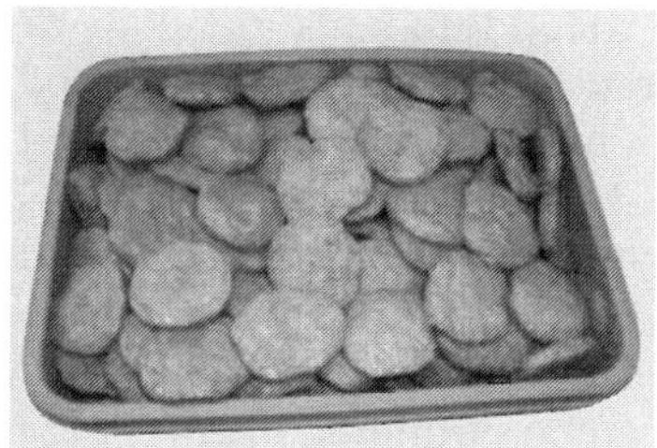

**Fig. 9.8:** Mutton patties.

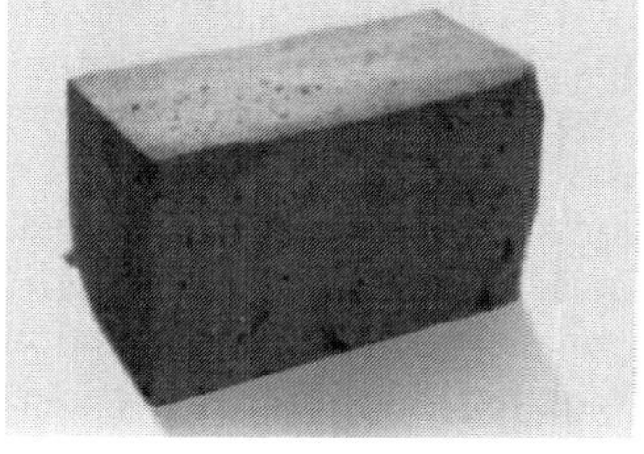

**Fig. 9.9:** Meat loaf.

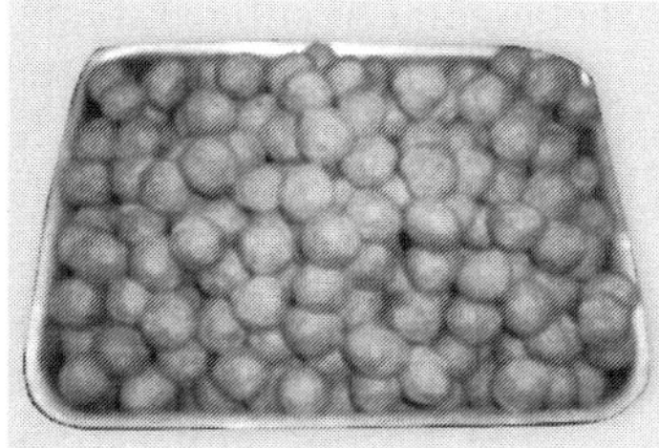

**Fig. 9.10:** Meatballs.

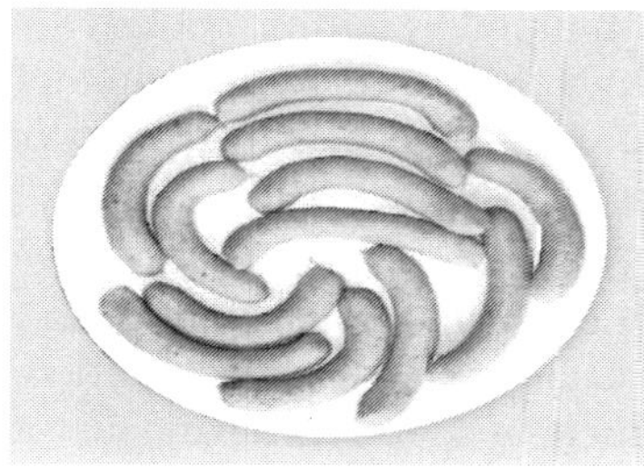

**Fig. 9.11:** Pork sausages.

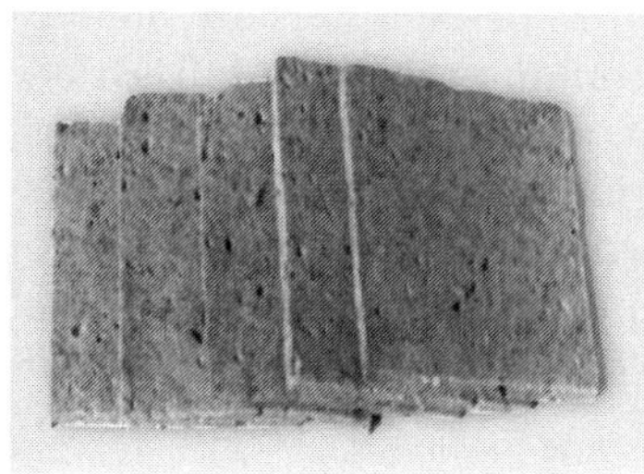

**Fig. 9.12:** Meat slices.

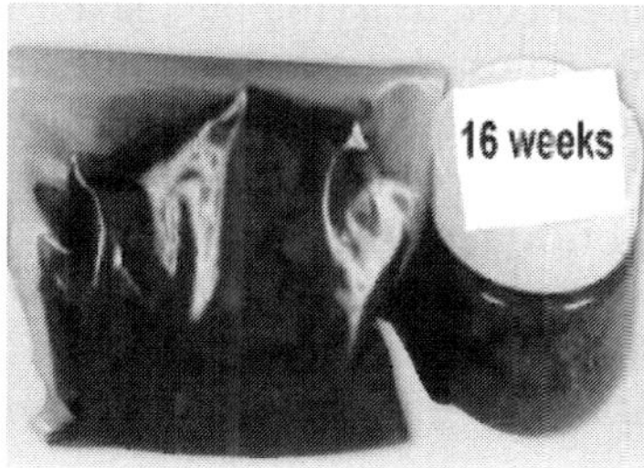


**Fig. 9.13:** Meat pickle.

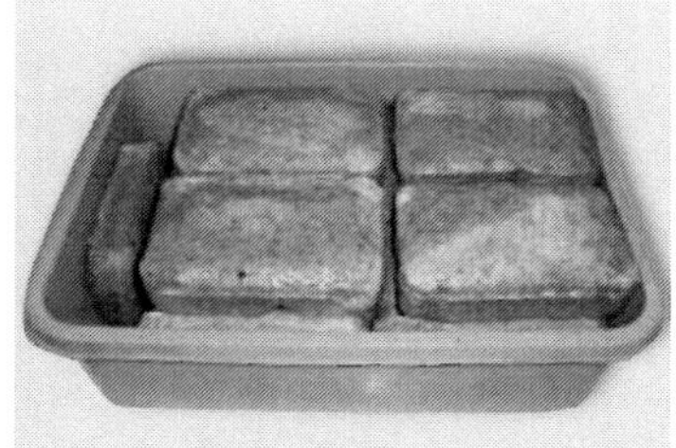

**Fig. 9.14:** Meat blocks.

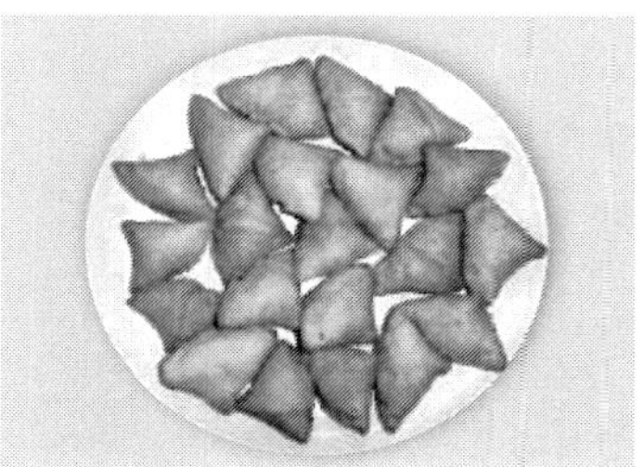

**Fig. 9.15:** Meat samosa.

The dough portions of 15–20 g are rolled into balls manually or mechanically. These are either stored raw or deep fat fried in refined vegetable oil at 135°C for three minutes to get brown color and fried flavor. Alternatively, these are cooked in hot water maintained at 80°C for 10 minutes to get an internal temperature of 65–70°C. Water cooked balls may be subjected to light frying to get golden brown color. These are packed in polyethylene pouches and can be kept at 4°C for a week. Whenever required, the cooked balls can be simmered in gravy for a few minutes and enjoyed with rice or bread.

**Meat nuggets:** It is a ready-to-eat convenient product which is obtained by cutting cooked and cooled rectangular or cubical shape meat loaves into approximately 4 cm × 1.5 cm × 1.5 cm pieces. The product is packed in unit pouches and can be stored at 4°C for a week. It is usually shallow fat-fried before serving for breakfast or refreshment.

**Meat pickle:** Pickling is a process of preserving food items by reducing the moisture and keeping at a pH range of 4 to 4.8. Indian pickles are usually spiced and suspended in mustard oil **(Fig. 9.13)**. To prepare meat pickle, extra fat and fascia is removed from the meat and it is cut into small chunks. Now 3 to 4 percent table salt is properly mixed in chunks which are pressure cooked for 8 to 10 minutes. Cooked pieces are taken in frying pan, shallow fried in 15 percent mustard oil and then put in a vessel for some time. Now onion-garlic mix (3:2) is fried in the same pan till it is brown and then 3.5 percent ground spices and 1 percent table salt is added and fried for some more time. This condiment-spices mix is added to fried chunks followed by some vinegar and citric acid. This pickle is put in a glass or PET jar in a mustard oil cover. It will become edible in one week and keep well for 5 to 6 months at room temperature.

# 10 CHAPTER

# Microbial and Other Deteriorative Changes in Meat and their Identification

Meat is a highly perishable food item. Hence, utmost precautions must be taken to safeguard it right from bleeding of slaughter animals till final consumption. Though muscle tissue of living animal is free of microorganisms, it gets contaminated by the body surface and visceral contaminants during slaughter and dressing operations. These organisms are bound to proliferate and cause deteriorative changes in meat unless proper measures are employed to retard their growth. Besides deteriorative changes can also be brought about by endogenous enzymes, lipid oxidation and improper storage conditions.

Microbial activity plays a major role in deterioration and spoilage of meat. We should, therefore, concentrate our efforts to check the initial invasion of microbes during slaughter and subsequent handling as well as processing.

## SOURCES OF MICROBIAL CONTAMINATION OF MEAT

There are a number of potential sources of contamination of meat within the abattoir itself. These include:

- Hides/skins and feet
- Gastrointestinal contents
- Instruments such as knives, cleavers saws, hook, etc.
- Water used for washing carcasses and instruments
- Airborne contamination
- Hands and clothing of the personnel

Contamination of meat may also take place during chilling, ageing, processing, packaging and distribution.

## GROWTH OF MICROORGANISMS IN MEAT

The microorganisms that occur in meat may be bacteria or fungi. Fungi may be multicellular filaments (mold) or large single cells with buds (yeast). Molds are capable of producing minute spores under unfavorable conditions. Fungi gain upper hand over bacteria in meat when it is semi-dry. Bacteria are unicellular microorganisms which are spherical or ovoid or rod shaped and may occur in chains or clusters. Bacterial growth or multiplication takes place in phases:

| | | |
|---|---|---|
| Lag phase | : | Bacterial cells increase in size under favorable conditions |
| Log phase | : | Bacterial cells multiply and increase in number |
| Stationary phase | : | Growth rate becomes relatively constant due to environmental limitations |
| Decline or death phase | : | There is destruction of bacterial cells either due to nutritional depletion or application of some preservation technique |

An understanding of growth curve **(Fig. 10.1)** enables the meat technologists to apply suitable preservation technique to prolong the lag phase so that bacterial multiplication is retarded or if conditions have already favored some growth, then to hasten the death phase.

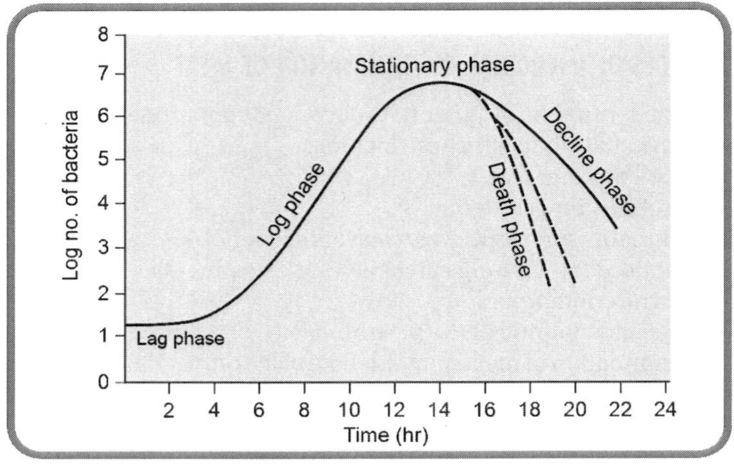


**Fig. 10.1:** A typical bacterial growth curve in meat.

Microbial growth activity in meat depends on various extrinsic and intrinsic factors. The extrinsic factors are temperature, oxygen and physical stage of meat. Different groups of bacteria have their own growth optima. Psychrophiles have their optimum growth temperature below 20°C, thermophiles above 45°C and mesophiles an optima ranging between these two. A refrigerated temperature of nearly 50°C greatly retards the growth of most psychrophilic organisms responsible for the spoilage of meat. These bacteria generally belong to genera *Pseudomonas, Achromobacter, Flavobacterium* (G- rods), *Micrococcus, Streptococcus* (G+ cocci) in fresh meat and *Lactobacillus* (G+ rods), in cured or vacuum packed meat products. The growth of bacteria on meat is usually characterized by slime formation. It should be noted that total bacterial population is above $10^7$ when most signs of spoilage appear on meat. Effective freezing damages or kills most of the bacteria present on meat. It may be remembered that meat spoilage molds are also psychrophiles. On the contrary, food pathogens generally belong to the thermophilic group of bacteria.

Oxygen environment around the meat will determine the type of microflora that will find favorable conditions for growth. Bacteria found in meat may be either aerobic or anaerobic or sometimes facultative. Bacteria that grow on the surface of fresh meat are generally aerobes, whereas it is a different flora in the interior of meat. All molds and yeast that grow in meat are aerobic in nature. Use of different barrier packaging films restricts the activity of aerobic microorganisms. Physical state of meat such as whole carcass or primal cuts or retail cuts or comminuted form also influence the rate of microbial growth. Microbial load increases with the increase in exposed surface area of meat.

Important intrinsic factors which affect the growth of microorganisms in meat are water activity, pH and redox potential. The amount of water available in a food system for the growth of microorganisms is generally expressed in terms of water activity. In fact, water activity ($a_w$) is defined as vapor pressure of the solution (p) in a food system divided by vapor pressure of pure solvent or water ($p_0$). Fresh meat generally has a water activity of 0.99 or more. Most meat spoilage bacteria can grow only up to a water activity of 0.91 but most spoilage mold and yeast can growth up to a water activity of 0.86. This factor is commercially exploited in the production of intermediate moisture meat products. Meat pH is yet another intrinsic factor which influences the growth of microorganisms. Bacterial growth is best at neutral pH (i.e., pH 7.0). It keeps on diminishing as meat pH goes down. If ultimate pH is 6.0 or so, a large number of bacteria can still grow in meat. However, when normal ultimate pH of nearly 5.5 is achieved in meat, bacterial growth is reduced to a large extent and the growth of mold and yeast is favored. Redox potential refers to the reducing or oxidizing conditions prevailing in meat and this factor also influences the growth of microorganisms.

## DETERIORATIVE CHANGES IN MEAT

When meat depicts signs of decomposition and putrefaction, it is referred as spoiled and becomes unfit for human consumption. Besides microorganisms, intrinsic enzymes and insects also contribute to the spoilage of meat. Microbial spoilage of fresh chilled meat is generally on the surface, whereas it is within meat at higher temperature. The causative agents and deteriorative changes are quite different in aerobic and anaerobic spoilage. Under aerobic conditions, most significant symptoms of meat spoilage by bacteria and yeast is the slime formation on the surface which results due to coalescence of a large number of individual colonies. There may be discoloration of meat due to oxidizing agents produced by bacteria or growth of colonies of colored organisms. The production of off-odors is also usually encountered. Bacterial action causes proteolysis of meat proteins and lipolysis of meat lipids. The end products of proteolysis are simple peptides and amino acids under aerobic conditions whereas sulfur dioxide, ammonia and other obnoxious compounds like amines and ketones under anaerobic conditions. Residual carbohydrates yield skatole and indole. Molds may grow on semi-dried meats causing surface stickiness and whiskers.

Under anaerobic conditions, meat decomposition is more offensive. There may be putrefaction in the deep tissues such as lymph nodes and bone joints, which is always accompanied by foul odors or taints. Souring may also develop due to accumulation of organic acids.

Canned meats may suffer chemical or biological spoilage or both. In the event of spoilage unopened cans may show distortion (swell) due to souring and putrefaction.

## IDENTIFICATION OF MEAT SPOILAGE

The identification of meat spoilage is based on the deteriorative changes brought about microorganisms, intrinsic enzymes and insects. During spoilage process, several utilizable substrates are consumed by microflora and new products are formed which can be measured or determined in meat. Thus, meat spoilage can be detected by any of the following physical and chemical methods:

- Some physical observations such as discoloration, slime formation, stickiness, whiskers, etc., give a clear indication of spoiled meats.
- At low temperature, meat spoilage is accompanied by the formation of many off-flavor compounds. Many of them owe their origin to free amino acids and related substances. The production of $H_2S$ and mercaptans can be measured to ascertain meat spoilage. Chemical determinations for the presence of ammonia, indole, skatole, di- and trimethylamine, etc., can be carried out to detect microbial spoilage in meats.
- The extract release volume (ERV) determination is particularly helpful in detecting the incipient spoilage in meats. ERV refers to the volume of aqueous extract, released by a meat homogenate when it is passed through a filter for a given period of time. As meats undergo microbial spoilage, there is a complete hydrolysis of proteins which significantly decrease the ERV.
- Dye (usually resazurin) reduction test is many times used to detect spoilage in meats. Spoiled raw or cooked meat homogenate prepared from stomacher could bring about resazurin reduction within 2 hours. This method shows a very good correlation with bacterial numbers.
- Incipient spoilage in meat shows a simultaneous rise in pH, bacterial counts and water holding capacity of meat proteins. At the time of incipient spoilage, pH value is more than 6.5 in ground meat but it may even increase to 8.5 in putrid meats.
- High thiobarbituric acid and peroxide values indicate chemical spoilage of meat and meat products.

# 11
# CHAPTER
# Standards and Quality Control Measures for Meat and Meat Products

Meat being a highly perishable commodity requires strict quality control right from slaughter operations till ultimate consumption. The basic objectives of quality control are:

- Protection of public health
- Extension of product shelf life
- Provision of consumer satisfaction
- Compliance of regulatory legislation
- Competitive edge in the trade

The general principles of meat product quality control involve:

- Raw material control
- Control of processing operations
- Finished product inspection and control

It is very difficult to examine meat and meat products for every pathogenic, toxigenic and spoilage microorganisms. However, a product cannot be improved unless some objective assessment of its quality is available. But the methods adopted should be simple with quick results. Hence, the following indicator organisms are relied upon to determine the sanitary and safety status of these items:

1. **Total Viable Counts**

   These are estimates of mesophiles and psychrophiles and serve as useful indicators of handling history and state of freshness or spoilage of meat. These counts provide meaningful guidance to streamline the processing operations. However, if these counts are less, most probable number (MPN) are enumerated.

2. **Coliforms**

   These consist of *E. coli* and *Enterobacter aerogenes*. Their presence indicate faecal contamination due to unhygienic handling during or after processing of meat products. Coliforms can be distinguished because of their property to produce gas from lactose at 44°C.

However, out of two organisms in this category, *E. coli* is a better indicator of faecal contamination.

3. **Enterococci**

   These are members of faecal streptococci (group D) which consist of:

   - S. faecalis (and its varieties)
   - S. faecium (var durans)
   - S. bovis
   - S. equinus

   These organisms indicate poor hygienic quality of frozen meats and inadequate heat treatment of canned meats.

4. **Other Indicators**

   Besides above indicators, specific organisms like *Staph. aureus, Salmonella,* Yeast and Mold counts are also important. Heat treated meats should also be screened for the presence or absence of *B. cereus* and *Clostridia*.

   Canned meat products are generally subjected to sterility test. For this purpose, cans are incubated at 30°C and 55°C for 15 days. Swollen or disfigured cans show the product spoilage.

## STANDARDS IN MEAT INDUSTRY

Quality control departments frequently utilize the reliable methods and techniques for establishing the standards. A standard can be referred as carefully drawn specification with respect to a food product. The specifications give comprehensive instructions to ensure correct and reliable process control. The compliance of specifications increases the confidence of top executives in the production and marketing of perishable food items.

Bureau of Indian Standards (BIS), established in 1947 as Indian Standard Institution (ISI) as a joint venture of Government of India and Industry took up the responsibility of preparing and promoting the general adoption of standards in the country. The erstwhile ISI constituted the Meat and Meat Products Sectional Committee, AFDC-18 under the Agricultural and Food Products Division Council in 1958 to prepare Indian Standards for the meat industry. This committee represents the scientists, technologists, manufacturers, government agencies and consumers. The standards are prepared keeping in mind the needs of industry protecting the interests of both producers and consumers and are reviewed periodically. A list of relevant standards is given below:

| | |
|---|---|
| IS: 4393–1979 | Basic requirements for an abattoir (first revision) |
| IS: 1982–1971 | Code of practice for antemortem and postmortem inspection of meat animals (first revision) |
| IS: 1723–1973 | Specifications for pork (first revision) |
| IS: 2474–1979 | Specifications for smoked bacon (first revision) |
| IS: 2476–1963 | Specifications for ham |
| IS: 2536–1995 | Specifications for mutton and goat flesh—fresh, chilled and frozen |
| IS: 2537–1995 | Specifications for beef and buffalo flesh—fresh, chilled and frozen |
| IS: 11748–1986 | Specifications for meat extract |
| IS: 3060–1979 | Specifications for pork sausages, canned (under revision) |
| IS: 3061–2001 | Specifications for pork sausages, fresh (under revision) |
| IS: 4352–1967 | Specifications for pork luncheon meat, canned |
| IS: 3044–1973 | Specifications for mutton and goat meat, curried and canned (first revision) |
| IS: 4674–1975 | Specifications for dressed chicken (first revision) |
| IS: 4951–1975 | Specifications for ham, canned (first revision) |
| IS: 5558–1970 | Specifications for chicken essence |
| IS: 13400–1992 | Specifications for chicken sausages |
| IS: 6659–1972 | Code of practice for antemortem and postmortem inspection of poultry |
| IS: 12541–1988 | Specifications for chicken curry, canned |
| IS: 8182–1976 | Code of hygienic conditions for processed meat products |
| IS: 5960 (Parts)–1996 | Methods of test for meat and meat products (Parts) 2000 |

These BIS specifications are voluntary but an adherence to these guidelines definitely improves the quality of processed products.

Food Safety and Standards Authority of India (FSSAI) has in 2018 notified the Food Safety and Standards (Foods Products Standards and Food Additives) Amendment Regulation, 2018 have prescribed standards for:

- Fresh/Chilled/Frozen Chevon (Goat Meat)
- Fresh/Chilled/Frozen Mutton (Sheep Meat)

- Fresh/Chilled/Frozen Pork (Pig Meat)
- Fresh/Chilled/Frozen Poultry Meat

## Fresh/Chilled/Frozen Chevon or Goat Meat Chevon

*Chevon* will be of the following three types:

1. Fresh or chilled or frozen carcasses or carcass halves or carcass quartes
2. Fresh or chilled or frozen cuts; bone-in or boneless, true to its type
3. Fresh or chilled or frozen edible offal

*Boneless meat* shall have:

- Moisture content between 74 to 76%
- Protein content between 22 to 22%
- Fat content between 2 to 4%

Chevon shall be stored at 4°C for short term storage and at –18°C for long term storage. The chilled chevon should be consumed within 2 to 4 days under normal chilling conditions of storage and frozen chevon shall be consumed within 12 months.

## Fresh/Chilled/Frozen Mutton or Sheep Meat

*Mutton* will be of the following three types:

1. Fresh or chilled or frozen carcasses or carcass halves or carcass quartes
2. Fresh or chilled or frozen cuts, bone-in or boneless, true to its type
3. Fresh or chilled or frozen edible offal

*Boneless meat* shall have:

- Moisture content between 68 to 72%
- Protein content between 20 to 22%
- Fat content between 4 to 10%

Mutton shall be stored at 4°C for short-term storage and at –18°C for long-term storage. The chilled mutton should be consumed within 2 to 4 days under normal chilling conditions of storage and frozen mutton shall be consumed within 12 months.

## Fresh/Chilled/Frozen Pork or Pig Meat

*Pork* may be categorized of the following three types:

1. Fresh or chilled or frozen carcasses or carcass halves or carcass quartes

2. Fresh or chilled or frozen cuts or bone-in or boneless, true to its type
3. Fresh or chilled or frozen edible offal

*Boneless meat* shall have:

- Moisture content between 70 to 72%
- Protein content between 20 to 22%
- Fat content between 5 to 6%

Pork shall be stored at 4°C for short term storage and at –18°C for long term storage. The chilled pork should be consumed within 2 to 4 days under normal chilling conditions of storage and frozen pork shall be consumed within 10 months.

Food Safety and Standard Authority of India has notified Food Safety and Standards (Food Products Standards and Food Additives) First Amendment Regulations 2020 relating to microbiological requirement as "Microbiological Standards of Food Products" with respect to meat and meat products in their **Table 5A** (Process Hygiene Criteria) and **Table 5B** (Food Safety Criteria) which are being presented here in **Tables 11.1** and **11.2**.

Microbiological standards help to improve plant sanitation, ensure safety of the products and prevent losses due to microbial spoilage. Establishment of microbiological specifications is a very expensive and cumbersome task. Lot of database is required in practical conditions at different locations, with a very good degree of reproducibility.

The concept of quality control at few points in the entire production chain is now giving way to integrated quality management systems. HACCP and ISO-9000 series are of particular interest to meat processors.

## HAZARD ANALYSIS CRITICAL CONTROL POINT SYSTEM

HACCP is a comprehensive food safety system right from the point of production to the point of consumption. This system analyses the hazards of raw material, identifies the points of potential contamination, monitors the processing operations and checks the risks arising from consumer abuse. It is a systematic approach to the production of microbiologically safe foods. It consists of the following steps:

1. Assessment of hazards and risks associated with raw materials, ingredients, processing, packaging, distribution and consumption of meat product on the basis of flowchart.
2. Identification of critical control points (potential contaminants and their sources) to control and minimize a hazard.

**Table 11.1:** Microbiological standards for meat and meat products—process hygiene criteria.

| S. No. | Product category | *Aerobic plate count* | | | | *Yeast and mold count* | | | | *Escherichia coli* | | | | *Staphylococcus aureus (coagulase +ve)* | | | |
|---|---|---|---|---|---|---|---|---|---|---|---|---|---|---|---|---|---|
| | | *Sampling plan* | | *Limits (cfu/g)* | | *Sampling plan* | | *Limits (cfu) g* | | *Sampling plan* | | *Limits (cfu/g)* | | *Sampling plan* | | *Limits (cfu/g)* | |
| | | n | c | m | M | n | c | m | M | n | c | m | M | n | c | m | M |
| 1. | Fresh meat/ chilled meat | 5 | 3 | $1\times10^6$ | $5\times10^6$ | 5 | 2 | $1\times10^4$ | $5\times10^4$ | 5 | 2 | $1\times10^2$ | $1\times10^3$ | 5 | 2 | $1\times10^2$ | $1\times10^3$ |
| 2. | Frozen meat | 5 | 2 | $1\times10^5$ | $5\times10^6$ | 5 | 2 | $1\times10^3$ | $1\times10^4$ | 5 | 2 | 1×10 | $1\times10^2$ | 5 | 2 | 10 | $1\times10^2$ |
| 3. | Raw marinated/ minced/ comminuted meat | 5 | 2 | $5\times10^5$ | $5\times10^6$ | 5 | 2 | [$1\times10^4$] | [$5\times10^4$] | 5 | 2 | $1\times10^2$ | $1\times10^3$ | 5 | 2 | $1\times10^2$ | $1\times10^3$ |
| 4. | Semi-cooked/ smoked meat/meat food product | 5 | 2 | $1\times10^4$ | $1\times10^5$ | 5 | 2 | 10 | $1\times10^2$ | 5 | 2 | 10 | $1\times10^2$ | 5 | 2 | 10 | $1\times10^2$ |
| 5. | Cured/ pickled meat | 5 | 2 | $5\times10^2$ | $5\times10^3$ | 5 | 2 | $1\times10^2$ | $1\times10^3$ | 5 | 2 | 10 | $1\times10^2$ | 5 | 1 | $1\times10^2$ | $1\times10^3$ |
| 6. | Fermented meat products | NA | NA | NA | NA | NA | NA | NA | NA | 5 | 2 | 10 | $1\times10^2$ | 5 | 1 | $1\times10^2$ | $1\times10^3$ |
| 7. | Dried/ dehydrated meat products | 5 | 2 | $1\times10^3$ | $1\times10^4$ | 5 | 2 | $1\times10^2$ | $1\times10^3$ | 5 | 2 | 10 | $1\times10^2$ | 5 | 1 | 10 | $1\times10^2$ |
| 8. | Cooked meat products | 5 | 2 | $1\times10^3$ | $1\times10^4$ | 5 | 1 | 10 | $1\times10^2$ | 5 | 2 | 10 | $1\times10^2$ | 5 | 1 | 10 | $1\times10^2$ |
| 9. | Canned/ retort pouch meat products | NA | NA | NA | NA | NA | NA | NA | NA | 5 | 0 | Absent | NA | 5 | 0 | Absent | NA |
| | **Test methods** | **IS: 5402/ISO: 4833** | | | | **IS: 5403/ISO: 21527** | | | | **IS: 5887, Part 1 or ISO: 16649-2** | | | | **IS: 5887, Part 2 or IS: 5887, Part 8 (Sec 1)/ISO: 6888-1** | | | |

n, Number of sample to be tested; c, Maximum allowable number of sample units having microbiological counts between m and M for 3-class sampling plan and above m for 2-class sampling plan; m, Maximum permissible number of relevant bacteria; M, Level at or above which the lot has to be rejected.

**Table 11.2:** Microbiological standards or meat and meat products—food safety criteria.

| S. No. | Product category | *Salmonella* | | | *Listeria monocytogenes* | | | *Sulphite reducing Clostridia* | | | | *Clostridium botulinum* | | | | *Campylobacter spp** | | | |
|---|---|---|---|---|---|---|---|---|---|---|---|---|---|---|---|---|---|---|---|
| | | *Sampling plan* | | *Limits (cfu/25 g)* | *Sampling plan* | | *Limits (cfu/25g)* | *Sampling plan* | | *Limits (cfu/g)* | | *Sampling plan* | | *Limits (cfu/g)* | | *Sampling plan* | | *Limits (cfu/g)* | |
| | | *n* | *c* | *m M* | *n* | *C* | *m M* | *n* | *c* | *m* | *M* | *n* | *c* | *m* | *M* | *n* | *c* | *m* | *M* |
| 1. | Fresh meat/chilled meat | 5 | 0 | Absent | NA | NA | NA | NA | NA | NA | NA | NA | NA | NA | NA | NA | NA | NA | NA |
| 2. | Frozen meat | 5 | 0 | Absent | NA | NA | NA | NA | NA | NA | NA | NA | NA | NA | NA | NA | NA | NA | NA |
| 3. | Raw marinated/ minced/ comminuted meat | 5 | 0 | Absent | NA | NA | NA | NA | NA | NA | NA | NA | NA | NA | NA | NA | NA | NA | NA |
| 4. | Semi-cooked/ smoked meat/meat food product | 5 | 0 | Absent | NA | NA | NA | NA | NA | NA | NA | NA | NA | NA | NA | 5 | 0 | Absent | |
| 5. | Cured/pickled meat | 5 | 0 | Absent | 5 | 0 | Absent | 5 | 2 | $5\times10^2$ | $5\times10^3$ | NA | NA | NA | NA | NA | NA | NA | NA |
| 6. | Fermented meat products | 5 | 0 | Absent | 5 | 0 | Absent | 5 | 2 | $5\times10^2$ | $5\times10^3$ | NA | NA | NA | NA | NA | NA | NA | NA |
| 7. | Dried/dehydrated meat product | 5 | 0 | Absent | 5 | 0 | Absent | 5 | 2 | $5\times10^2$ | $5\times10^3$ | NA | NA | NA | NA | NA | NA | NA | |
| 8. | Cooked meat product | 5 | 0 | Absent | 5 | 0 | Absent | 5 | 1 | $1\times10^2$ | $1\times10^3$ | NA | NA | NA | NA | 5 | 0 | Absent | |
| 9. | Canned/retort pouch meat product | 5 | 0 | Absent | 5 | 0 | Absent | 5 | 0 | Absent | | 5 | 0 | Absent | | 5 | 0 | Absent | |
| | **Test methods** | **IS: 5887, Part 3/ISO: 6579** | | | **IS: 14988, Part 1 & 2/ISO: 11290-1 & 2** | | | **ISO: 15213** | | | | **IS: 5887, Part 4 or ISO: 17919** | | | | **ISO: 10272-1&2** | | | |

*, Applicable for poultry meat; n = Number of sample to be tested, m = Maximum permissible number or relevant bacteria; c = Maximum allowable number of sample units having microbiological counts between m and M for 3-class sampling plan and above m for 2-class sampling plan; M = Level at or above which the lot has to be rejected.

3. Establishment of critical limits or tolerance levels (standards) at each control point.
4. Outlining the procedures to monitor the critical control points.
5. Defining the corrective action if a deviation is noticed during monitoring.
6. Maintenance of proper records or documents of HACCP plan.
7. Verification of methods, procedures and tests to oversee the compliance of the plan.

HACCP system has proved very effective in identifying and preventing contamination. It is designed to check each step critically along the processing line to ensure the safety of a food instead of testing at the end.

## ISO-9000 STANDARDS

International Organization of Standardization (ISO), Geneva has issued ISO-9000 series of quality standards to facilitate world trade. In this series.

| | |
|---|---|
| ISO-9000 | Provides guidance on the choice of specific model to be adopted for quality assurance in an organization. |
| ISO-9001 | Is meant for manufacturers having their own product research and development (R&D). |
| ISO-9002 | Is for contract manufacturers without any product research and development. |
| ISO-9003 | Is meant for commodity suppliers, having only final product inspection and testing. |

Thus, ISO-9000 is a very detailed quality management system. It has twenty elements for compliance by the manufacturers. Some of the important ones are management responsibility, design control, purchasing, product identification, process control, inspection and testing, corrective action, packaging, proper documentation and internal audit. ISO-9003 requirements are comparatively less strict. Many food processing and packaging companies in the developed world have sought ISO-9003 certification. This certification can open up global market for food product suppliers. It has the potential for obtaining competitive advantage in the world food trade.

## CODEX STANDARDS

Codex Alimentarius is a Latin word meaning Food law or Food Code. Codex Alimentarius Commission is joint FAO/WHO Food Standard body which protects the health of the consumers by ensuring safe and quality food, provides guidelines for industries towards production, manufacture and sell of safe and quality food products, facilitates harmonization through adoption of Codex Standards into national guidelines and facilitates international food trade by accepting the Codex Standards as bench marks. It has 176 member nations.

Codex Alimentarius Commission consists of ten committees on General subjects dealing with standards which are applicable to all foods regardless of the category viz. General Principles, Pesticide Residues, Residues of Veterinary Drugs in Foods, Food Import and Export Inspection and Certification Systems, Nutrition and Food for Special Dietary Uses and Contaminants in Food.

Finalization of any Codex standard or text follows a definite protocol in which a draft proposal is prepared, circulated to member countries and all interested parities for comments, then comments are reviewed and referred to Executive Committee for critical review and adaptation as a draft. The approved draft is sent again to governments and interested parities for comments which are again looked into by the relevant committee before adoption. At times Codex prefers to farm working groups on certain issues before laying down standards and formulating codes of practices. Typical components of a commodity standard includes Name of the Standard, Scope, Description of the product, Essential Composition and quality Factors, Food Additives, Contaminants, Hygiene, Weights and Measures, Labeling and Methods of Analysis and Sampling.

Codex standards are globally accepted standards which are used as the benchmark by most of the countries to set their own national standards. The consumers in the country gain confidence about the safety and quality of the food available for consumption by them. The Codex standards facilitate international trades. Most of the countries prefer to adopt the Codex standards as common benchmark. These standards and guidelines provide a ready reference for the food manufacturers throughout the world.

## ISO-22000

It is a standard developed by the International Organization for Standardization dealing with food safety. This is a general derivative of ISO-9001. Thus, ISO-22000 is globally harmonized and process-oriented standard for food safety that may be applied by any organization in the entire food supply chain. This international standard specifies the requirement for a food safety management system that involves the following key elements:

- Interactive communication along the food chain
- Structured system management
- Integrates prerequisite programs
- HACCP principles

The increased demand for safe food, as well as a result of globalization and international trade, led the food processing industry to implement food safety management systems based on HACCP (Hazard Analysis and Critical Control Point). A number of standards have been developed in different countries, and organizations in the food sector used their own codes to audit their suppliers. The sheer number of standards and the cost involved in conforming to all of them made it nearly impossible to keep up with the different requirements in the global food market.

The International Organization for Standardization (ISO) has developed ISO-22000 as a way to systematically ensure safety and control in all links of the food chain. Organizations implementing ISO-22000, which include the principles of the HACCP system, can now cover the key requirements of the various global standards by using a single document and since ISO-22000 is designed to be fully compatible with ISO-9001, a food supply company with an established quality management system, will find it easy to extend their system to include this new standard.

The major advantages of ISO-22000 (2018) are systematic identification and management of food safety hazards, greater confidence in customers and suppliers about sustainable food safety and its integration with ISO-9001 (quality management), the principles of HACCP system and application steps developed by Codex Alimentarius Commission. It gives holistic consideration in respect of food product hygiene and health protection.

# 12 CHAPTER

# Food Safety Laws Governing Trade of Meat and Meat Products in India

The creator God has shaped human being as the most efficient and intellectual biomachine. The survivability and proper functioning of this creature totally depend upon the fuel that in this case is "food". The most indispensable component food determines the healthiness and expectancy of human life. The quality of the food needs to be up to the mark, so that the nutritional, physiological and esthetic requirements of human body can be satisfied properly. Food and water are the most indispensable for the survival of human being. Therefore, safety of food is the major concern of today's health-conscious consumer population. Food safety refers to the conditions and practices that preserve the quality of food to prevent contamination and food-borne illnesses. The safety issues are always tagged with all those hazards which make food injurious to health. These hazards related to food especially animal food arise from the malpractices engaged in food production chain viz., improper production practices, manufacture and processing, poor hygiene at various stages of the food production, processing and handling, lack in preventive controls in food processing operations, unjustifiable use of chemicals for more profit generation, unaware contaminated inputs, or inappropriate storage and further handling, etc.

Presently the most specific concerns about food hazards are microbiological contaminants to food, chemical and biological toxins, pesticide residues, veterinary drug residues, and allergens. Various governmental and non-governmental organizations are engaged in the controlling the contamination of food and its products from any types of hazards. It is important that the national food control system is liable to protect the consumer from unsafe food. So far, the Prevention of Food Adulteration Act prescribed food standards and also established an inspection system for marketed products. However, the production chain and distribution system are so vast and well spread, it did not seek to identify and prevent the sources of contaminants. With elongated food chain, rapidly changing technologies and greater consumer awareness, it has become necessary to modernize the food control system. The food safety and inspection service of the different organizations educate consumers about the importance of safe food handling and to reduce the risks associated with food-borne illness.

Food and food products are the largest consumption category in India, with a market size of ₹ 9,100 billion. Domestically, the spending on food and food products amounts to nearly 21% of the gross domestic product of the country and constitutes the largest portion of the Indian consumer spending more than a 31% share of wallet. Going forward, the Indian domestic food market is expected to grow by nearly 40% of the current market size, to touch ₹ 12,900 billion by 2015 (FICCI–EY report, 2009). In this background, the crucial role of the national food control system can be perceived, therefore, it can play a great role for securing safe and healthy food supply to the ultimate users, and should be effective and comprehensive with science-based food law and regulations and a compact institutional structure which is active and responds to the needs of food safety management. The Central, State and local authorities have complementary and interdependent roles in the implementation of the national food safety system with the ultimate objective of protecting the consumer.

In the present situation, the Prevention of Food Adulteration Act offered some safety of food materials for the consumers. However, the Act did not make available a holistic approach to ensure overall food safety. Therefore, in recognition of the need to modernize the Food Control System the Food Safety and Standards Act, 2006 was passed by the Parliament. This Act brings together different valuable parts of legislation pertaining to food safety and its control under a single law and under a single authority. Efficient and beneficial national food control systems are essential to protect the health and safety of domestic consumers. They are also critical in enabling countries to assure the safety and quality of their manufactured foods entering international trade and to ensure that imported foods conform to national requirements and benefits. The new global environment for food trade places considerable obligations on both importing and exporting countries to strengthen their food control systems and to implement and enforce risk-based food control strategies for their own safety. Consumers are taking unprecedented interest in the way food is produced/procured, processed and marketed and are increasingly demanding from their Governments to accept greater responsibility for the food safety and consumer protection.

The Food and Agriculture Organization of the United Nations (FAO) and the World Health Organization (WHO) have a strong agenda in promoting national food control systems that are based upon scientific principles and guidelines and which address all components of the food chain. This is particularly important for developing countries like India, as they seek to achieve improved food safety, quality and nutrition for their nations' health but will require a high level of political and policy commitment to make it into a hard reality.

## FOOD SAFETY LAWS

In India, multiple regulations for food have been enacted at different points of time to supplement each other. This incremental approach has led to incoherence and inconsistency in the food sector regulatory scenario. The food sector in India has been governed by a multiplicity of laws under different ministries. A number of committees, including the Standing Committee of Parliament on Agriculture in its 12th Report submitted in April 2005, have emphasized the need for a single regulatory body and an integrated food law. To this effect, the Food Safety and Standards Act, 2006, consolidated eight laws governing the food sector and established the Food Safety and Standards Authority of India (FSSAI) to regulate the sector. This Act aimed to integrate the food safety laws in the country in order to systematically and scientifically develop the food processing industry and shift from a regulatory regime to self-compliance.

## FOOD SAFETY AND SANITARY AND PHYTOSANITARY SITUATION IN INDIA

In the recent past, awareness regarding importance of health measures and fear of health hazard has shown a definite upward trend even in developing countries like India. As a result an elaborate system of inspection and certification has evolved over the years. This system becomes more rigorous if the goods in question are to be sent to foreign markets. The required legal structure has been in place in India for a long time now. There are some organizations concentrating their efforts towards formulation and implementation of SPS standards. Some important standard setting organizations are:

## Bureau of Indian Standards (BIS)

This is a premier organization for setting standards. So far it has set more than 17,000 standards. 150 of these are mandatory and others voluntary. The procedure adopted by BIS is same as in other countries. A suggestion coming from a consumer or an organization is considered by a committee for its viability before formulation of a final draft. BIS provides various services to the firms. These include product certification, training on ISO 9000 and ISO 14000, list of Indian and international standards for different products and also some general information required by the firm.

## Ministry of Food Processing Industry (MFPI)

The ministry formulates the procedures and standards for the food processing industries. Thus rules are put together regarding the following thrust areas:

- Material to be used for the machine and equipment that come in contact with food.
- Quality of water used for production and for other purposes like washing and cleaning.
- Requirements of in-house laboratories.
- Assessment of the quality by food technologists.
- Standards pertaining to chemical content, physical characteristics, contaminant levels, and additive levels allowed in food.

## Export Inspection Council (EIC)

This is an apex agency that facilitates exports of SPS compliant commodities. It also gives advice to the government regarding measures to be taken for enforcement of quality control and inspection. Further, it also makes arrangement for pre-shipment inspection of commodities to ensure compliance of all specified standards. EIC provides three kinds of inspection and certification viz.,

- Consignment-wise inspection.
- In-process quality control.
- Food safety management system-based certification.

## Codex Alimentarius

This is an international organization that brings together all the interested parties, scientists, technical experts, governments, consumers and industry representatives. The standards set by codex are becoming increasingly acceptable world over, and thus are used as a benchmark by the domestic organizations. They even play a vital role in trade negotiations and settling of disputes.

## EVOLUTION OF FOOD SAFETY OBJECTIVES

### Planning for the National Food Control Strategy

The changing socioeconomic condition of Indian health-conscious consumer population making it necessary to develop some national level food control strategies to meet up the assurance of hygienic food.

### Gathering of Information

This is achieved through correlation of relevant data which help in strategy development, with stakeholders reaching consensus on objectives, priorities, policies, roles of different ministries/agencies, industry responsibilities and timeframe for implementation.

### Outlining of Strategy

The preparation of a national food control strategy enables the country to develop an integrated, coherent, effective and dynamic food control system and to determine priorities which ensure consumer protection and promote the country's economic development. The strategy should be based on multisectoral inputs and focus on the need for food security and consumer protection from unsafe adulterated or misbranded food.

## FOOD SAFETY AND STANDARDS AUTHORITY OF INDIA

The Food Safety and Standards Act, 2006 has come into force with effect from 5th August, 2011. The enabling Rules and Regulations have been notified and have become effective from the date.

The existing Acts, orders, rules, regulations as mention hereunder have been repealed simultaneously:

1. Prevention of Food Adulteration Act, 1954
2. Fruit Products Order (FPO), 1955
3. Solvent Extracted Oil, De-oiled Meal and Edible Flour (Control) Order, 1967
4. Meat Food Products Order, 1973
5. Edible Oils Packing, 1998

6. Vegetable Oil Products Order, 1988
7. Milk and Milk Products Amendment Regulations, 2009

Besides, for the first time, water has been recognized as a food. This Act consolidates the laws relating to Food and to establish the FSSAI for laying science-based standards for articles of food and to regulate their manufacture, storage, distribution, sale and import to ensure availability of safe and wholesome food for human consumption and for matters connected therewith. The new law puts in place a unified structure for all food safety-related matters in the form of FSSAI at the Center and Commissioners of Food Safety at the State level. Other new functionaries defined by the statute are Designated Officer at the district level, Food Safety Officer at cutting edge level, Adjudicating Officer, Special Courts and Appellate Tribunal for speedy disposal of cases.

Under the new law, the food business operators, term denoting all businesses that deal with food in any manner, are responsible for supply of safe food to the consumers. The emphasis is on 'food safety' that focuses on the entire food chain and not just the final product as was the case under the PFA Act. The food testing laboratories in the country will be upgraded to NABL standards besides drafting the services of private NABL-accredited lab for testing food samples. The new regulatory framework emphasizes on transparency and accountability besides aiming at achieving high degree of consumer's confidence in quality and safety of food. It also empowers consumers to take samples and get it tested and in case of samples being found adulterated, prosecution can be launched by the Designated Officer. For the first time, the new law also covers Nutraceuticals, health food, food supplement, functional food, etc. Designated Officer has to dispose of the application for license within 60 days from the date of application. Where an existing establishment for starting food licenses is found deficient, the Designated Officer has to give improvement notice before launching any prosecution. There are heavy penalties on selling substandard, misbranded or unsafe food with time limit for prosecution within one year.

FSSAI has been following up with the State/UT Governments regarding preparatory action to be taken for the implementation of the Act. The State Governments have taken steps for smooth transition from the PFA Act to the FSS Act.

## FOOD BUSINESS OPERATOR (FBO)

The FSS Act defines a Food Business Operator (FBO) as a person engaged in the business of food manufacture, processing, packaging, transportation, distribution, storage and import, etc. and includes food services, catering services and sale of food or food ingredients.

## REGISTRATION FOR PETTY FOOD BUSINESS OPERATOR (PFBO)

A producer, whose production capacity of the milk and meat products is less then 100 kg/liter per day or is handling milk less than 500 liters per day, meat or meat products producer in the capacity for slaughter of maximum 2 large animals or 10 small animals or 50 poultry birds per day or any other FBO where annual turnover is less than ₹ 12 Lakh is termed as Petty Food Business Operator (PFBO) and is required to be registered.

## LICENSING FROM LOCAL DISTRICT DESIGNATED OFFICER OF THE STATE

All those producers whose production capacity of the Milk is more than 500 liters up to 50,000 liters per day, meat or meat products producer in the capacity for slaughter of more than 2 up to 50 large animals or more than 10 up to 150 small animals or more than 50 up to 1000 poultry birds per day. It will also cover Meat Processing Units producing up to 500 kg. meat per day or 150 MT per annum. The FBO should be operating in one state only.

## CENTRAL LICENSING

All those producers whose production capacity of the milk is more than 50,000 liters per day or 2500 MT of milk solid per annum, meat or meat products producer in the capacity for slaughter of more than 50 large animals or more than 150 small animals or more than 1000 poultry birds per day. It will also cover Meat Processing Units producing more than 500 kg. per day or more than 150 MT per annum. The FBO operating in more than one state has to apply for Central Licensing.

Besides, FBOs with 100% export-oriented units, all importers importing food items including food ingredients and additives for commercial use, food catering services in establishment and units under central government agencies like railways, air and airport, seaport, defence, etc., have also to apply for Central Licensing.

## OFFENCES AND PENALTIES

- Designated officer to be sanctioning authority for launching prosecutions.
- Designated officer to decide whether contravention is punishable with imprisonment or fine only.
- Commissioners of food safety may delegate powers to designated officers for compounding the cases of retailers, hawkers, vendors or temporary stall holders (cases not involving imprisonment may be compounded).
- Renalties graded according to gravity of offence but more stringent than the existing one.

| *Offence* | *Punishment* |
|---|---|
| Selling substandard food | Fine up to 5 lakh |
| Misbranded | Fine up to 3 lakh |
| Misleading advertisement | Fine up to 10 lakh |
| Extraneous | Fine up to 1 lakh |
| Unsafe | Imprisonment + fine |

- Appointment of adjudicating officers/tribunals/special courts for speedy trial.
- Time limit for prosecution—within one year.
- In case punishment is with imprisonment then commissioner to decide whether to refer to court of ordinary jurisdiction (offences punishable with imprisonment up to three years).

Offence punishable with imprisonment exceeding three years to be referred to special courts.

New information on food safety is constantly emerging. Recommendations and precautions for people at high risk are updated as scientists learn more about preventing food-borne illness. Individuals in high-risk categories should seek guidance from a healthcare provider. The application of newly invented technologies instead of our traditional food production and processing techniques can bring phenomenal changes. We can assure the public health by controlling the supply of hygienic and safe food to them, therefore, the proper implementation and monitoring of rules and regulation regarding safe food production is to be materialized. Proper government policy can promote this for overall development. Time-to-time transfer of knowledge of safe food and water to the consumers and efforts to upgrade their life expectancy can only bring our national health to the summit where the developed countries already reached.

13

CHAPTER

# Packaging of Meat and Meat Products

## PACKAGING OF RAW MEAT

Packaging refers to the scientific method of containing a food for optimum protection till it reaches the ultimate consumer. Modern concept treats packaging as an important marketing tool also. Proper packaging helps in maintaining the keeping quality of a product during storage, transport and provides convenience for easy handling by the consumers.

### Packaging Objectives and Requirements

- To prevent moisture loss during storage.
- To offer meat in a most desirable color to the consumers.
- To prevent further microbial contamination.
- To check the pick-up of foreign odor by meat
- To prevent lipid oxidation.

### Packaging Materials and Techniques

The following packaging materials and techniques are in vogue for primal and retail cuts of fresh meats:

#### *Overwraps*

Primal and subprimal cuts of fresh meat are overwrapped with thermoplastic films having excellent optical properties. Low density polyethylene (100 gauge) is the most widely used and cheapest film for this purpose. However, rubber hydrochloride, nylon-6 or 11 film, highly plasticized PVC film (70 gauge) can also serve this purpose. Cellophane coated with nitrocellulose on one side has been in use for wrapping fresh meat for a considerable period. The uncoated side is kept in contact with meat. Another grade of cellophane coated with polyethylene can be used for irregular-shaped meat.

### *Tray with Overwrap*

The most common packages for retail fresh meat cuts in Western countries are polystyrene foam or clear plastic trays overwrapped with a transparent thermoplastic film. These trays offer an esthetically appealing background. Provision of absorbent cotton within the pack eliminates the chances of excessive meat juice accumulation. This meat has a shelf-life of 10 days at 0°C. However, it can retain the desirable bright red color for 5 days only.

### *Shrink Film Overwrap*

These films are biaxially oriented to stay stretched at room temperature but shrink on exposure to hot air or hot water for a few seconds. Shrink films are good water vapor barriers and have high structural strength. These films are used for wrapping large and uneven cuts of fresh meat. These are also frequently recommended for storage of carcass quarters under frozen condition. Shrink films offer neat appearance, contour tight package and are easy to handle. Heat shrinkable polypropylene, irradiated polyethylene or polyvinylidene chloride (PVDC) can be used for this purpose.

### *Vacuum Packaging*

This technique is recommended for long-term storage of primal and subprimal cuts of buffalo meat and beef. It ensures a shelf-life of 8–10 weeks at 0°C **(Figs. 13.1A and B)**. Vacuum packaging of lamb and pork is avoided for different reasons. Lamb may have a shelf-life of 3 weeks only because of comparatively high pH. Pork starts with a large load of bacteria and pork cuts are reported to have a shelf-life of 2 weeks only at 1°C.

Vacuum shrink packaging in cryovac barrier bags may provide a means of storage and transport of frozen carcasses, sides or quarters to overseas destinations. Vacuum packaging is done either in laminates or co-extruded films. Typical laminates in use are:

- Aluminium foil/Polyethylene
- Polyester/Polyethylene
- Polyamide/Polyethylene
- PVDC/Polyester/Polyethylene

### *Modified Atmosphere Packaging*

In this technique, atmosphere inside the package is modified to extend the shelf-life of meat while retaining its color, flavor and weight. The package air can be suitably replaced by gases usually nitrogen, oxygen or carbon dioxide alone or in combination **(Figs. 13.2A to C)**. Different

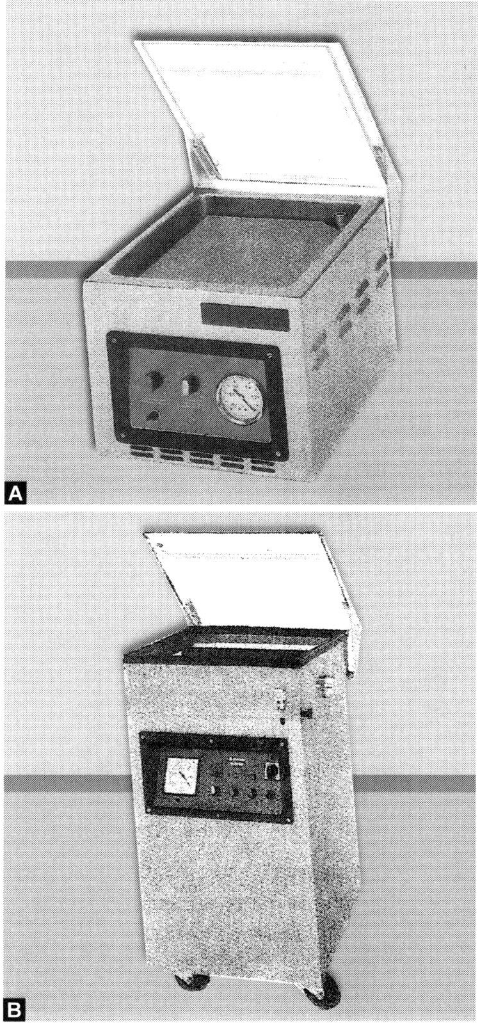

**Figs. 13.1A and B:** Vacuum packaging machines.

meats have varying modified atmosphere requirements. Buffalo meat and beef need high oxygen content to maintain a bright red color. Pork needs less oxygen due to high fat content. Nitrogen serves as an inert filler to balance a gas mixture. However, its use increases the cost of packaging.

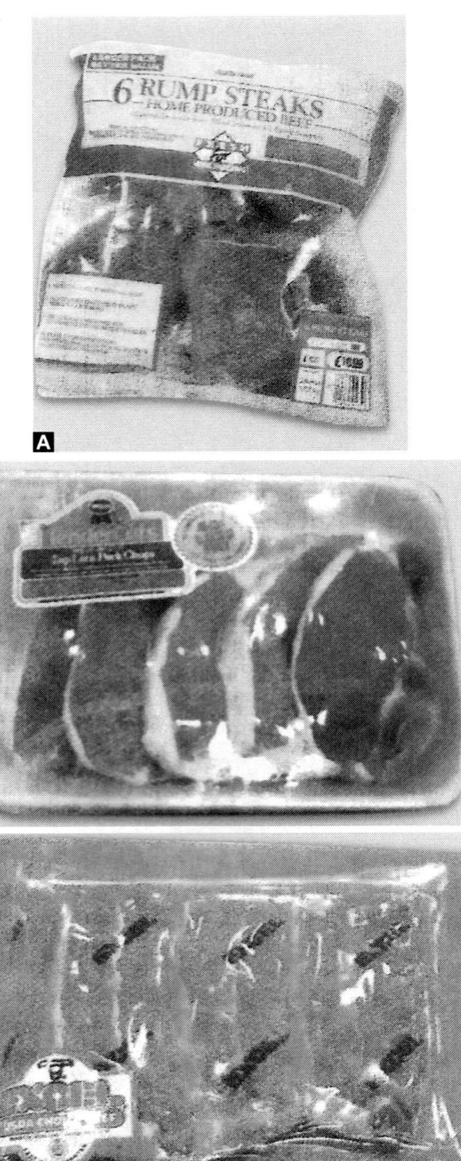


**Figs. 13.2A to C:** (A) Modified atmosphere and skin packaging; (B) Modified atmosphere pack; (C) Vacuum packaging.

## PACKAGING OF FROZEN MEATS

Freezing of meat becomes practically inevitable at home as well as in industry. Meat undergoes slow freezing in the freezer cabinet of the household refrigerator whereas in industry it is quickly frozen by blast freezers. On thawing, the latter results in very little drip loss and nearly fresh texture is maintained. If frozen meat is not properly packed there is a continuous dehydration from the surface resulting in freezer burn. This condition markedly affects the surface texture and color. Meat fat is also prone to the development of oxidative rancidity if a good oxygen barrier is not used. Temperature fluctuation during storage may cause expansion and contraction of the meat cuts.

### Packaging Objectives and Requirements

- To prevent loss of moisture from meat surface or dehydration.
- To protect meat from loss of surface texture.
- To preserve the desirable meat color.
- To check rancidity development in fatty meat.

The packaging for frozen meat should have a very low water vapor permeability, good strength and grease resistance.

### Packaging Materials and Techniques

#### *Overwrap*

Low density polyethylene (150–200 gauge) is the least cost protective film which can withstand low temperatures and maintain clarity. Polyester or nylon/PE laminates can also serve as ideal overwrap.

#### *Shrink Packaging*

Heat shrinkable low-density polyethylene and PVC/PVDC copolymer films provide required functional properties, besides giving neat appearance to the frozen meat cuts. Shrink packaging also allows convenient handling of the product.

## PACKAGING OF MEAT PRODUCTS

Meat and its products are not just commodity for the purpose of packaging. They differ in physicochemical properties including nature of pigments, sensory attributes and microbial flora. The selection of packaging materials is done very carefully to protect these qualities of meat and its products. The purpose is to retard or prevent the main deteriorative changes and make the products available to the consumers in the most attractive form. However, initial quality of meat has to be very good because packaging can at best maintain the existing quality of meat. It cannot improve it.

Packaging requirements are basically regulated by the type of meat, nature of processing it has been subjected to and the channel of merchandising to be adopted. The packaging material should essentially be of good grade and it should not alter the specific attributes of meat and meat products.

## PACKAGING OF CURED MEATS

Cured meat products like ham, bacon, luncheon meat and frankfurters have a shelf-life of 12–15 days at 4°C depending upon the level of nitrite in the cured brine. Much sought after pink color of these products is due to nitrosomyoglobin—a pigment which is formed as a result of action of nitrite with myoglobin. This nitrosomyoglobin is not a very stable pigment. It is susceptible to oxidation into metmyoglobin (dull brown) in a high oxygen environment. This oxidation can be further influenced by an increase in light and temperature of storage. A decrease in pH can also enhance the oxidation of nitrosomyoglobin to metmyoglobin.

Long-term storage of unpacked meats at ambient temperature in tropical countries may favor the growth of bacteria, yeasts and molds resulting in slimy surface. Proper curing and adequate heat processing brings down the initial bacterial load to a large extent. However, lactic acid bacteria are frequently encountered in the cured meats. *Lactobacillus* may cause green cores in the interior of the product. *Streptococcus* and *Micrococcus* may cause souring. An overcure or reuse of brine enhances the growth of halophilic bacterial flora.

### Packaging Objectives and Requirements

- To prevent further microbial contamination.
- To check dehydration or moisture loss, thus avoiding the concentration of color on the surface.
- To prevent the fading of attractive pink cured color.
- To retain cured flavor.

The packaging material should be a good oxygen and water vapor barrier. It should be flexible enough to make a close surface contact with meat. The packaging film should be capable of lamination or coextrusion and hermetical sealing. The package must be able to withstand refrigeration and freezing and to present an attractive appearance. This objective can be achieved by storing the products away from the light and heat. Intensity of light in the storeroom should not exceed 15 watt and should be switched on only when required.

## Packaging Materials and Techniques

### *Overwrapping*

Short-term storage of cured meats can be done by overwrapping the product with various plastic films. Polyethylene (PE) can very well serve this purpose. Some other plastic films viz., polyvinyl chloride (PVC), polyvinylidene chloride (PVDC) and rubber hydrochloride provide tight-fitting overwraps. Coated cellophane can also be used.

Aluminium foil/paper laminate overwrap can protect the cured meats against light and add to eye appearance of the product due to good printability.

### *Shrink Packaging*

Ham and other large irregular cuts of cured meats can be packaged in shrinkable (PVDC/PVC copolymer film where the air is evacuated and the contour overwrapped or bagged product is either immersed in hot water (90–95°C) or passed through hot air tunnel to effect shrink.

Besides contour fitting, shrink packaging also gives clean appearance, package rigidity and an appealing display.

### *Vacuum Packaging*

It is advisable for long-term storage of bacon blocks, luncheon meat, etc. which could be packaged in bags or pouches of the following laminations:

- Cellophane/PVDC/LDPE
- Polyester/PVDC/LDPE
- Polyamide/PVDC/LDPE
- Metallized polyamine/Ethylene-vinyl acetate (EVA)
- EVA/PVDC/EVA
- Polyamide/LDPE/Ionomer

Recent trend is towards the use of semirigid all-plastic vacuum packaging for sliced luncheon meat. Polyvinylchloride alone or a suitable laminate like PVC (2.00 mm)/PVDC (0.025 mm)/LDPE (0.5 mm) can very well serve this purpose. Semirigid all-plastic vacuum packages have very good strength properties, decrease the chances of leaning packages, add to consumer preference due to their attractive look and can be easily stacked in the storeroom or display cabinets.

It is a general practice to have a vacuum level of 25–29 inches in vacuum packages. Vacuum-packed sliced bacon could be kept in a good condition for 3 months at 0–4°C and for 6–8 months at still lower temperature (–18 to –21 and –27°C). Vacuum packaging offers a neat compact package to meat products because the film is pushed against the product by the vacuum from inside and by the positive pressure from outside.

*Controlled Atmosphere Packaging (CAP)*

It is also practiced for long-term storage of cured meats in laminates to make the package completely free of oxygen. Nitrogen alone or a mixture of nitrogen (85–90%) and carbon dioxide (10–15%) can be flushed either through displacement of air or conducting the filling and sealing operation in a gaseous atmosphere.

If the processed meat slices are very thin, it is difficult to separate them in vacuum packaging. But controlled atmosphere packaging or gas flushing is the answer for such a problem. It is general practice to have less than one percent oxygen level in controlled atmosphere packages. The residual oxygen within the package is exhausted in biological respiration in a day or two, thus extending the shelf-life of cured meats upto three months.

## PACKAGING OF THERMO-PROCESSED MEATS

Most thermo-processed meat products are cooked to an internal temperature of 65–70°C to bring about pasteurization. This treatment kills most of the microorganisms in meat products, besides trichinae sometimes encountered in pork. It also causes heat setting due to protein coagulation, denaturation and partial dehydration. The products become tender and its refrigerated shelf-life is also enhanced. Thermal processing over 100°C, usually accomplished by applying pressure is done to prepare commercially sterile meat products.

### Packaging Objectives and Requirements

- To prevent contamination of the product.
- To prevent weight loss.
- To maintain the delicate flavor of cooked meat.
- To hold the desired texture.
- To preserve the typical appearance.
- To provide heat sustainability during long-term storage.

The packaging material should be very good oxygen barrier. It must be in a position to give a hermetic seal for long storage life. It should allow high speed filling and closure. It has to be puncture and deformation resistant **(Fig. 13.3)**.

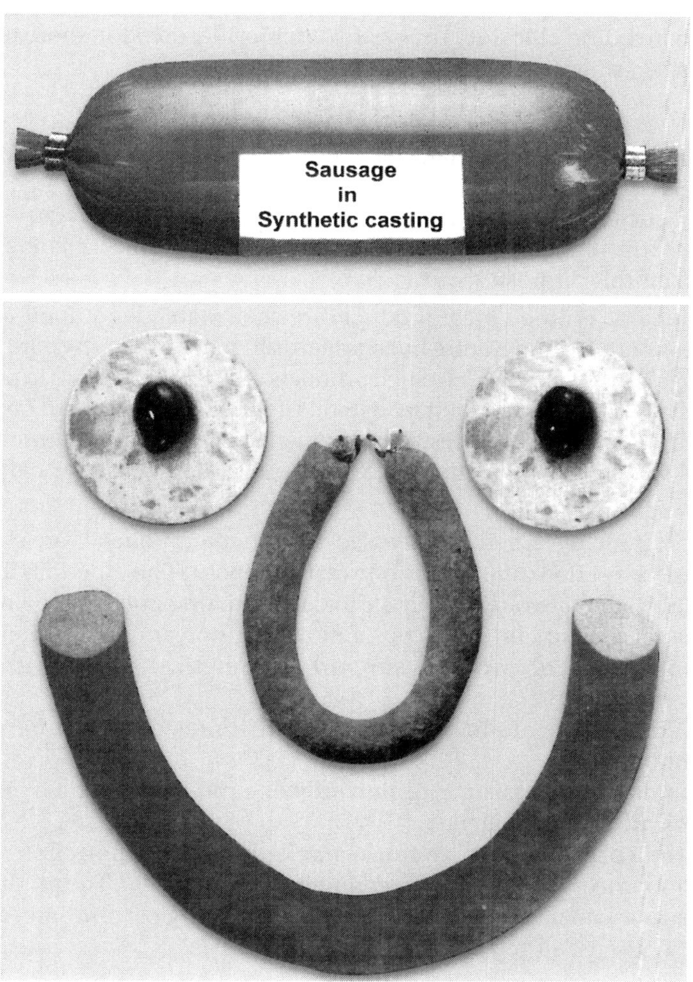


**Fig. 13.3 :** Sausages in synthetic casing.

## Packaging Materials and Techniques

### *Short-term Storage*

Meat products like patties, sausages, nuggets, meat balls, etc., can be packaged in pouches made up of polyethylene, polypropylene, polyvinylidine chloride, rubber hydrochloride, etc., for short-term storage lasting 10–12 days at 4°C.

### *Long-term Storage*

Meat products like corned beef, corned pork, meat gravies, meat soups, liver sausages, chicken curry, boneless chicken, etc., are hermetically sealed and cooked to make commercially sterile for long-term storage at room temperature. Two types of containers are used for this purpose:

**Meat cans:** Canned meat products are shelf-stable for a number of years at room temperature but standards in many Western countries recognize the storage life of such products only for two years. Tin plate cans have maintained their lead in this field. These are coated on the inner side with a sulfur-resistant lacquer. Shallow drawn aluminium cans with internal lacquer have been successfully used for certain meat products.

**Retort pouches:** Thermoprocessed meat in retort pouches are shelf-stable for a period of minimum one year. Composite film especially film/foil/film laminates are used in the making of retort pouches as follows:

a. Outer plastic film made up of polyester, polyamide or oriented polypropylene provides support and physical strength to the composite.
b. Middle layer of aluminium foil contributes excellent barrier properties.
c. Inner layer consisting of polyethylene, polypropylene or PVC provides heat sealability.

Meat products are vacuum packed in these pouches and thermoprocessed in retorts for commercial sterilization. The products have good consumer appeal due to transparency, gloss and agreeable feel. These are stored in printed board cartons.

## PACKAGING OF DEHYDRATED MEATS

Dehydration is a successful means of preserving many meats with proper packaging. Light weight of these meats and stability at ambient temperature renders them the best choice as military rations. While hot air-drying of cooked ground meat was found to have only little success, freeze-drying and accelerated freeze-drying are widely accepted methods for drying all types of meats. Proper packaging is vital for stability of these products because there is a marked susceptibility of dehydrated meats to oxidation resulting in rancid odor.

### Packaging Objectives and Requirements

- To prevent the ingress of moisture into the product.
- To protect the product against oxygen and light.
- To check the absorption of foreign odors.
- To maintain the integrity of the crisp product.
- To help in convenient and safe transport of the product.

An important requirement of packaging dehydrated meats is the need to compress it in order to increase its density and exclude air from the open texture of dry particles.

### Packaging Materials and Techniques

*Tin Plate Cans*

The best packaging technique for freeze-dried meats and their products is vacuum sealed in plate cans.

*Metal Foil/Plastic Film Laminates*

These are widely used for the packaging of dehydrated meat products:

a. Compressed bars of dehydrated minced meat with inner cellophane and outer paper/Alu foil/PE laminate wrap are reported to be shelf-stable for one year.
b. Flexible pouches most suitable for vacuum and modified atmosphere packaging consist of Polyester/PE/Alu foil/PE or Cellophane/PE/Alu foil/PE laminates.

In modified atmosphere packaging, nitrogen as an inert gas keeps the product under sufficient pressure to restrict its movement within the package. It also improves the package shape.

## NEW TECHNOLOGIES IN FOOD PACKAGING

Processors are not satisfied even with the present main function of protection and a major role in marketing of food products. They have as well started assigning specific functions to packaging which requires its active involvement in the extension of shelf-life. Such a packaging has been named as ***active or smart packaging***. In dehydrated and hurdle treated shelf-stable foods, humidity build-up in the package due to carbohydrate and fat metabolism can be checked by moisture scavengers such as diatomaceous pad in the packaging system. It restricts the growth of yeast and molds. In oxygen-sensitive foods, head space oxygen can be eliminated by incorporating oxygen scavengers. Similarly, carbon dioxide build-up in a pack can be checked by carbon dioxide scavengers. On the contrary, carbon dioxide can be regularly generated in the package by placing a carbon dioxide-filled sachet to control oxygen concentration. Ethylene scavenger may be placed in the packages of fruits and vegetables to retard maturity and enhance their shelf stability.

Plastic packaging materials and polymers of synthetic origin have posed the problem of after-use disposal throughout the world. This is adding to the misery of environmental pollution. In Indian cities, the problem of blockage of sewer lines has acquired a stupendous proportion and many municipal corporations have banned their use to overcome this problem. Hence, efforts are being made to come up with ***environment-friendly biodegradable*** packaging. The natural biopolymers are films of vegetable origin. Polysaccharide films may be derived from starch and its derivatives, cellulose and its derivatives, gelatin, gum, gluten, etc. These have good mechanical and optical properties but their limitations are susceptibility to moisture and low water vapor barrier properties. On the contrary, biopolymer films made up of lipids and waxes or their derivatives are a good barrier to water vapor but are fragile, opaque and prone to rancidity. Such a situation has forced the technologies to look for viable alternatives.

Hence, the concept of mixing synthetic polymers and biopolymers has been invented. Starch is the base of most of these mixtures. A potential example of these types of composite packaging materials is gelatinized starch/hydrophobic copolymer/polyethylene. Another alternative is the use of starch hydrolysates along with polyesters which are prone to microbial degradation. Yet another example is thermoplastic corn starch incorporating the use of plasticizers such as glycerol, sorbitol, etc.

We are familiar with the sugar and chocolate coatings on certain candies for a long time. With the development of all vegetable biopolymers, the area of edible films and coatings has acquired a new dimension. Now ***edible packaging*** is an emerging field and improved starch and pectin films have been proposed for coating red meats also. These films and coatings help in maintaining the desired color without affecting their sensory attributes.

People wish to buy and consume perishable livestock products in as much fresh condition as possible. They look forward to the labeling with shelf-life dating on the food product itself as an assurance of quality, nutrition and safety. Quality indicators are now being proposed to be inbuilt in packaging material or fastened on packages. The indicators can respond to storage temperature fluctuations with a color change and give an idea about the probable loss of shelf-life. Further, intensive research work is required in this area to come up with reliable time-temperature on packaged livestock products.

# 14 CHAPTER

# Basics of Sensory Evaluation of Meat Food Products

Consumers are the ultimate users of a food item. So, their perception and satisfaction is of paramount importance for the success of any food product. If a product is very palatable, it makes an excellent eating. Some of the important eating quality attributes are flavor, texture and tenderness, appearance or color, juiciness, etc. A knowledge of these attributes is of prime importance for their subjective and objective assessment.

## FLAVOR

Flavor is a complex sensation comprising mainly taste and odor. It is sensed jointly by the oral and olfactory senses. There are only four basic tastes-sweet, salty, sour, and bitter **(Fig. 14.1)**. Some researchers believe in 5th basic taste called umami (savory or meat like). The

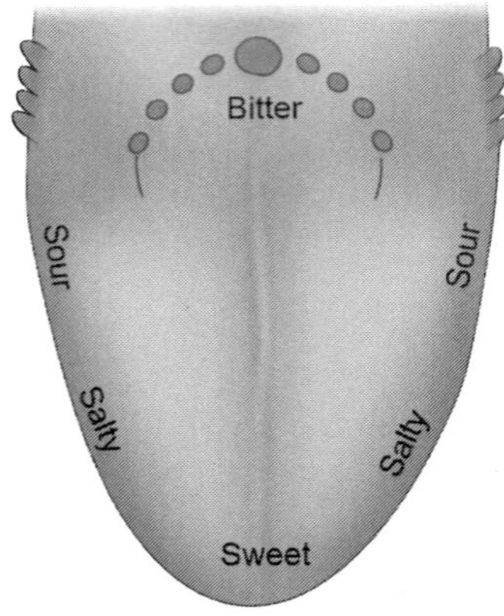


**Fig. 14.1:** Concentration of taste papillae on the tongue.

receptor taste buds for each of these tastes are located on the tongue and the upper palate. These taste buds are small structures which are situated on the raised protrusions of the tongue surface called papillae. These are involved in the taste perception. The taste receptor cells send information detected by the clusters of receptors and ions channels to the gustatory areas of the brain via 7th, 9th, and 10th cranial nerves. A human tongue has about 1,000 taste buds. Odor is sensed at the regio olfactoria inside the nose. Meat sample should be smelled first followed by tasting for a rational and sound flavor perception of several volatile components present in meat. These components are significantly marked when meat is cooked. Flavor has been shown to have a profound effect on the overall acceptability of meat product.

Flavor of meat depends on species, sex, age, and method of cooking. In general, flavor of fresh raw meat is weak, salty, and serum-like. Fresh meat fat also has almost indistinct taste and odor. It is during cooking that flavor get pronounced and becomes meaty. Fresh cooked beef is metallic and astringent. Veal flavor is sweet and flat. Pork flavor is regarded sweet and bland. Sex odor is more pronounced in male. Pork from boar has a definite piggy odor or boar taint. During long term storage, most meats develop rancid odor due to fat oxidation. It may be muttony for mutton, tallowy for beef and stale, cheesy or fishy for pork. In case, meat is spoiled during storage, it emanates putrid odor due to protein decomposition. When cooked meat is stored for a long time, myoglobin catalyzed fat oxidation takes place yielding a distinct warmed-over flavor. Canning imparts canned-meat flavor to meat products due to severe heat treatment.

## TEXTURE AND TENDERNESS

Texture is one of the most important eating quality attributes in the acceptance of meat. The overall impression of texture is perceived by the senses of touch, sight and hearing. The texture of animal foods has different components. The mechanical component relates to the effect of stress, e.g., hard, brittle, gummy, chewy, elastic, cohesive etc. The geographical component relates to size, shape and arrangement of fibers in meat, e.g., coarse, grainy, gritty, fibrous etc. Some other components relate to the moisture and fat perception of meat, e.g., greasy, oily, watery, dry, moist, etc. In general, three factors are considered to get an overall impression of meat tenderness. These are the ease with which teeth sink into meat, the ease with which the meat breaks into fragments and the leftover residue after chewing.

The texture of meat is affected by many preslaughter factors like sex, age, heredity, diet, carcass grade, etc. Several post slaughter factors like postmortem glycolysis, fat deposition, connective tissue, conditioning, freezing, cooking, etc., have a profound influence on the texture of meat.

Several tenderizing agents like salt, weak acids (vinegar and citric acid) and some enzyme preparations are used to make the meat tender. Plant enzymes like papain, bromelain and ficin have a proven tenderizing effect on meat. During cooking, connective tissue (including collagen) becomes more tender.

## APPEARANCE AND COLOR

Appearance is a wider term than color because it is influenced by other factors also. Appearance and color have a definite appeal when a consumer goes out to buy meat or meat products. The color of fresh meat is species specific. It is determined by the concentration of principal meat pigment - myoglobin and its derivatives (oxymyoglobin and metmyoglobin). Consumers relate the appearance and color of meat with safety and healthfulness.

The color of cooked meat is related by consumers to doneness. The final color of cooked meat is dependent upon the pigment changes brought about by temperature, time and method of cooking. When meat is cooked, there is gradual change of color from dark red or pink to a lighter shade and finally at higher temperatures to gray or brown color, Pressure cooked or boiled meat will discern a gray color whereas roasted, broiled or canned meat turns brown. The brown color of thoroughly cooked meat is due to denaturation of heme pigments and polymerization of some proteins and fats. The color of fresh pork, mutton, and buffalo fat is white and undergoes very little change during cooking. The color of cured meats is due to nitric oxide myoglobin which is heat stable.

## JUICINESS

The juiciness of cooked meat comprises of two components - the first impression of juiciness comes from rapid release of meat fluids during initial chews, whereas sustained juiciness is due to slow release of serum and stimulatory effect of fat on salivation. A good quality meat is more juicy than that of poor quality because of higher content of intramuscular fat. Fresh frozen meat with high ultimate pH is quite juicy.

Cooking temperature has a profound effect on the juiciness of meat. The degree of shrinkage on cooking is inversely proportional to the juiciness of meat. Juiciness and tenderness are closely related to meat attributes. In a tender meat, the juices are quickly released on chewing and leftover residue is less.

Besides these, certain other eating quality attributes also influence the overall palatability of a meat product. Some meat products have a residue coating the mouth after swallowing. Mouth coating has been observed in chicken frankfurters, buffalo sausages, patties etc. Overall acceptability of a meat product is not the sum average of all the eating quality attributes. This is so because some attributes influence the overall acceptability of the product more as compared to others. Lawrie (1985) rated texture and tenderness as the most important eating quality attributes whereas Rartholonew and Osulao (1986) reported that compared to texture and appearance, flavor had more effect on the overall acceptability of processed mutton products.

## SENSORY EVALUATION

Sensory evaluation of foods including meat refers to their scientific assessment through the use of human senses. This evaluation is necessary for:

a. New product development
b. Analysis of competitive products
c. Product shelf-life studies
d. Market level consumer tests
e. Aroma research, etc.

Modern instruments available these days can analyze usually one and at times two eating quality parameters at a time but almost all attributes and the total impression of a food product can be properly assessed only by human sensory perception.

## SPECIALIZED PANEL

The sensory evaluation of meat and meat products may be product oriented or consumer oriented. Product oriented evaluation is done by specialized panel. When new products or formulations are being developed or earlier ones are being altered, specialized panel testing usually precedes consumer panel testing. In specialized panel testing, small number of trained panelists use their senses as biological detectors. Such panelists can easily identify even minor differences in the eating quality attributes of similar meat products.

Sensory panel members are selected on the basis of general health, appetite, sensitivity, willingness, availability etc. They are invited to attend an orientation session where testing facilities are shown and importance of this work is explained to them. Their sensitivity is tested by conducting recognition test and threshold test for four basic tastes. Selected individuals are then trained by making them familiar with the important meat traits and conducting serial dilution tests till they attain good performance on hedonic scale.

The sensory panel members are presented test meat samples along with a control in a random order after assigning suitable codes **(Fig. 14.2)**. The ideal time for conducting sensory evaluation of meat and meat products is late morning or late afternoon. It is necessary to rinse the mouth between successive samples. Difference tests are usually applied for product testing. In paired difference test, there is direct comparison of a control sample and an analytical sample for a single attribute. In a triangle test, three meat samples are offered - two similar and one different. The odd sample has to be identified. In hedonic scoring or rating test, the degree of acceptance is inferred on the basis of numerical rating of meat samples **(Table 14.1)**. In a ranking test, panel members are assigned to rank the samples according to their preference.

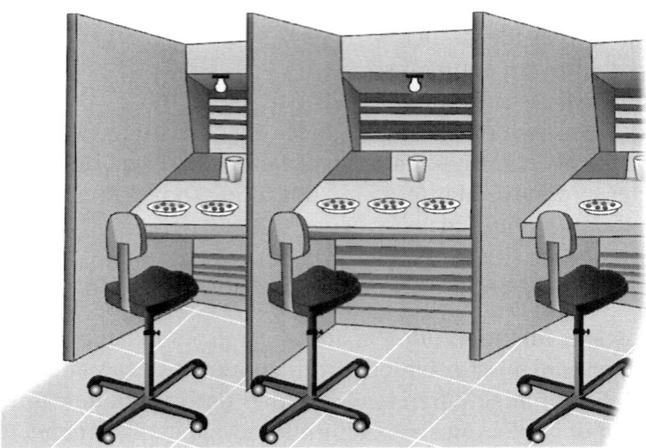

**Fig. 14.2:** Individual booths in the sensory evaluation laboratory.

**Table 14.1:** Proforma for sensory evaluation of meat products based on hedonic scale.

Name: ____________ Expt. No.: ____________ Product: ____________ Date: ____________

| *Scoring guide* | | | | | | | | |
|---|---|---|---|---|---|---|---|---|
| *Attributes* | *Scale of descriptive attribute of product* | | | | | | | |
| | 8 | 7 | 6 | 5 | 4 | 3 | 2 | 1 |
| Appearance/ Color | Excellent | Very good | Good | Fair | Slightly poor | Moderately poor | Very poor | Extremely poor |
| Flavor | Extremely desirable | Very desirable | Moderately desirable | Slightly undesirable | Slightly undesirable | Moderately undesirable | Very undesirable | Extremely undesirable |
| Juiciness | Extremely juicy | Very juicy | Moderately juicy | Slightly juicy | Slightly dry | Moderately dry | Very dry | Extremely dry |
| Texture | Extremely desirable | Very desirable | Moderately desirable | Slightly undesirable | Slightly undesirable | Moderately undesirable | Very undesirable | Extremely undesirable |
| Saltiness | Extremely desirable | Very desirable | Moderately desirable | Slightly undesirable | Slightly undesirable | Moderately undesirable | Very undesirable | Extremely undesirable |
| Mouth coating | None | Practically none | Traces | Slight | Moderate | Slightly abundant | Moderately abundant | Abundant |
| Overall acceptability | Extremely acceptable | Very acceptable | Moderately acceptable | Slightly acceptable | Slightly unacceptable | Moderately unacceptable | Very unacceptable | Extremely unacceptable |
| Sample | Appearance | Flavor | Juiciness | Texture | Saltiness | Mouth coating | Overall acceptability | |
| 1 | | | | | | | | |
| 2 | | | | | | | | |
| 3 | | | | | | | | |
| 4 | | | | | | | | |

Remarks: Signature:

## CONSUMER PANEL

Consumer panel generally consists of 100 or more persons drawn from the geographical area proposed to be the market of a particular meat product. The panel members need not have any formal education or training. They may be factory workers, laboratory attendants or any body from the consumer population. This panel is of practical utility in predicting the future market performance. The consumer panel members may be selected from the target population on random basis. Their likes and dislikes, eating habits, income group, psychological state or environment, etc., are allowed to play its natural or justifiable role, since they are the potential product users. Consumer panel can be conducted at any central location supermarket, retail outlet or even consumer's homes. With little instructions and guidance, panelists can easily be involved in ranking test or hedonic score test. The data obtained from specialized as well as consumer panel is statistically analyzed to enable proper interpretation and application of results.

# 15

CHAPTER

# Chemical Composition and Nutritive Value of Poultry Meat

Poultry meat is a good source of protein. It has a balanced lipid content and low calorific value. It is palatable, tender and easily digestible. It is easy to prepare and can be served in a variety of ways.

## CHEMICAL COMPOSITION

A quantitative proximate composition of poultry meat is presented in **Table 15.1**. The composition of meat tissue varies according to the age of the bird.

### 1. Moisture

This is the largest component of muscle tissue. It dissolves nutrients and serves as a medium for their transport. Raw chicken meat contains 70–74% moisture. In general, younger birds have a higher moisture to skeletal muscle ratio as compared to older ones. The fat content of meat is inversely proportional to the moisture content. So, as the fat increases, the moisture content decreases.

**Table 15.1:** General composition of raw poultry meat.

| *Species* | *Moisture (%)* | *Protein (%)* | *Fat (%)* | *Ash (%)* | *Food Energy (Cal/100 g)* |
|---|---|---|---|---|---|
| **Chicken** | | | | | |
| (i) Broiler (8 weeks) | 74.0 | 18.5 | 6.0 | 0.80 | 125 |
| (ii) Spent hen | 72.0 | 19.0 | 6.5 | 1.25 | 120 |
| Quail (8 weeks) | 70.5 | 20.5 | 5.5 | 1.20 | 125 |
| Duck (8 weeks) | 58.0 | 20.0 | 19.8 | 0.50 | 300 |
| Turkey (medium fat) | 60.0 | 19.5 | 18.0 | 1.00 | 270 |

## 2. Protein

Poultry meat has higher protein content than most of the red meats. This protein is of very superior quality with respect to biological value and essential amino acid contents **(Table 15.2)**. Male birds generally have higher protein content as compared to their female counterparts. Protein content of the body is less prone to change in comparison to moisture and fat contents.

**Table 15.2:** Detailed composition of raw chicken meat.

| *(i) Amino acid content (Percent of protein)* | |
|---|---|
| Lysine | 7.5 |
| Methionine | 1.8 |
| Arginine | 6.7 |
| Cystine | 1.8 |
| Tryptophane | 0.8 |
| Tyrosine | 2.5 |
| Leucine | 6.6 |
| Isoleucine | 4.1 |
| Histidine | 2.0 |
| Valine | 6.7 |
| *(ii) Mineral content (mg/100 g)* | |
| Calcium | 5.8 |
| Phosphorus | 407 |
| Iron | 0.7 |
| Sodium | 46 |
| Potassium | 248 |
| Magnesium | 29 |
| Sulphur | 268 |
| *(iii) Vitamin content (per 100 g)* | |
| Vitamin A | 730 IU |
| Thiamin ($B_1$) | 0.07 mg |

*Contd...*

*Contd...*

| | |
|---|---|
| Riboflavin ($B_2$) | 0.38 mg |
| Niacin | 5.6 mg |
| *(iv) Lipid contents (percent of total lipids)* | |
| Phospholipids | 48 |
| Neutral lipids | 52 |
| *(v) Cholesterol content (mg/100 g)* | *60* |

*Sources:*

i. Scott, M.L. (1958). J. American Dietetic Assoc. 34(2).
ii. McCancc and Widdewson (1960). World's Poult. Sci. J. 36:25.
iii. and v. Wall and Merril (1963). USDA Handbook no. 8.
iv. Katz et al. (1966). J. Food Sci. 31:717.

## 3. Fat

Most fat in poultry remains confined underneath the skin in contrast to red meats where it is generally distributed throughout the tissues. The content varies widely depending on the species, age, sex and diet of poultry. The carcass fat invariably increases with a raise in dietary fat or high energy diet. The proportion of desired unsaturated fatty acids—oleic and linoleic acid is more than 60 percent of the total meat fat. Poultry meat contains less cholesterol, a fatty alcohol associated with atherosclerosis, as compared to most other animal-based foods.

## 4. Carbohydrate

Poultry meat has very little carbohydrate content, hardly 1–2 percent of total edible tissue. Inositol, glucose and fructose are the major whereas mannose and ribose are the minor constituents of carbohydrate.

## 5. Vitamins

Poultry meat is a good source of many vitamins. Niacin is present in good quantity whereas thiamin (vitamin $B_1$), riboflavin (vitamin $B_2$) and ascorbic acid (vitamin C) are also present in fair quantity. Poultry liver is a rich source of vitamin A, vitamin B complex and vitamin C.

## 6. Minerals

Poultry meat contains nearly one percent desired minerals. Some of the important ones are sodium, potassium, calcium, magnesium, iron, phosphorus, sulfur, chlorine, etc.

## NUTRITIVE VALUE

Poultry meat is a food of high nutritional value. It is higher in protein content as compared to red meats. Poultry meat proteins are classified under first class category because it contains all the essential amino acids in balanced proportion. Such high protein diet ensures overall development of the body and plays an important role in tissue repairs.

Chicken meat with low fat content offers good quality food to the consumers **(Table 15.3)**. It provides the much-desired essential fatty acids which form necessary constituents of the cell wall, mitochondria and other cell constituents. Thus, it helps in maintaining the health of the consumers. Due to its low energy value, chicken meat is a good food for weight control diets. Chicken meat contains more phospholipids and low cholesterol than other meats, which minimizes risks due to diabetes and heart diseases.

Chicken meat is a good source of vitamins and minerals in human diet. It is rich in niacin and moderately rich in thiamin, riboflavin and ascorbic acid. Chicken meat is also a good source of iron and phosphorus. Due to high biological value and easy digestibility, it is a choice food for aged persons as well as children. Chicken meat carries a high-class image because of its product variety and healthful nature.

**Table 15.3:** Nutritive value of roasted chicken meat (per 100 g).

| | |
|---|---|
| Protein | 24.5 g |
| Fat | 6.2 g |
| Ash | 1.04 g |
| Food energy | 154 Calories |

[*Source:* Scott, M.L. (1956). J. American Dietetic Assoc., 32(10)]

In general, poultry meat contains all the essential amino acids, fatty acids and minerals in an appropriate quantity. It has the ability to alleviate the nutritional stress conditions in the human beings. It has a good aesthetic appeal. Poultry meat has no religious inhibition and its many products satisfy the variety quest of the consumers.

16

CHAPTER

# Preslaughter Handling, Transport and Dressing of Poultry

Several modern poultry dressing plants have come up in the country and many more are in the offing where large number of birds are to be handled and processed every day. These birds should be handled properly before slaughter. It reduces the changes of bruises, cuts and tears on the dressed birds. In fact, preslaughter care contributes a good deal to the wholesomeness of dressed chickens.

## PRESLAUGHTER CARE AND HANDLING

In the intensive housing system, a great care has to be exercised in catching and crating the birds. All feeders, waterers and other accessory equipment should be moved to one corner of the house before catching and assembling is undertaken. The broilers are generally caught at night under very dim light. Culled and spent hens are caught in the cooler hours of the day, preferably in the afternoon. The birds are caught manually by the shank in a humane way.

## TRANSPORT

Crates, coops or cages are used to transport birds in vans from the farm to poultry dressing plant. Special attention is paid to prevent overcrowding and suffocation. The loading of birds is carried out in dim light either early morning or late evening to avoid excitement and transported in the cool period without much exposure to sun to prevent excessive shrinkage.

Bulk weighing of birds in crates is the general practice at the large-sized dressing plants. A shrinkage of 3–4 percent takes place during preslaughter handling and transport. Birds should be kept off feed for 12 hrs before slaughter but enough drinking water should be made available. This practice not only helps in early evisceration but risk of contamination of meat by the intestinal contents is also minimized.

## DRESSING OF POULTRY

### Slaughtering

Slaughtering involves stunning and bleeding:

a. **Stunning:** Stunning prevents struggling and relaxes the muscles holding the feathers. However, it is generally not practiced in case of chicken. A low-voltage electric stunning of 50 volts AC for 1 minutes has been found to be satisfactory.

b. **Bleeding:** This process is carried out in an inverted cone-shaped equipment to rest the body of the bird and keep the head out and down. There are several techniques of slaughtering poultry in order to seek proper bleeding. The technique most commonly used these days is "Modified Kosher Method" in which jugular vein is severed just below the jowl taking care not to cut trachea and esophagus. Another technique for slaughtering the birds is decapitation which is not so common. Still another method which involves piercing knife through the brain has become obsolete. In general, a bleeding time of 1.5–2 minutes is allowed. Incomplete bleeding retards the keeping quality of dressed chicken.

### Scalding

Scalding refers to immersion of birds in hot water for loosening the feathers. It should be done when all reflexes have ceased. The birds are transferred into the scalding tank. Broiler and young birds are scalded at 55°C for 1.5 minutes, whereas culled birds and spent hens are scalded at 60°C for 2 minutes.

### Defeathering

The process is carried out in a feather plucker consisting of two drums with rubber fingers which revolve in opposite directions pulling of feathers from the carcass. Any remaining feathers are picked up manually.

### Singeing

The carcasses are now singed over a blue flame for 5–10 seconds to remove hair-like appendages called filoplumes.

## Washing

The singed carcasses are washed with spray water to remove dirt and reduce the microbial load.

## Removal of Feet and Oil Gland

The next step involves cutting of feet from tarsometatarsal joint with a sharpen knife and removal of oil gland.

## Evisceration

The carcasses are hung by hocks to the shackles for evisceration. By a slit opening from the tip of breast bone, abdominal cavity is opened by means of a transverse cut. A circular cut is made around the vent. The viscera is drawn outside but allowed to remain attached to the carcass for postmortem inspection. Meanwhile, a slit is made in the skin of the neck for easy removal of crop and neck. After postmortem inspection, inedible offals, including trachea, lungs, esophagus, crop, intestines, gall bladder and kidneys are removed whereas giblet consisting of heart, liver and gizzard should be collected, cleaned and packed in a wrapper.

## Chilling and Draining

After washing, the dressed birds are chilled in a chilling tank containing slush ice or crushed ice for 30–45 minutes in order to cool the carcasses to an internal temperature of about 4°C. The chilled birds are kept on the draining rack for 10 minutes to remove the excess water.

## Washing

Dressed birds are thoroughly washed again with clean spray water preferably maintained at 15 ± 5°C. Special care should be taken to wash the interior and sides.

## Grading

Dressed chickens are graded on the basis of conformation, degree of fleshing, bruises, cuts, and other quality tributes. Indian standards for dressed chicken are given in **Table 16.1.**

**Table 16.1:** Indian standards for dressed chicken.

| | *Grade 1* | *Grade 2* |
|---|---|---|
| (a) Conformation | Free of deformities that detract from its appearance or that affect the normal distribution of flesh. Slight deformities such as slightly curved or dented breast bones and slightly curved backs may be present. | Slight abnormalities such as dented curved or crooked back or mis-shapen legs or wings which do not materially affect the distribution of flesh or the appearance of the carcass or part. |
| (b) Fleshing | The breast is moderately long and deep, and has sufficient flesh to give it a rounded appearance with the flesh carrying well up to the crest of the breast bone along with its entire length. | The breast has a substantial covering of flesh, with the flesh carrying up to the crest of the breast bone sufficiently to prevent a thin appearance. |
| (c) Fat covering | The fat is well distributed so that there is a noticeable amount of fat in the skin in the areas between the heavy feather tracts. | The fat under the skin is sufficient to prevent a distinct appearance of the flesh through the skin, especially on the breast and legs. |
| (d) Defeathering | Free of pin feathers. Diminutive feathers and hair which are visible to the inspector or grader. | Not more than an occasional protruding pin feather or diminutive feathers shall be in evidence under a careful examination. |
| (e) Cuts and tears | Free of cuts and tears on the breast and legs. | The carcass may have very few cuts and tears. |
| (f) Discoloration | Free from discoloration due to bruising, free of clots; flesh bruises and discoloration of the skin such as "blue back" are not permitted on the breast or legs. | Discoloration due to bruising; free of clots; moderate areas of discoloration due to bruises in the skin or flesh. |

*Contd...*

*Contd...*

| | *Grade 1* | *Grade 2* |
|---|---|---|
| (g) Freezer burn | May have an occasional pock marks due to drying of the inner layer of skin (derma), provided that none exceeded the area of a circle 0.5 cm in diameter on chickens. | May have a few pock marks due to drying of the inner layer of skin (derma), provided that no single area exceeds that of a circle 1.5 cm in diameter |

## Packaging

Before packaging, dressed chickens having gizzard without mucosal layer, heart without pericardium and liver without gallbladder are placed in the abdominal cavity of the carcass and packed in polyethylene bags (200 gauge). Shrink packaging may be adopted if dressed chickens are to be stored in a frozen condition.

## Storage

Dressed chicken can be stored in a refrigerator at 2°C for 7 days and deep freezer at –18 to –20°C for a period of 4–6 months.

**FSSAI** has notified the Food Safety and Standards (Food Products Standards and Food Additives) Amendment Regulation, 2018, wherein Standards have been prescribed for poultry meat as follows:

## Fresh or Chilled or Frozen Poultry Meat

*Dressed Chicken* shall be of the following *three* types:

1. Fresh or chilled or frozen carcasses
2. Fresh or chilled or frozen cuts, bone-in or boneless, true to its type
3. Fresh or chilled or frozen edible offal

*Boneless meat* shall have:

- Moisture content between 60% and 74.86%
- Protein content between 19.5% and 23.20%
- Fat content between 3.50% and 18%

*Poultry meat* shall be stored at 4°C for short-term storage and at –18°C or below for long-term storage. The chilled mutton should be consumed within 2–4 days under normal chilling conditions of storage and frozen mutton shall be consumed within 12 months.

17

CHAPTER

# Antemortem and Postmortem Examination of Poultry

It is essential to conduct proper antemortem inspection of live poultry in order to ensure that they are not affected with any disease or condition which may render their meat unwholesome. Postmortem inspection becomes essential to detect dressed poultry which might have been diseased, thereby rendering them unfit for human consumption.

## ANTEMORTEM INSPECTION OF POULTRY

Live poultry should be subjected to antemortem inspection in the holding pens by a qualified veterinarian on the day of slaughter. Enough space and water should be provided in the holding pens. Adequate light is an essential requirement during inspection. The birds are carefully examined and those in good health and alert condition are declared fit for slaughter. In general, birds with abnormal conditions are categorized as follows:

### Unfit for Slaughter

Birds with morbid condition due to clinical evidence of a contagious disease, heat stroke or traumatic injury which cannot be treated are declared unfit for slaughter.

### Suspects

Birds affected with disease conditions not advanced enough to declare unfit are passed for slaughter as suspect. Such birds are slaughtered separately and both ante- and postmortem findings are considered while taking a final decision.

Various poultry diseases and their antemortem significance is presented in **Table 17.1**.

**Table 17.1:** Antemortem significance of poultry diseases.

| | *Disease* | *Unfit for slaughter* | *Passed for slaughter as suspect* |
|---|---|---|---|
| 1. | Ornithosis | All affected birds | — |
| 2. | Ranikhet disease | Birds in acute stage | All others |
| 3. | Chronic respiratory disease | -do- | Birds with slight respiratory distress |
| 4. | Infectious bronchitis | Birds in advanced stage | Recovered birds |
| 5. | Neural bronchitis | Birds in advanced stage with cyanosis | Birds with initial signs of disease or evidence of recovery |
| 6. | Infectious coryza | Acute stage of disease with debilitation | Highly affected birds |
| 7. | Neural lymphomatosis | All affected birds | — |
| 8. | Coccidiosis | Anemic birds | Highly affected birds |
| 9. | Infectious enterohepatitis (Black head disease of turkey) | Birds showing symptoms | Slight involvement and recovered birds |
| 10. | Fowl typhoid | All affected birds | — |
| 11. | Fowl pox | Birds in debilitated and febrile condition | All others |
| 12. | Fowl cholera | Birds with septicemic form | All others |
| 13. | Botulism (limber neck) | All affected birds | — |

## Postmortem Inspection

The body cavity of every dressed bird is opened through the transverse incision and visceral organs are drawn out. Now the carcass is inspected externally for signs of disease, bone abnormalities, wounds, muscular atrophy, tumors, etc., followed by body cavity. Liver is examined for consistency, texture, lesions and color changes. Spleen is also palpated for texture and abnormalities. A cut is given on the hock to see synovial fluid for sinusitis. Common diseases encountered during postmortem examination along with their importance are presented in **Table 17.2**. Pathological lesions may be referred in Diseases of Poultry by Hofstad et al. (1972).

**Table 17.2:** Postmortem significance of poultry diseases.

| | *Disease* | *Unfit for food/ condemned* | *Partially condemned/ passed for* |
|---|---|---|---|
| 1. | Avian leukosis complex | All affected carcasses | — |
| 2. | Erysipelas | -do- | — |
| 3. | Tuberculosis | -do- | — |
| 4. | Ranikhet disease | Carcasses with systemic involvement | If lesions are localized, only affected parts are condemned. Rest are passed for food |
| 5. | Infectious laryngotracheitis | -do- | |
| 6. | Infectious Coryza | -do- | |
| 7. | Chronic respiratory disease | -do- | |
| 8. | Fowl typhoid | -do- | |
| 9. | Pullorum disease | -do- | |
| 10. | Listeriosis | Carcasses with acute septicemia | |
| 11. | Salmonellosis | Carcasses with active septicemic lesions | In chronic cases, affected parts are condemned. Rest are passed for food |
| 12. | Fowl pox | Carcasses with progressive lesions and systemic changes | Recovered birds may be passed for food after removal of scabs |
| 13. | Fungal diseases | — | Only affected parts are condemned |
| 14. | Fowl cholera | All carcasses are condemned | — |

All the condemned carcasses and parts thereof should be destroyed by chemical denaturing with crude carbolic acid or any phenolic disinfectant or completely destroyed by incineration.

18

CHAPTER

# Preservation of Poultry Meat

The basic purpose of poultry meat preservation is to retard or prevent microbial spoilage and other physicochemical changes which cause deterioration in quality. Thus, proper preservation safeguards the sensory quality and nutritive value of poultry meat. Various methods employed for preservation of poultry meat are as follows:

## CHILLING

Chilling extends the shelf-life of dressed birds by retarding the microbial growth. The efficiency of chilling depends on temperature, air circulation and moisture control. It is advisable to prechill the carcasses at 15°C to remove body heat. Dressed birds are usually chilled by immersion in ice water or chill packed in crushed ice for delivery to stores. Poultry meat can be safely stored at a temperature of 1–4°C and relative humidity of 80–85 percent for a period of 5–7 days. The effectiveness of refrigerated storage can be enhanced to several weeks by applying vacuum packaging.

## FREEZING

Chilled poultry carcasses can be packaged and stored frozen for quite some time. Freezing of poultry meat can be accomplished either using refrigerated plates or in air. Slow still air-freezing generally accomplished in home freezer takes 4–10 hours to freeze depending on the size of the product. Quick air blast freezing is widely used for long-term storage in commercial enterprises. Here the prepackaged carcasses are frozen at an air velocity of 1400 rpm to –30 to –40°C in 1–2 hours. Quick freezing has distinct advantage over slow freezing because intracellular ice crystals formed in this case do not affect the appearance and other sensory attributes. In slow freezing, there is formation of extracellular ice crystals which distort the musculature.

## SMOKING

Smoking is generally practiced along with curing. Smoke obtained by the slow combustion of hardwood sawdust contains lower alcohols, aldehydes, organic acids, carbonyl compounds, phenols, etc., preserve meat by its bacteriostatic, bactericidal and antioxidant properties besides providing a protective film on the surface. Smoke also imparts characteristic flavor and stabilizes the cured color. The temperature of smoke chamber is maintained at 50°C to produce ready-to-cook chicken, whereas it is kept at 80°C for 4 hours at 30–35 percent relative humidity to produce ready-to-eat chicken. In order to eliminate the carcinogenic components obtained due to combustion of lignin especially benzpyrene, liquid smoke is produced these days through condensation. Liquid smoke can be directly sprayed over the cured chicken or added to meat emulsion to impart distinct flavor. Cured and smoked chicken has a shelf-life of 1 month under refrigeration (4°C) and 2–4 months in a freezer (–18°C).

## DEHYDRATION

Cooked chicken meat is sometimes dehydrated for specific supplies. Chicken chunks may be dried in a rotary air dryer at controlled temperature to a moisture content of 4%. Finely ground cooked meat may be spray-dried to yield chicken soup mix. However, the best results are obtained in freeze dehydration. In this process, chicken meat chunks are quick-frozen and vacuum-dried at 1.55 mm Hg at low temperature for 12–24 hours. The final product containing hardly 2% moisture is packed in tins under nitrogen and has a shelf-life of one year. The product retains its natural flavor and nutrients and can be reconstituted within minutes.

## CANNING

This process refers to extreme thermal processing of chicken meat in hermetically sealed cans. It involves precooking of chunks and gravy, filling in lacquered cans, exhausting, sealing under vacuum and cooking in retorts at 15 psi pressure for 35 minutes followed by rapid cooling. The canned chicken product has a shelf-life of two years at ambient temperature.

## RADIATION PRESERVATION

Poultry meat can also be preserved by using radiant energy. Radiation brings about lethal changes in the nuclear material of microorganisms and inactivates the enzyme system without raising the temperature. Cobalt-60 gamma radiation is generally utilized because of its adequate penetrating power. This method, usually called as cold sterilization, is used as a supplement to other preservation methods such as refrigeration and freezing. For poultry meat, radiation sterilization dose of 45 kGy alone and pasteurization dose of 5 kGy in combination with other preservation methods have been successfully used.

High radiation doses may initiate several undesirable changes in meat such as discoloration, off-flavor, loss of water-holding capacity, rancidity development and loss of nutrients like thiamine, vitamin $B_{12}$ and vitamin C. Off-flavor development may occur due to the production of ammonia, $H_2S$ and mercaptans from free amino acids. These undesirable effects can be prevented by undertaking irradiation when the meat is in frozen condition and packaged under vacuum or inert gas atmosphere. Radiation preservation has the advantage of speedy operation. However, high cost restricts its use as a commercial practice.

19

CHAPTER

# Processing of Some Convenience Poultry Products

Chicken is the major species of poultry in India. It is consumed far and wide in many forms of traditional and processed products. Convenience products do not require any preparation prior to consumption. The common traditional products are tandoori chicken, chicken seek kabab, chicken shami kabab, chicken curry, chicken kofta, chicken tikka, chicken samosa, etc. Other poultry products such as barbecue, chicken patties, chicken sausages, etc., also have a good market in urban areas. The methods of preparation of some convenience poultry products have been described in this chapter.

## TANDOORI CHICKEN

Broilers at 6 weeks of age are preferred for tandoori chicken because of their tender meat and ability to sustain roasting. Dressed chickens with intact skin are rubbed with 4% salt along with spices and seasoning and kept for 15 minutes. After draining, the carcasses are thoroughly marinated with sauce on the surface and in the interior. A marination time of 1–2 hours is allowed. The formulation of sauce depends on the consumers preference for taste and other sensory attributes. In general, dry and ground spices along with condiments are blended with vinegar (10%) and curd (10%).

The marinated chickens are roasted in a tandoori oven under smokeless, moderate and uniform heat for 20–30 minutes depending on the temperature of oven and size of the broilers. Care must be taken to keep the chickens away from the direct fire and avoid burning or blistering of the skin or extremities. During roasting, chickens

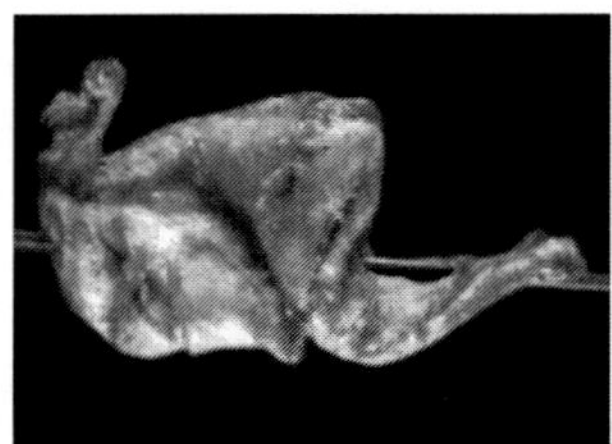

**Fig. 19.1:** Chicken tandoori.

are occasionally removed from the oven and pasted with sauce or fat with the help of a brush. The doneness of tandoori chicken is tested by twisting one of the drumsticks when it dissociates easily from the joint. By this time, it also acquires slightly smoked flavor **(Fig. 19.1)**.

## CHICKEN BARBECUE

Broilers with about 750 g dressed weight are preferred for barbecuing. The dressed chickens are longitudinally halved for this purpose after removing the neck portion. The chicken halves are marinated with sauce containing spices, salt and seasonings according to the consumers taste and preference and allowed to stay for an hour. The sides are then placed on the oven for barbecuing during which these are periodically turned and basted with sauce with the help of a brush to avoid drying. The cooking should proceed slowly at moderate temperature so that tender, golden brown and slightly smoked flavored barbecue is obtained.

## CHICKEN SEEK AND SHAMI KABABS

Culled or spent chicken meat can be utilized for preparing seek kababs. Lean meat is minced through 8 mm plate of a meat grinder. Wheat flour (3 percent) and whole egg liquid (5 percent) should be incorporated as binders to provide sufficient strength to the mince. Fat, salt, dry spices, and seasonings are added as per consumer preference. The mince is pasted around specially made iron bars (sheek) and cooked over moderate and uniform heat, turning the bars and basting with vegetable oil from time to time till doneness with brown color is achieved.

In the preparation of shami kababs, meat chunks, and water-soaked black gram dal are simmered in water for nearly 15 minutes before grinding. It is seasoned with salt, dry spices and condiment paste. Some people also add liquid egg to the mince. It is made into round cakes which are shallow fried with edible oil on a girdle till both the sides are brown.

## CHICKEN PATTIES

Raw deboned chicken meat and fat are minced twice through a meat grinder. Other ingredients like wheat flour or texturized soy protein (binding agent), salt, condiments, spices, etc., are mixed to the ground meat in an electrically operated meat mixer. The blended mass is divided into 100 g portions and moulded into patties. These are broiled in a hot air oven set at 200°C for 5–20 minutes to get a core temperature of about 72°C. Hot patties may be used to prepare burgers or chilled in a refrigerator for later use (**Fig. 19.2**).

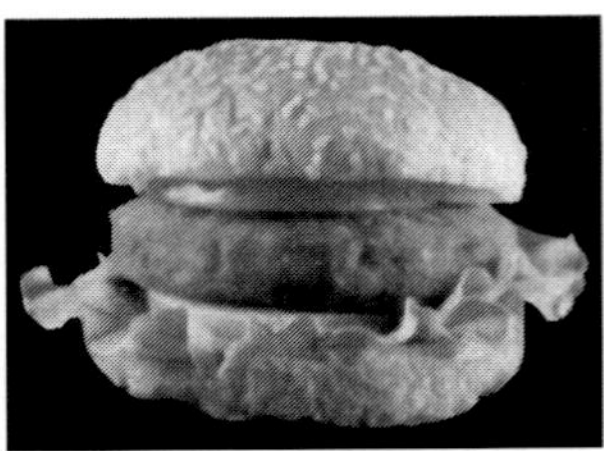

**Fig. 19.2:** Chicken patties.

## CHICKEN SAUSAGE

The tough meat from spent hens can be utilized for the preparation of chicken sausages. Deboned chicken meat is minced once through 9 mm and then through 4 mm plate of a meat grinder. Fat is minced separately through 4 mm plate. Lean meat, ice flakes (10%), salt and sodium nitrite are run along with fat in a bowl chopper to prepare a fine emulsion. Other ingredients like spices, condiments, etc., are added to the emulsion in the final run for a minute. Meat emulsion is filled into casings with the help of a sausage filler and suitable links are made. The sausages may be cooked in water at 80°C for 15–20 minutes or steam cooked. Smoking along with cooking stabilizes the color and imparts a characteristic flavor to the sausages (**Fig. 19.3**).

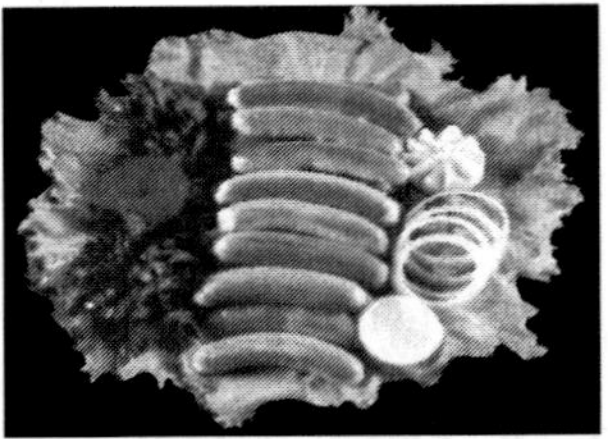

**Fig. 19.3:** Chicken sausages.

## CHICKEN KOFTA

Meat from spent or culled chicken can be utilised for preparing kofta (meatballs). Lean meat is coarse ground through 8 mm plate of a meat grinder. Ten to fifteen percent vegetable oil is added to it. Wheat flour (3 percent) in combination with whole egg liquid (5 percent) are incorporated to provide sufficient binding strength. Seasonings,

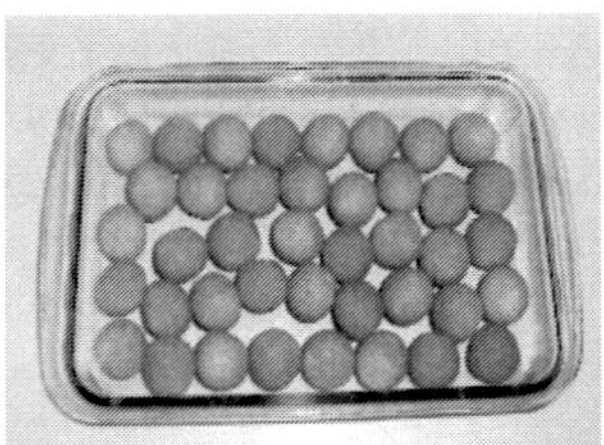

**Fig. 19.4:** Chicken meatballs.

salt and spices can be mixed as per consumer preference. The dough is rolled into 15 g balls with hands. The balls are deep fat-fried for 5 minutes. Cooked balls, packed in polyethylene pouches have a keeping quality of 8–10 days at 4°c **(Fig. 19.4)**.

## POULTRY PICKLE

Dressed chicken is trimmed off excess fat and deboned. Now meat is cut into 2.5 cm cubes, applied with 2% salt and pressure cooked for 8–10 minutes. Cooked meat is taken out and fried at medium heat in mustard oil to get brown color. Oil is decanted from the fried cubes and green curry stuff is fried in the same oil to get golden brown color. This is followed by addition of dry spices, remaining 2% salt and fried meat continuing frying for another 3–4 minutes. After some cooling, it is thoroughly mixed with 10% vinegar. The product has a shelf-life of 100 days at ambient temperature without any appreciable loss of quality attributes.

## CHICKEN SAMOSA

Lean chicken is minced through 5 mm plate of a meat grinder. Condiments are fried in vegetable oil to get a golden brown color and dry spices along with salt are added towards the end. Minced lean and cooked mashed potatoes are mixed with the fried spices and heating is continued for another 4–6 minutes. The fried stuff is ready for filling. Dough portions of about 30 g are rolled out and divided into two halves. Each half is moulded into a triangular pouch and the fried stuff (20–25 g) is filled in. The pouch is closed and samosas are deep fried in vegetable oil at medium heat to obtain a crispy product.

## CHICKEN TIKKA

Deboned chicken is minced in a meat grinder. Forty per cent of the mince is pressure cooked for 2 minutes. Besides, peeled and shredded potatoes are partially cooked in boiling water separately. Now, mince meat (60 raw: 40 cooked), shredded potatoes, rice powder, bread crumbs, salt, spices, and condiments are thoroughly mixed in an electrically operated meat mixer. The blended mass is divided into 70 g portions and moulded into tikkas. These are shallow fat-fried in a girdle to achieve an internal temperature of 70°C. The product has a unique texture and is consumed as a hot snack.

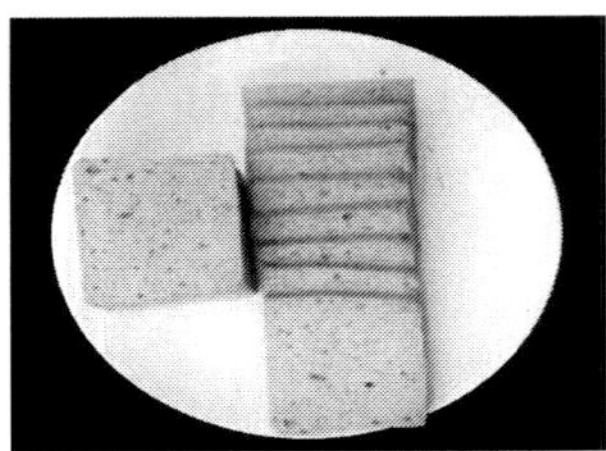

**Fig.19.5:** Chicken slices.

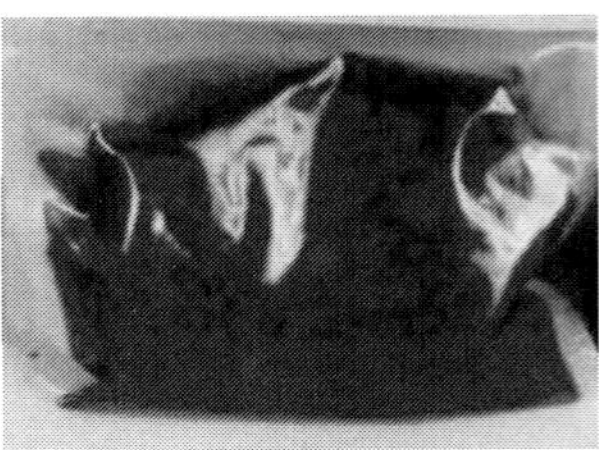

**Fig. 19.6:** Chicken curry.

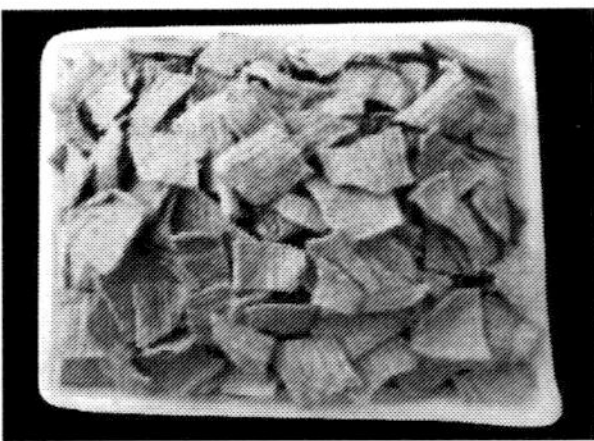

**Fig. 19.7:** Chicken chips.

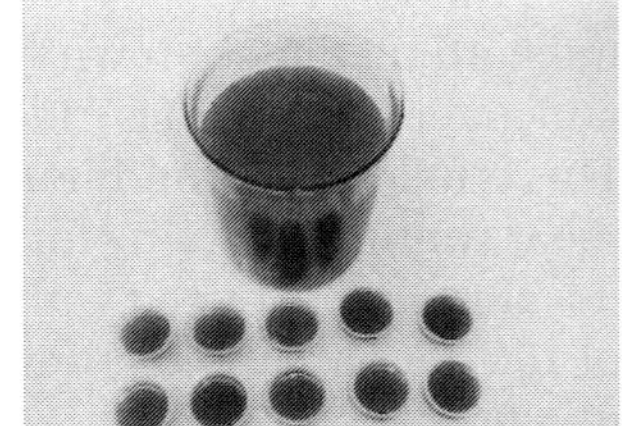

**Fig. 19.8:** Chicken soup.

The list of convenience chicken products is on the increase. These ready-to-eat products have a bright scope in India **(Figs. 19.5 to 19.8)**. These have already become quite common at the fast food corners and restaurants in the urban areas. With the vast availability of spent hens, comminuted chicken products are likely to surpass other meat products in near future.

# 20 CHAPTER

# Utilization of Poultry Industry Byproducts

Indian poultry industry has made rapid advances in the last two decades. A large number of poultry farms have come up as clusters resulting in the so called poultry pockets in various parts of the country. There is a growing realization to collect and beneficially utilize the byproducts of poultry industry which have so far been dumped as waste, except for poultry manure. Establishment of a **poultry byproduct processing plant,** within each cluster of farms having hatchery dressing units, etc., will generate substantial revenue, minimize environmental pollution and help to reduce the livestock feed cost. However, places where collection of poultry byproducts is not enough to warrant a separate plant, services of **carcass utilization plant** or renderer operating in the area can be requisitioned once or twice a week. Byproducts of poultry industry are:

A. Poultry dressing plant waste (on live weight)
   1. Feathers : 6%
   2. Blood : 3.5%
   3. Offal
      - Heads : 3%
      - Feet : 5%
      - Inedible viscera : 9%
        (intestines, lung, pancreas, spleen, etc.)

B. Hatchery waste: Infertile eggs, dead in germs, dead embryos, egg shells, unhatched chicks, unusable chicks, etc.

C. Egg processing unit waste: Unsound eggs and egg shells.

D. Poultry manure: Used-up deep litter and wet droppings from cage houses.

E. Dead birds

## FEATHERS

- **As livestock feed:** Poultry feathers are hydrolyzed to yield feather meal in byproduct processing plant or renderer at a steam pressure of 30 psi for 2 hours with continuous stirring. Feathers are sometimes crushed to break thick shanks and speed up the process. Since feather meal has a poor amino acid profile, feathers are generally processed with blood.
- **As bedding:** Soft and fluffy down feathers are used to make comfort pillows and mattresses. These bedding articles have good resilience and warmth besides being easy to handle and store.
- **As fertilizer:** Feathers are crushed and cooked under pressure to yield a good quality fertilizer. In places where cooking is not cost-effective but irrigation is not a problem, feathers can be ploughed in the soil to slowly decompose and release nitrogen.
- **Ornamental and sport use:** Feathers are used for making artificial flowers, toys and various decorative articles. Stiff feathers are used for making shuttle cocks.

## BLOOD

- **As livestock feed:** Blood collected in the poultry dressing plant can be processed in a simple cooker to yield dry blood meal with only 9% moisture. Since quantity of blood is generally inadequate and blood meal alone is not so palatable to the livestock, blood and feathers are usually cooked together in a byproduct processing plant or renderer. Caking of blood on the renderer wall is prevented by putting an iron can in the renderer. Blood and feather meal has a rich amino acid profile and very good digestibility.
- **As fertilizer:** Unwholesome or decomposed blood can be simply cooked for sometime to reduce moisture and used as a fertilizer in the fields.
- **As fish bait:** Blood can also be used as a bait during fishing operations.

## OFFAL

Poultry offal comprises heads, feet and inedible viscera. Inedible viscera include intestines, lungs, pancreas, spleen and the reproductive organs. Irrespective of end use, offals should be sufficiently cooked to destroy microorganisms. Generally, offals are processed for the following purposes:

- **As livestock feed:** Offals are cooked in the byproduct processing plant at 15 psi pressure for half an hour and allowed to dry. After cooling, fat is extracted and material is ground to yield offal meal. Some renderers first hydrolyze feathers and then add offals to yield offal and feather meal without any fat extract.
- **As pet food:** Poultry offal is utilized as a good quality pet food especially for dogs. For this purpose, offal is washed, cooked, ground and then mixed with other products to form pellets. Some processors prepare canned pet food from poultry offals.
- **As a feed for fur-bearing animals:** In cold countries, poultry offals have been conveniently used as a feed for fur-bearing animals as a replacement for costly meals. Mince has been specially found to relish poultry offal and record fast growth.
- **As fish food:** In fish hatcheries, poultry offal is cooked, ground and utilized as delicious fish food.

## MIXED POULTRY BYPRODUCTS MEAL

Poultry offal, blood and feathers are mixed in their natural proportion and dry rendered at a pressure of 15 psi for 3 hours to ultimately yield a meal with only 8% moisture. Dead birds can also be included in the charge. MPBM serves as a fairly balanced livestock and poultry feed. It can be used up to 5–7% in poultry ration.

## HATCHERY WASTE

Entire hatchery waste, other than egg shells, is utilized in the preparation of hatchery byproduct meal which is comparable to fish meal with respect to protein content. The meal can be used in poultry ration at 3% level.

The egg contents from infertile eggs, dead in germs, etc., are collected and cooked at a pressure of 10 psi for 15 minutes. After cooking, the material is allowed to dry and then ground. The yield of hatchery byproduct meal is about 25%. It contains nearly 35% crude protein, 40% crude fat and 4.5% total ash. Calcium and phosphorus contents are 0.05% and 1% respectively.

Egg shells are sterilized and powdered to pass through very fine sieve. Egg shell powder is used in mineral mixture as a calcium supplement. Unsterilized egg shells are sun-dried and ground for use as a fertilizer.

## POULTRY MANURE

- **As fertilizer:** Poultry manure has been traditionally used as a fertilizer. Its nutrient value depends on litter to manure ratio. In general, dried poultry manure contains 15–18% moisture, 25–30% total protein, 6–8% uric acid (nonprotein nitrogen), 15–25% ash, 3–6% calcium and 1.5–2% phosphorus besides many other essential trace elements. It has a good fertilizing value for crops, lawns and gardens. It also improves the soil structure because of high organic content.
- **As livestock feed:** Caged poultry manure can be used as feed for pigs and poultry whereas deep litter manure has been used as a feed for ruminants. For this purpose, the manure is spread in the sun for drying to moisture content of 10% or less. If facilities are available, it can be autoclaved at 15 psi pressure for 30 minutes and taken to hot air drier for drying. Dehydrated poultry manure has been successfully incorporated up to a level of 15% in layer poultry ration.

**Table 20.1:** Percent yield and composition of poultry byproducts meal.

| *Constituents* | *Feather meal* | *Blood meal* | *Offal meal* | *Mixed byproduct meal* |
|---|---|---|---|---|
| Yield | 33 | 18 | 55 | 33 |
| Moisture | 7 | 9 | 10 | 8 |
| Crude protein | 85 | 86 | 52 | 66 |
| Crude fat | 3 | 1 | 24 | 18 |
| Ash | 4 | 3 | 14 | 1.8 |

Thus, poultry industry byproducts in the form of poultry dressing plant waste, hatchery waste, egg processing unit waste, poultry droppings and dead birds should invariably be processed and utilized for a number of reasons. It will solve the waste disposal problem and reduce pollution in and around the farms and processing units. It will also economize the poultry production as such by yielding various byproduct meals for feeding poultry **(Table 20.1)**.

# 21 CHAPTER

# Structure, Composition and Nutritive Value of Eggs

An acquaintance with the formation and structure of eggs is necessary to effectively preserve its quality during storage and marketing. Egg is basically nature's device to produce a chick. So, it has the necessary infrastructure for the production and nutritional requirements of developing embryos and newly hatched chick.

There are four main components of hen's egg **(Fig. 21.1)**:

a. Shell
b. Shell membranes
c. Albumen or white
d. Yolk

The yolk develops in the functional left ovary of the hen as an ovum largely during the final 10 days before release. After ovulation or release, fully developed ovum or yolk is engulfed in the oviduct where a gel of albumin or egg white is secreted to surround the yolk for a few hours. Finally, the shell membranes and the calcareous shell are deposited in the oviduct for nearly 16 hours before the egg is laid.

## STRUCTURE

### Shell

The outer protective covering of an egg is shell which comprises around 11% of its total weight. It is mainly composed of calcium carbonate. The shell contains numerous minute pores on the entire surface, which are partially sealed by keratin. These pores allow loss of carbon dioxide and moisture from the eggs. However, a few of them (hardly 12–20) may permit bacterial penetration within the egg under specific circumstances. Thus shell structure consists of three basic units:

a. Outer cuticle made up of keratin
b. Middle spongy or calcareous layer
c. Inner mammary layer

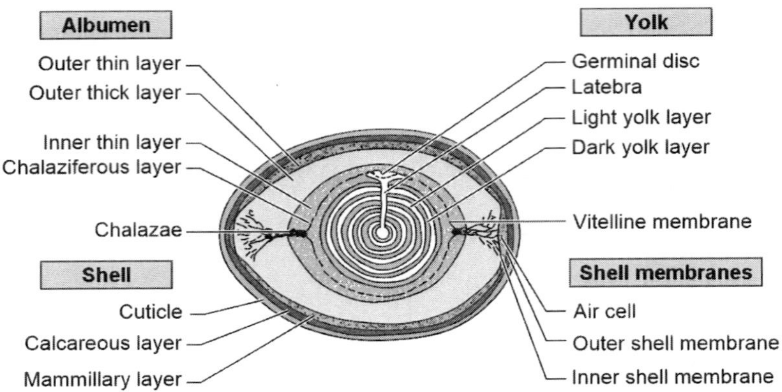


**Fig. 21.1:** Structure of an egg.

## Shell Membranes

The shell is attached to the shell membranes. The outer thick and inner thin membranes are usually inseparable except at the broad end of the egg forming an air cell. The shell membranes are a part of in-built defence mechanism in the egg because of their role as an effective barrier against bacterial invasion. The air cell continues to increase in size during storage due to loss of moisture and shrinkage of egg contents.

## Albumen

The white or albumen portion of egg constitutes about 58% of the total weight of an egg. It occurs in four layers as follows:

a. Outer thin layer
b. Outer thick layer
c. Inner thin layer
d. Inner thick white or chalaziferous layer

The proportion of thin and thick white varies according to the breed and age of the hen. Thick content is comparatively more. The inner thick white layer surrounds the vitelline membrane of the yolk and its firm mucin like fibers continue as chalazae which has the specific function of keeping the yolk in the center.

## Yolk

The yolk constitutes nearly 31% of the total egg weight. It consists of the following four structures from outside:

a. Vitelline membrane

b. Concentric rings of light and dark yolk material
c. Latebra (cone like portion extending to the center of yolk)
d. Germinal disc (located in the cone of latebra)

## CHEMICAL COMPOSITION

As mentioned earlier, an egg consists of 11% shell, 58% albumen and 31% yolk. The cuticle of eggshell is composed of a foaming layer of proteinaceous matter especially keratin. It covers the calcified portion of the shell which is made up of calcium carbonate (94%) with minor quantities of calcium phosphate (1%), magnesium carbonate (1%) and proteinaceous material especially keratin **(Table 21.1)**. The true cell membrane consist of protein fibers. The inner membrane is comparatively thick.

**Table 21.1:** Chemical composition of egg.

| *Component* | *Total (%)* | *Water (%)* | *Protein (%)* | *Fat (%)* | *Ash (%)* |
|---|---|---|---|---|---|
| Whole egg | 100 | 65.5 | 11.8 | 11.0 | 11.7 |
| Albumen | 58 | 88.0 | 11.0 | 0.2 | 0.8 |
| Yolk | 31 | 8.0 | 17.5 | 32.5 | 2.0 |
| | | Calcium carbonate (%) | Calcium phosphate (%) | Magnesium phosphate (%) | Organic matter (%) |
| Shell | 11 | 94 | 1 | 1 | 4 |

*Source:* USDA.

Egg albumen or white contains approximately 88% water. Most of the solid content is protein. Lipid content is virtually absent. However, very minute quantity of carbohydrate (0.5%) may be present. Albumen may be regarded as a protein system consisting of microscopic fibers in a solution of numerous globular proteins. Some important albumen proteins and their characteristics are presented in **Table 21.2**.

**Table 21.2:** Important proteins in egg albumin.

| *Protein* | *Relative amount in albumen (%)* | *Characteristics* |
|---|---|---|
| Ovalbumin | 54 | Phospho-glycoprotein |
| Conalbumin | 13 | Binds metals especially iron |
| Ovomucoid | 11 | Inhibits trypsin |

*Contd...*

*Contd...*

| *Protein* | *Relative amount in albumen (%)* | *Characteristics* |
|---|---|---|
| Lysozyme (Globulin G1, G2, G3) | 10 | Lyses some bacteria |
| Ovomucin | 1.5 | Sialoprotein |
| Flavoprotein | 0.8 | Binds riboflavin |
| Ovoinhibitor | 0.1 | Inhibits several proteases |
| Avidin | 0.05 | Binds biotin |

*Source:* Baker (1968).

Egg yolk contains more than 50% solids, which are mainly lipids (32%) and proteins (16%). Yolk lipid is composed of mostly triglyceride (65%), good amount of phospholipid (28%) and controversial cholesterol (5%). The ash content of yolk is about 1%. A little of carbohydrate, usually less than 0.5%, may also be present.

## NUTRITIVE VALUE

**Table 21.3** shows the nutritive value of a chicken egg. An egg contains about six grams of protein. Egg protein is of such a high quality that its biological value has been taken as 100 and it acts as a standard for evaluating the biological value of other food proteins. All the essential amino acids required in human diet are present in egg proteins. An egg also provides five to six grams of easily digestible fat, wherein the proportion of much desired unsaturated fatty acids (especially oleic acid) is more as compared to most other livestock products. Egg is an important source of fat soluble vitamins (A, D, E and K) and water soluble vitamins of B-complex group. However, it does not contain vitamin C.

With very little carbohydrates, egg has a remarkably low caloric value which justifies its inclusion in the food for people on restricted diet. Egg is a very good source of important minerals such as iron, phosphorus, potassium and trace elements which are necessary for the formation of blood, bone and soft tissues. Though cholesterol content of egg yolk is comparatively high, it is not likely to significantly influence the blood cholesterol level unless taken indiscriminately because cholesterol is found in blood, nerve tissues and other parts of the human body as a normal constituent of the cell.

**Table 21.3:** Nutritive value of edible portion of a chicken egg.

| | *Fresh raw egg* | | |
|---|---|---|---|
| *Component* | *Whole* | *Albumen* | *Yolk* |
| Weight (g) | 50 | 33 | 17 |
| Water (%) | 73.7 | 87.6 | 51.1 |
| Food energy (Cal) | 81.5 | 16.83 | 59.16 |
| Protein (g) | 6.45 | 3.60 | 2.72 |
| Fat (Total lipids g) | 5.75 | trace | 1.65 |
| Total saturated FA (g) | 1.65 | - | 1.65 |
| Total unsaturated FA (g) | 3.30 | - | 3.30 |
| Oleic (g) | 2.2 | - | 2.2 |
| Linoleic (g) | 0.5 | - | 0.5 |
| Cholesterol (mg) | 230 | - | 230 |
| Carbohydrate (g) | 0.36 | 0.264 | 0.1 |
| Fiber (g) | 0 | 0 | 0 |
| Ash (g) | 0.5 | 0.231 | 0.289 |
| Calcium (mg) | 27.0 | 2.97 | 23.97 |
| Iron (mg) | 1.15 | 0.033 | 1.117 |
| Magnesium (mg) | 5.5 | 2.97 | 2.72 |
| Phosphorus (mg) | 102.5 | 4.95 | 96.73 |
| Potassium (mg) | 64.5 | 45.87 | 16.66 |
| Sodium (mg) | 61.0 | 48.18 | 8.84 |
| Vitamin A (IU) | 590 | 0 | 590 |
| Choline (mg) | 253.4 | 0.4 | 253.0 |
| Inositol (mg) | 16.5 | - | - |
| Niacin (mg) | 0.05 | 0.033 | 0.017 |
| Riboflavin (mg) | 0.15 | 0.089 | 0.076 |
| Thiamine (mg) | 0.055 | - | 0.037 |
| Ascorbic acid (mg) | 0 | 0 | 0 |

*Source:* American Egg Board (1974).

Food Safety and Standard Authority of India has in 2018 specified the following standards for the fresh shell eggs:

- Fresh eggs mean eggs which have not been washed or dry-cleaned and which are collected at least once weekly and shall be packed and graded not later than the first working day after arrival at the packing station.

- The standard specified in this clause shall be applicable to eggs in shell other than broken, incubated or cooked eggs, laid by poultry species or birds meant for direct human consumption or for the preparation of egg products.
- Eggs shall have a clean and sound shell and free from cracks, leaks, and fecal contamination.
- Minimum requirements of major chemical constituents in the whole egg contents of chicken, quail and duck shall be:

| *Chemical constituents (%)* | *Chicken* | *Quail* | *Duck* |
|---|---|---|---|
| Water (%) | 72.8–75.6 | 73.1–76.4 | 68.2–71.4 |
| Proteins (%) | 12.8–13.4 | 12.5–13.4 | 13.1–14.2 |
| Fat (%) | 10.5–11.8 | 10.6–11.7 | 13.8–15.0 |
| Carbohydrates (%) | 0.3–1.0 | 0.8–1.0 | 1.1–1.3 |
| Ash (%) | 0.8–1.0 | 1.0–1.2 | 0.9–1.0 |

The FSSAI guidelines to consumers mention that egg quality is best maintained when these are stored at cold temperatures preferably under refrigeration and consumed within few days.

22

CHAPTER

# Microbial Spoilage of Eg

It was widely believed in nineteenth century that contents of fresh eggs were always sterile. Studies conducted afterwards revealed that microorganisms can gain entry into the egg congenitally. However, most of the contaminants of eggs are of extragenital origin and come in contact with egg shell at oviposition from the dust, soil and fecal matter adhered to the nesting material. Since the cuticle and pores of the egg shell are moist at this stage, the possibility of invasion of the shell by some contaminants through a few pores cannot be ruled out. The microorganisms on the shell surface usually belong to a mixed roup, but those causing spoilage of egg (generally called rot) are gram-egative in nature which have very simple nutritional requirements.

The microorganisms have to pass through a series of in-built ysico-chemical barriers in the egg—the shell, the shell membranes l the albumen before reaching the yolk where they could easily tiply causing rot. The mechanism of microbial spoilage can, thus, ivided into three serial steps:

netration of microorganisms through the egg shell and shell mbranes.

onization of microorganisms on the shell membrane.

rpowering of the antibacterial factors present in the albumen.

## RATION OF MICROORGANISMS THROUGH THE EGGSHELL AND MEMBRANES

cquires a diverse microflora at the time of oviposition. mal conditions of handling and storage, shell gets dried ost of these microorganisms fail to survive. An eggshell re than 17,000 pores. However, only ten to twelve pores roorganisms to pass through. The microorganisms either hen the egg contents contract on cooling or gain entry due to capillary action through pore canals when the shell surface is oist. The role of microorganisms remains passive in both situations. due to capillary action that incidence of rotting are comparatively in washed eggs which have been subjected to dry abrasion. The cular plugs on the pore canals are opened during the process of asion of eggs.

After gaining entry through the shell pores, microorganisms come across shell membranes. These membranes act as bacterial filters and offer maximum resistance to the offending organisms which have succeeded in penetrating the shell. Some researchers believe that membrane lysozyme also has a limited role. Mold may also cause rot in eggs under humid storage conditions. In such case shell is generally covered with mycelium (whisker) and hyphae penetrate the pores to reach shell membranes.

## COLONIZATION OF MICROORGANISMS ON THE SHELL MEMBRANE

Once the microorganisms have an access to shell membrane, are able to multiply and form colonies. However, the coloni is not instant. In the early stages, there is preferential sele gram-negative organisms having low iron requirement from population dominated by gram-positive organisms which iron requirement. Thus initially there is a decline in th numbers. In the later stages, multiplication of organisms a faster rate because by this time albumen becomes he The pH of egg contents move towards neutrality an contact with inner shell membrane.

## OVERPOWERING THE ANTIBACTERIAL FACTORS ALBUMEN

Egg white or albumen provides an unfavorabl growth because of the defensive role played proteins which have been listed under co role played by lysozyme and conalbume Lysozyme of albumen causes lysis of gram-positive organisms. This enzym cell wall of gram-negative bacteria h lipopolysaccharide over mucopepti

Conalbumen which is uniforml than 10% of albumen chelates i bacteria. Conalbumen is the pri the egg and its inhibitory action is more on gram-positive as compared to gram-negative organisms. This inhibition definitely delays the spoilage of eggs to some extent. However, as yolk contents migrate into albumen or get mixed, multiplication of organism is very fast which results in the rotting of eggs. Some general types of rots may be summarized in **Table 22.1**.

**Table 22.1:** Some general types of egg rots.

| *Types of rot* | *Changes in egg* | *Organisms* |
|---|---|---|
| Green rot | Albumen becomes green | *Pseudomonas fluorescens* |
| Black rot (Type I) | Blackening of yolk with "fecal odor" | *Proteus* sp. |
| Black rot (Type 2) | Green colored albumen but yolk is black with "cabbage odor" | *Pseudomonas* sp. |
| Red rot | Albumen stained red throughout, yolk surrounded by custard like material | *Serratia* sp. |
| Fungal rot | Pink spots on egg contents<br>Black spots on contents<br>Yellow or green spots on contents | *Sporotrichum*<br>*Cladosporium*<br>*Penicillium* |

Besides rots, eggs may develop various types of off odor due to bacteria without any apparent signs of spoilage. These off-odors may be musty or earthy (*Achromobacter* sp.), hay like (*Enterobacter* sp.), fishy (*E. coli*) or that of cabbage water (*Pseudomonas* sp.).

# 23 CHAPTER

# Preservation and Maintenance of Eggs

A freshly laid egg can be assumed to have a highest quality. Since egg is full of essential nutrients, deteriorative changes soon start taking place which may pose a danger to the excellent sensory attributes of this nourishing and satisfying food item. Cleanliness and soundness of shell is the first step to assure the quality of egg to the consumers. The shell quality deficiencies mostly relate to the production practices adopted at the farm. Proper handling of eggs can delay the decline in the quality.

Following precautions should be taken during handling of eggs:

- Eggs should be collected 3 to 4 times per day. This will result in less dirty eggs and fewer breakage.
- After collection, eggs should be shifted to holding room maintained at a temperature of about 15°C and 70 to 80% RH at least for 12 hours.
- Eggs should be properly packed in filler flats with broad end up. Bulk packing should be done in fiber board cartons.
- Eggs should be rapidly moved through the marketing channel so as to reduce the period between production and consumption.

All preservation methods for shell eggs have been designed to retard one or more of the following physico-chemical alterations which lower the quality of egg as it ages:

- As the surface of egg dries, the keratin cuticle shrinks and size of shell pores increase rendering it easier for gases and microorganisms to pass in and out of the shell.
- As the warm egg cools down, the egg contents also contract, resulting in the formation of air cell.
- The breakdown of carbonic acid causing loss of carbon dioxide from the albumen is rapid during the first few hours after an egg is

laid. The alkaline pH acts on the mucin fibers to disturb the thick gel of albumen making it thin or watery.

- As the egg ages, water migrates from the albumen to the yolk which may overstretch, weaken or even rupture the vitelline membrane.

Following preservation methods are employed to maintain the quality of shell eggs:

## EGG CLEANING

Earlier, it was a general practice to dry clean dirty egg shells by abrasive mounting on a mechanical wheel. This practice has now become obsolete because it weakens the shell. These days washing in warm water containing a detergent sanitizer is an effective way of cleaning the eggs with dirty shells. A temperature difference of 10–15°C between eggs and wash water is ideal, otherwise there may be problem of crack shells. Besides eggs should not be immersed in warm water for more than 3–4 minutes. After washing, the eggs should be dried promptly. Wash water should be changed after washing every five to six baskets of eggs. It should be emphasized that only dirty eggs are subjected to washing. It not only reduces the microbial load on the egg shell surface but also improves the appearance and consumer appeal.

## OIL TREATMENT

Oil coating spray of eggs has become very popular for short-term storage of this commodity. Coating oil forms a thin film on the surface of the shell sealing the pores. It should be done as early as possible, preferably within first few hours after laying of eggs because loss of $CO_2$ is more during this period and evaporation of moisture is also more during the first few days. Egg coating oil should be colorless, odorless and conform to food grade. Coating is done by dipping the eggs in the ground nut oil whereas for oil spray, the eggs are arranged in the filler flats with their broad end up. If the eggs need washing, oil coating should be done after washing. It is important to drain out excess oil before packaging. The temperature of oil should be in range of 15 to 30°C for ideal results. Oil treatment safeguards the quality of albumen for at least 7 days because it effectively seals the shell pores.

## COLD STORAGE

This method of preservation is suitable for long-term storage of clean eggs in the main laying season and abundant availability. The temperature of cold store is maintained at 0°C (32°F) and relative humidity between 80 to 85 percent. An anteroom with intermediate temperature is generally provided to check condensation of water vapor on the eggs during removal. Use of new egg packing trays are advised for cold storage. Like all other animal products, eggs also pick up strong odor, so the same cold store can not be used for storing onion, garlic or any other commodity with strong odor. The quality of shell eggs can be maintained for about 6 months in a cold storage. Oil coating of eggs prior to cold storage can further enhance their keeping quality. Such eggs could keep well at 14°C and 90% RH for a period of 8 months.

## THERMOSTABILIZATION

This preservation method involves stabilization of albumen quality by holding the eggs in an oil bath maintained at 55°C for 15 minutes or 58°C for 10 minutes. This process brings about coagulation of thin albumen just below the shell membranes, thereby blocking the passage of air and moisture. In addition, oil coating of shell pores also takes place. Thus, keeping quality of eggs is maintained for sometimes and thinning of egg white is retarded. Alternatively, eggs are immersed in hot water at 71°C for 2 to 3 seconds. In this flash heat treatment, bacteria present on the surface of the shell are destroyed and a thin film of albumen just below the shell membrane is coagulated sealing the egg shell from inside.

## IMMERSION IN LIQUIDS

Under rural conditions, lime-water or water-glass immersions are most useful. In lime-water treatment, a liter of boiling water is added to 1 kg of quick lime and allowed to cool. Now 5 liters of water and 250 g of table salt are added to it. The solution is strained through a fine cloth when the mixture settles down. Eggs are dipped in the clear fluid overnight and then dried at room temperature. In this process, an additional thin film of calcium carbonate is deposited on the egg shell and seals the pores. Such eggs can be stored for a month at ambient temperature. In water-glass treatment, one part of sodium silicate is mixed in 10 parts of water and eggs are dipped overnight. In this process, a thin precipitate of silica is deposited on the egg shell and partially seals the pores.

It is clear from the above discussion that eggs should be collected frequently, held initially at low temperature and then a suitable preservation method be employed to maintain its keeping quality for anticipated consumer acceptance.

## EGG QUALITY INDICATORS

External quality of an egg is measured by egg size, shell color, shell thickness and texture whereas internal egg quality is measured by albumen viscosity, yolk color and air space. Albumen and yolk indexes provide indication of the freshness of egg.

1. **Albumen index:** It is the ratio of height of albumen/width of albumen when the egg is broken onto the flat surface.
   It should range between 0.08–0.1. As the egg ages or deteriorates, the albumen keeps thinning and this value decreases.
2. **Yolk index:** It is the ratio of height of Yolk/diameter of yolk when the egg is broken onto the flat surface.
   It should range between 0.35–0.45. As the egg ages or deteriorates, the vitelline membrane loosens and this value decreases.
3. **Haugh unit (HU):** It is a commonly used measure to check the internal quality of an egg.

$$\text{HU} = \text{Height of albumen/Weight of egg}$$

Higher the number, better is the quality. A good quality egg has HU of 72 and above while HU of about 30 to 60 indicates poor quality.

**Air cell size** should be 2–3 cm. It increases as the egg ages.

## FUNCTIONAL PROPERTIES OF EGG CONTENTS

Egg contents possess several functional properties which make them desirable ingredients of many food products. Some of them are summarized below:

| | *Property* | *Applications* |
|---|---|---|
| 1. | Coagulation | Egg proteins coagulate irreversibly upon heating. So act as thickening agent in custard, cakes, etc. Heat coagulated proteins help to hold the shape to act as binding agent in cutlets, chops, etc. |
| 2. | Foaming | On whipping, egg proteins trap air and produce large foam volume to give fluffy and spongy product. Egg white is extensively used as leavening agent in baked products |

*Contd...*

*Contd...*

| | *Property* | *Applications* |
|---|---|---|
| 3. | Emulsification | Phospholipids and certain proteins present in the egg act as excellent emulsifying agent. In mayonnaise, egg yolk acts as emulsifier |
| 4. | Coating | Egg white and egg yolk provide surface coating, gloss or finishing to several baked products |
| 5. | Clarification | Egg white can clarify various fluid products such as broth, wine, etc. |
| 6. | Browning | Egg products can contribute to product color such as browning of exterior in baked food products |
| 7. | Flavoring | Egg contents contribute to the taste and flavor of several food products |
| 8. | Fortification | Egg proteins have essential amino acids, hence used to fortify several foods |
| 9. | Edible packaging | Egg white has been used to prepare edible packaging films |
| 10. | pH stability | Egg white is naturally alkaline, so it has uses in balancing pH of food products |

## PREPARATION OF EGG POWDER

Fresh eggs play an important role as an ingredient of wide range of food products. However, egg powder can be a good alternative at industrial level. The manufacture of egg powder involves the following steps:

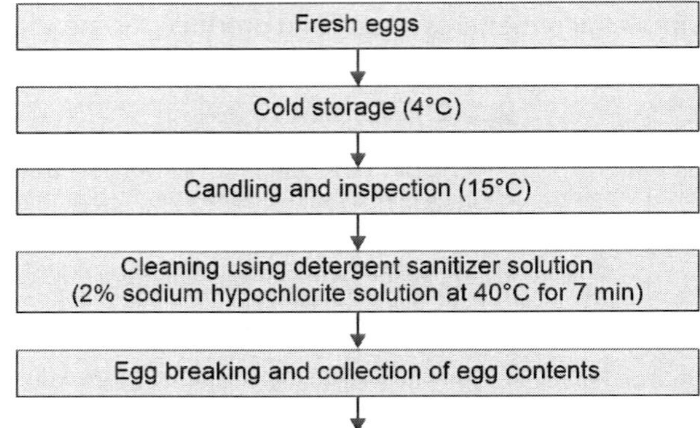


*Contd...*

*Contd...*

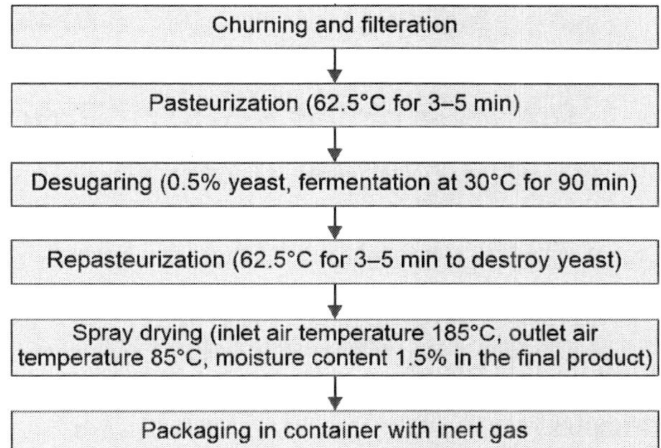


Egg powder has all the nutritional benefits of a fresh egg. It has the advantage of a long shelf life and does not require any refrigeration. It requires very less storage space. It is comparatively cheaper in cost and easier to use.

# 24 CHAPTER

# Packaging of Poultry Products

## PACKAGING OF SHELL EGGS

### Product Attributes

Egg has been bestowed with a natural package—the shell and shell membrane by the nature. In spite of the strength provided by shell, egg still remains a fragile commodity and needs protection against breakage. Eggs are susceptible to loss of moisture, deterioration from ageing and attack by bacteria and fungi. Eggs are also susceptible to the absorption of foreign odors.

### Packaging Objectives and Requirements

- To protect against breakage.
- To safeguard against attack from bacteria and fungi.
- To check deterioration due to ageing.
- To prevent loss of moisture.
- To prevent absorption of foreign odors.

Shell eggs can be safely stored for a period of 4–5 months at 0°C and 85–90% RH.

### Packaging Materials and Techniques

- **Molded pulp fillers flats:** In India, eggs are traditionally stored and transported in moulded pulp filler flats. Each filler flat contains 30 eggs which are kept with broad end up. It is cheap but lack strength and is unattractive.
- **Plastic filler flats:** These are strong, attractive and washable. These can be easily stacked in wooden crates. However, since eggs are sold with trays in wholesale markets, plastic filler flats are yet to replace moulded pulp trays.

- Paper board cartons with dividers.
- Folded paper board cartons with shrink film overwrap of PE, PVC or PVDC.
- Expanded polystyrene foam egg cartons or trays—provide excellent cushioning and strength besides being light weight.
- **Bulk packaging:** In Indian conditions, it is advisable to keep 210 eggs per carton (7 trays of 30 eggs each) during shipment. For export purpose, all white paper board shipping cartons—each containing 360 eggs are used. Lately, these cartons have been upgraded to make them stronger and printable.

## PACKAGING BROKEN-OUT EGGS

Broken-out eggs are generally sold frozen—either whites or yolks separately or whole after homogenization. Before freezing, salt or sugar (10% by weight) is added to prevent rubberiness due to coagulation.

Broken-out eggs are very much susceptible to bacterial contamination and require proper packaging to protect them from contamination and check their deterioration till end use.

Polyethylene pouches, paper canisters or larger cans serve as satisfactory packaging material for broken-out eggs.

## PACKAGING OF WHOLE EGG POWDER

### Product Attributes

Whole egg powder is manufactured either by spray drying or foam mat drying or accelerated freeze drying. Commercially, spray drying is the most widely used process wherein desugaring is usually done by yeast fermentation.

Moisture content of the product is restricted to a maximum of 2 percent. The spray dried whole egg powder is highly hygroscopic and its shelf life is influenced considerably by storage conditions, packaging materials and packaging techniques.

### Packaging Objectives and Requirements

- To prevent the ingress of moisture into the product.
- To prevent the product against oxygen and light.
- To retain the characteristic color and flavor of the product.
- To maintain the thickening, leavening and emulsifying properties.
- To check the absorption of foreign odors.
- To help in safe transport and convenient dispensing of the product.

Economy in space during storage and transport is of paramount importance for providing rations to the troops. So egg powder is usually compressed in blocks. In this process, air/oxygen trapped in between particles of egg powder is also excluded, eliminating the necessity of packaging under nitrogen.

### Packaging Materials and Techniques

- Egg powder is placed inside MST cellophane (300 gauge) pouch with an opening in one corner. This is placed in a laminate pouch consisting of Brown casing (BC) paper/Alu foil (0.04 mm)/PE (150 gauge) which is sealed after flushing with nitrogen.
- Egg powder blocks (30 g each) are made by compressing the powder at ambient temperature in blocks of 4 cm × 4 cm size under pressure. These are wrapped in MST cellophane (300 gauge) and then heat sealed in BC paper/Alu foil (0.02 mm)/PE (150 gauge) laminate. Pouch protects the whole egg powder from exposure to atmospheric air or oxygen. In this way, a shelf life of more than 3 months is ensured.
- Thirty gram each of egg powder is packed in 202 × 307 plain sanitary cans under nitrogen gas. In this way, a shelf life of minimum 1 year is ensured.
- Bulk packaging of egg powder is done in 2 lb and 14 lb capacity plain sanitary cans which are hermetically sealed under vacuum or 100% nitrogen.

## PACKAGING OF DRESSED AND CUT-UP POULTRY

### Product Attributes

Poultry meat has a very good protein content of high biological value. It has low calorific value because of low fat content. The fat mostly runs beneath the skin, only very little being inside the muscle tissues. By nature, poultry fat is unsaturated and is very prone to the development of oxidative rancidity. Dressed poultry has a shelf life of 5–7 days during refrigerated storage.

Packaging of poultry meat should be undertaken immediately after the dressing operations are over. Unpackaged refrigerated storage may result in surface dehydration whereas frozen storage may give rise to freezer burn, characterized by surface discoloration, tough texture and diminished juiciness as well as flavor. Evisceration during dressing operations exposes meat to many microorganisms. Among them,

*Pseudomonas* and *Salmonella* are comparatively more conspicuous by their presence in raw meat. Like other meats, poultry meat is also susceptible to the absorption of foreign odors.

## Packaging Objectives and Requirements

- To contain dressed or cut up poultry and thus provide a convenience means of dispensation.
- To prevent moisture loss or surface dehydration.
- To preserve natural color, flavor and texture.
- To check the development of rancidity.
- To prevent further microbial contamination.
- To help in marketing by persuasive and informative labeling.

Flexible packaging materials—monofilms, co-extruded films or laminates are most suitable for the packaging of poultry meat. The specific use of these materials vary on the basis of type of product to be packaged whether dressed whole birds or halves or quarters, cut up parts, bulk shipments or frozen storage and whether it is for short-term or long-term.

## Packaging Materials and Techniques

### *Overwraps*

Packaging of dressed whole birds, halves or cut up parts for retailing and early use can be done in plastic films such as polyethylene, polypropylene, PVDC, rubber hydrochloride or Nylon-6 films of 150 to 200 gauge. These films are transparent to translucent and have good water vapor and gas barrier properties along with grease resistance. Polyethylene is the most widely used packaging material in our country because of its low cost and easy availability. These thermoplastic film sheets can be fabricated into bags. Each dressed eviscerated bird is inserted into a bag. Giblet or individual bird is wrapped in waxed paper or parchment paper and placed into the body cavity before bagging. The problem of body fluid accumulation is avoided by putting an absorbent pad or blotter on the back of each bird to soak up the liquid. The bag can now be heat sealed or twist tied or clipped shut.

### *Tray with Overwrap*

The common packages for retail dressed small whole fryers, broilers, roasting chicken or even cut up parts in western countries are polystyrene foam trays overwrapped with a transparent plastic film.

These trays offer an aesthetically appealing background. A blotter underneath absorbs the excessive meat juice accumulation. Printed decorative labels may be applied on the outside of the packages or slipped onto the bird before over wrapping. Chickens thus wrapped have a shelf life of 7 days at 4°C in a refrigerator.

### *Shrink Film Overwrap*

These films are especially useful for wrapping dressed poultry because of their ability to form contour tight package over uneven surface. These are also frequently recommended for storage of dressed birds under frozen condition. Many thermoplastic films such as polyethylene, polypropylene, polyvinylidene, hydrochloride can be biaxially-oriented to stay stretched at ambient temperature. Dressed birds are overwrapped with such films and passed through hot air tunnel or dipped in water tub maintained at 90°C for few seconds to effect shrinkage of the film. The shrink film overwraps offer neat appearance and are easy to handle. Such packaging film should have a high structural strength and be a good water vapor barrier. It should be capable of withstanding storage temperature down to –45°C.

### *Vacuum Packaging*

This technique is recommended for long-term storage of dressed whole or halved poultry because it ensures a shelf life of 5–6 weeks at 2°C. Vacuum packaging reduces the volume of air sealed with meat. The residual oxygen, if any, is quickly consumed by meat. Thus, vacuum packaging provides a good avenue for keeping the product at a better level of quality. The advantages of vacuum packaging can be enumerated as follows:

- There is saving of space and energy during storage, transport and distribution.
- There is no loss in weight.
- The natural flavor of the product is preserved.
- The product has better keeping quality.
- The display of the product is better which help in better marketing and fetching better price.

A suitable film for vacuum packaging must have a good mechanical strength and barrier properties, besides making perfect seals. Some of the typical laminates in use are:

- Polyester/Polyethylene (PE)
- Polyamide/Polyethylene
- PVDC copolymer film

- Copolymer coated cellulose/PE film
- Nylon/EVA

Vacuum packaged product is stored in a refrigerator at 0–2°C. Storage of chilled meat in gas impermeable packs restricts the growth of *Pseudomonas* sp., thus extending the shelf life of meat. The most common bacteria on stored vacuum packaged poultry meat are the lactic acid bacteria mainly *Lactobacillus* sp. However, a puncture or slit or loose seal in vacuum pack may result in blue of green discoloration.

*Modified Atmosphere Packaging*

In this technique, the atmosphere surrounding the perishable commodity is modified. The manipulation of package atmosphere is done by flushing carbon dioxide, nitrogen and oxygen alone or in combination. This packaging technique has been adopted in many developed countries for storage of meats requiring shipment to long designation or in anticipation of hike in prices. Modified atmosphere packaging offers several advantages:

- It greatly extends the shelf-life of muscle foods during refrigerated storage (6–8 weeks).
- The sensory quality of poultry meat such as color, texture and flavor are preserved.
- There is active inhibition of bacteria and post harvest respiration.
- There is decrease in distribution cost due to extended transit time and bulk deliveries.
- There are no losses in weight during storage.

Studies have shown that a mixture of 60% nitrogen and 40% carbon dioxide or 50% nitrogen and 50% carbon dioxide is ideal for modified atmosphere packaging of chicken meat. Carbon dioxide provides anaerobic conditions whereas nitrogen serves as an inert filler to balance the gas mixture. However, its use adds to the cost of packaging.

*Bulk Packaging*

Birds from dressed plants, after unit packaging, can be transported to retail outlets in wire baskets, metal containers or plastic crates. Plastic crates have become popular as bulk containers due to many advantages. These are tough, light weight, dent proof and easy to stack, handle and clean. These plastic crates in various dimensions are easily available even in moderate cities. These are able to withstand a temperature range of –40°C to 75°C.

## PACKAGING OF MECHANICALLY DEBONED POULTRY MEAT (MDPM)

### Product Attributes

Mechanically deboning involves grinding meat and bone together and forcing the meat through the fine sieves of a mechanical deboner. Bone particles are left behind in the waste residue, which increases the calcium content of MDPM. The meal is obtained as a finely ground paste in which myofibrils are in a highly fragmented form. It contains considerable quantities of lipid (15–22%) and heme component. Heme pigment acts as a catalyst in the auto-oxidation of lipids and may cause flavor problems.

The process of mechanical deboning causes maceration of tissue. So, microbial contamination may be easily blended throughout the deboned tissue. Further, heat evolved during the deboning process may also enhance bacterial growth. *Pseudomonas, Achromobacter* and *Flavobacterium* are the predominant flora.

MDPM is susceptible to soft texture, unstable color and rapid microbial deterioration during storage. Freezing of meat at –20°C reduces the microbial counts.

### Packaging Objectives and Requirements

- To stabilize the color.
- To check lipid oxidation.
- To inhibit further microbial deterioration.
- To maintain the texture.

The shelf-life of MDPM can be maintained during storage only if proper packaging techniques are adopted. The packaging material should have good moisture and gas barrier properties.

### Packaging Materials and Techniques

#### *Vacuum Packaging*

Application of this technique in suitable laminates is a low cost proposition to achieve the desired objectives. It eliminates the volume of air around the meat and restricts further entry of oxygen during storage. The residual air is quickly consumed by meat respiration and partial pressure of oxygen drops below 10 mm Hg within two days of packaging. Further, meat respiration allows the accumulation of carbon dioxide in the packaging which limits the growth of *Pseudomonas* and favor lactic acid bacteria which do not produce putrid odor.

Vacuum packaging extends shelf life of meat while retaining the desired flavor. It saves the refrigerated space during transport and storage which indirectly reduces the labor cost. Besides, there is no weight loss during storage. However, since meat and package, both are subjected to mechanical stress, there may be problem of purge and increased drip loss.

*Modified Atmosphere Packaging (MAP)*

In this technique, atmospheric composition surrounding the meat is changed by manipulation of $CO_2$, $O_2$ and $N_2$ levels. In MAP, only initial change is made whereas in controlled atmosphere packaging (CAP) selective atmospheric composition of gases is maintained by constant monitoring the same throughout the storage period. Nitrogen flushing in meat packaging effective inhibits lipid oxidation. Besides, there is also a slight increase in the redness of meat during 10 minutes exposure to atmosphere. $CO_2$ packaging selectively inhibits gram-negative bacteria such as *Pseudomonas* and related psychrotrophs, although lactic acid bacteria are not much affected. An effective atmospheric composition for mechanically deboned poultry meat may be 20–30% oxygen and 70–75% nitrogen. A combination of carbon dioxide and sorbate treatment provides the most effective inhibitory system against poultry spoilage organism. It reduces the oxidation rate and stabilizes the meat color.

Modified atmosphere packaging extends the shelf life of MDPM to a considerable extent (up to 400%). It maintains the color, texture and flavor of meat during storage. However, it adds to the cost of packaging.

25

CHAPTER

# Role of Meat and Poultry Products in Human Nutrition

We have already discussed the nutritive value of fresh meat and chicken in Chapters 2 and 15 respectively. Meat is a very well-recognized nutritious food due to abundant high quality protein, B-complex vitamins and important minerals especially iron. However, all the nutrients contained in fresh meat do not reach the consumer. Several of them could be partially lost in the processing. The extent of nutrient loss will depend on the processing steps undertaken during the manufacture of a particular product. Hence, there is a need to have a fresh look at the nutritive value of meat and poultry products. Although variety range of processed meat products is very high, relevant information is available only generally prepared products **(Tables 25.1 and 25.2)**.

Most processing procedures involve cooking which brings about a number of changes in meat. Cooking coagulates and denatures the meat proteins altering their solubility. It inactivates or destroys the indigenous proteolytic enzymes. Cooking invariably decreases the water content of meat lowering the water activity level. It intensifies the flavor and modifies the texture. In addition, considerable numbers of microorganisms are killed enhancing the storage life of meat.

Smoking and cooking take place simultaneously in most cured meat products. During smoking, carbonyl groups present in smoke react with amino groups of protein whereas phenols and polyphenols in smoke, could react with sulfhydryl group of protein. Both the reactions cause some loss of available amino acids, thereby decreasing the nutritive value of protein. Water soluble vitamins may also be affected to some extent. In fact, some destruction of thiamine (vitamin $B_1$) is inevitable, although effect on riboflavin (vitamin $B_2$) and niacin may be very little. Smoking process can be nutritionally advantageous because it helps to stabilize the fat soluble vitamins due to antioxidant properties. Canning process is particularly detrimental to the water soluble vitamins present in meat. In canning, about 20–40% of thiamine, 10% each of riboflavin and niacin, 20% of biotin and 20–30% pantothenic acid are destroyed.

Processing changes the nutritional characteristics of fresh meat to some extent. The percentage of protein is slightly decreased whereas that of fat and minerals is increased. The percentage of minerals is generally increased due to added salt and seasonings. Besides, processed meats have more caloric values as compared to fresh meat due to the addition of fillers, binders and other extenders in the form of cereal flours or skimmed milk powder and frequently some fat.

**Table 25.1:** Proximate composition and caloric value of some processed meat and poultry products (per 100 g edible portion).

| *Product details* | *Calories* | *Water* | *Protein* | *Fat* | *Carbo-hydrate* | *Ash* |
|---|---|---|---|---|---|---|
| Chicken, boneless, canned | 198 | 65.2 | 21.7 | 11.7 | - | 1.4 |
| Chicken with vegetables, canned | 100 | 79.6 | 7.4 | 4.6 | 7.2 | 1.2 |
| Turkey with vegetables, canned | 86 | 81.3 | 6.7 | 3.2 | 7.6 | 1.2 |
| Egg yolks with ham or bacon, canned | 208 | 70.3 | 10.0 | 18.1 | - | 1.3 |
| Lamb, strained, canned | 107 | 79.3 | 14.6 | 4.9 | - | 1.2 |
| Lamb, junior, canned | 121 | 76.0 | 17.5 | 5.1 | - | 1.4 |
| Liver, strained, canned | 97 | 79.7 | 14.1 | 3.4 | 1.5 | 1.3 |
| Pork, strained, canned | 118 | 77.7 | 15.4 | 5.8 | - | 1.1 |
| Bacon, cured, cooked and drained | 611 | 8.1 | 30.4 | 52.0 | 3.2 | 6.3 |
| Ham, cured, medium fat, cooked | 289 | 53.6 | 20.9 | 22.1 | - | 3.4 |
| Pork with gravy (90% pork 10% gravy), canned | 256 | 56.9 | 16.4 | 17.8 | 6.3 | 2.6 |
| Beef, corned, boneless, medium fat, canned | 216 | 59.3 | 25.3 | 12.0 | - | 3.4 |

*Source:* USDA Handbook no. 8.

**Table 25.2:** Mineral and vitamin content of some processed meat and poultry products (per 100 g edible portion).

| *Product details* | *Ca (mg)* | *P (mg)* | *Fe (mg)* | *Na (mg)* | *K (mg)* | *Vit B (mg)* | *Vit $B_2$ (mg)* | *Niacin (mg)* | *Vit A (IU)* |
|---|---|---|---|---|---|---|---|---|---|
| Chicken, boneless, canned | 21 | 247 | 1.5 | 250 | 138 | 0.04 | 0.12 | 4.4 | 230 |
| Chicken with vegetables, canned | 22 | 85 | 0.9 | 265 | 71 | 0.09 | 0.15 | 1.6 | 100 |
| Egg yolks with ham or bacon, canned | 71 | 185 | 2.8 | 313 | 82 | 0.10 | 0.23 | 0.5 | 1900 |
| Lamb, strained, canned | 9 | 124 | 2.1 | 241 | 181 | 0.02 | 0.17 | 3.3 | - |
| Liver, strained, canned | 6 | 182 | 5.6 | 253 | 202 | 0.05 | 2.00 | 7.6 | 24000 |
| Pork, strained, canned | 8 | 130 | 1.5 | 223 | 178 | 0.19 | 2.0 | 2.7 | - |
| Bacon, cured, cooked and drained | 14 | 224 | 3.3 | 1021 | 238 | 0.51 | 0.34 | 5.2 | 1021 |
| Ham, cured, medium fat, cooked | 9 | 172 | 2.6 | - | - | 0.47 | 0.18 | 3.6 | - |
| Pork with gravy (90% pork, 10% gravy), canned | 13 | 183 | 2.4 | - | - | 0.49 | 0.17 | 3.5 | - |
| Beef, corned, boneless, medium fat, canned | 20 | 106 | 4.3 | - | - | 0.02 | 0.24 | 3.4 | - |

*Source:* USDA Handbook no. 8.

In fact, meat products could meet a major portion of recommended dietary allowance (RDA) of 56 g protein per day as prescribed by the National Research Council. Since protein is needed to make up the day-to-day wear and tear of body tissues in adults and large amount of protein can be stored in the body. Consumption of meat products can ensure its availability to a large extent. Besides, protein supports the growth in children and pregnant ladies. Consumption of enough protein products with high biological value becomes an absolute necessity. Since meat products contain ample amount of fatty acids that are essential in the diet of human the recommended dietary allowance of fat is relatively less, it can be easily met. However, it should be emphasized that people with genetic disposition for obesity should restrict the consumption of animal fat.

Meat products contain enough of vital minerals such as iron, sodium, potassium and phosphorus. However, these are particularly deficient in calcium. Much of the requirement of iron which is an absolute necessity for health upkeep, can be made available by the meat products. Anemic patients are usually recommended a liver diet because of its high iron content. A regular intake of iron is must for the proper synthesis of hemoglobin, myoglobin and certain enzymes due to very limited capacity to store iron in the body. All the water soluble vitamins are present in meat products but thiamine, riboflavin and niacin are present in significant quantities. Liver containing meat products are extremely rich in vitamin A content.

Though processed products vary in the relative proportion of nutrients, 100 g serving of most meat products can supply 50% of recommended dietary allowance for protein, 25–50% of B-complex vitamins, 35% of recommended iron and 10% of the calorie requirement of an adult person. The nutritional attributes of meat products are highly acclaimed by the dieticians for a healthy living.

In spite of some processing losses, meat and poultry products are rich sources of vital nutrients. Meat products depict a lot of variation in the amount of the protein but most of the products are rich in protein content which is of very high quality due to the availability of essential amino acids.

# 26
CHAPTER

# Fish Products Technology

During ancient period and even before the advent of cultivation, man used to depend on hunting, wherein fish was the most easily available prey. As the civilization dawned, man started giving preference to consumption of fish in diet and started taking interest in proper handling and preservation of fish. These days, India is exporting fish and fish products to several foreign countries.

## INDIAN FISHERIES SECTOR

India has a coastal length of 8,118 kilometer and an exclusive economic zone of 2.02 million sq. kilometer, ponds 2.26 million hectare, reservoirs 2.05 million hectare whereas it has a river and canal length of 1,91,024 kilometer which is contributing to the production of fish.

According to statistical figures of 2019–20, India had a fish production of 14.15 million tons wherein marine and inland fisheries contributed to 3.72 million tonnes and 10.43 million tonnes, respectively. After independence, fisheries sector has had a tremendous growth in India and is still poised for further development. Presently, India is the second largest producer of fish in the world and accounts for nearly 6% of global fish production. It is the largest producer of shrimps in the world. This sector is providing employment and means of livelihood to more than 28 million people. It has an important place in Indian economy and contributes to the valuable foreign exchange also. Fish production of India is contributing 1.25% to national economy and 7.2% of agricultural sector of the country. This sector earned 46,662 crores from export in 2018–19.

The inland water bodies like rivers, canals, lakes, ponds, etc., are very rich in nutrients and these resources have a lot of production potential. The inland fisheries sector is poised for further exploitation and growth. Marine capture fisheries has provided lot of employment in coastal areas for countries and presently contributes a fish catch of about 3.72 million tonnes. The commercial exploitation of marine fisheries sector is almost static for the last few years. Coastal aquaculture production is largely based on shrimp farming.

The per capita consumption of fish in India has been worked out as 10 kg per annum on the assumption that 56% of the population is fish eating. Almost two-third (67%) of the entire fish production is used as fresh whereas 23% is consumed in preserved and processed form which includes dried (16%), frozen (6.5%) or canned (0.5%). About 6% of the fish harvest is converted into fish meal for use by the livestock sector.

Japan and China are major destinations of seafood export (>50 %) from India. There are several other important markets like European Union, USA, Belgium, Italy, Korea, Hong Kong, Malaysia, Singapore, etc., for our seafood. Fresh water fish such as major carps are in demand from West Asia. Indian seafood industry should exploit the big demand of surimi products in overseas market.

## FISH MUSCLE STRUCTURE AND MEAT COMPOSITION–DISTINGUISHING FEATURES

The muscular and fatty tissue of fish are also similar in structure and composition to livestock meat. Fish muscle occupies the same place in human diet as livestock meat and is similar in nutritive value but it has a much different texture and flavor. In fish, the phenomena of rigor mortis is accomplished faster than livestock meat and fish muscle soften again after initial stiffing. Fish meat is more perishable than livestock meat.

Fish also has the same three types of muscle as that of livestock. Fish meat is also basically striated muscle similar to livestock meat. Thus, fish muscle can be divided into ordinary constituting white meat and dark muscle constituting dark meat. White muscle fibers contain much less fat than dark muscle fibers.

Sarcoplasmic proteins are water soluble and some amount of this important component is lost during water washing of fish meat. Myofibrillar proteins form myofibril which contains myosin, actin and regulatory proteins like tropomyosin, troponin and actin. Tropomyosin is a heat stable protein which can be extracted even from heat treated fish products. Stroma proteins form the connective tissues. Fish meat contains less stroma proteins than livestock meat. Studies on fish myosin revealed that it was comparatively unstable as compared to that of livestock muscle.

In general, edible portion of fish varies from 45 to 50% of the whole fish on weight basis. It may go up to 60% in elliptically shaped fish like salmon and may be as less as 35 to 40% in large head or bellied fish like cod or Pollack fish.

Broadly, fish meat contains 65–80% moisture, 15–24% protein, 1 to 15% fat and 1 to 1.5% ash. Amount of crude fat in fish meat varies accordingly to species, age, body part, pre or post spawning and the food condition. In general, there is a negative correlation between crude fat and moisture. In deep sea fish, water content is comparatively more and fat content is less. Proximate composition of raw fish is presented in **Table 26.1,** whereas that of processed fish is given in **Table 26.2**.

**Table 26.1:** Composition of raw fish (%).

| *Species* | *Moisture* | *Protein* | *Fat* | *Ash* |
|---|---|---|---|---|
| Carp | 75.4 | 18.2 | 6.0 | 1.3 |
| Seabass | 79.3 | 19.8 | 0.5 | 1.4 |
| Cod | 82.6 | 16.5 | 0.4 | 1.2 |
| Herring | 72.5 | 19.0 | 7.0 | 1.5 |
| Lamprey | 71.1 | 15.0 | 13.3 | 0.7 |
| Mackerel | 73.9 | 18.7 | 7.1 | 1.2 |
| Pollock | 76.0 | 21.6 | 0.8 | 1.5 |
| Salmon | 64.6 | 22.0 | 12.8 | 1.4 |
| Sardine | 71.0 | 18.2 | 6.0 | 1.3 |
| Trout | 70.8 | 17.8 | 10.3 | 1.2 |

**Table 26.2:** Composition of processed fish (%).

| *Species* | *Moisture* | *Protein* | *Fat* | *Ash* |
|---|---|---|---|---|
| Cod; boneless and 10% salted | 55.0 | 27.3 | 0.3 | 19.0 |
| Mackerel, dressed and 10% salted | 43.6 | 17.3 | 26.4 | 13.0 |
| Herring, 10% salted and smoked | 34.6 | 36.9 | 15.8 | 13.2 |
| Salmon, canned | 63.5 | 21.8 | 12.1 | 2.6 |
| Sardine, canned | 52.3 | 23.0 | 22.4 | 5.6 |
| Lamprey, canned | 63.3 | 16.9 | 12.2 | 4.0 |
| Minogy, pickled | 56.5 | 22.0 | 18.6 | 3.0 |
| Bluefish, broiled | 68.2 | 25.9 | 4.5 | 1.2 |
| Cod fish, fried | 64.0 | 22.13 | 10.2 | 1.2 |

Fish oil contains comparatively large amount of highly unsaturated fatty acids. It oxidizes easily in air and color changes to brown or dark red with a distinctive rancid smell. Fresh water fish has higher content of potassium whereas marine fish has more of sodium.

## NUTRITIVE VALUE OF FISH AND FISH PRODUCTS

Fish is a highly nutritious, tasty and easily digestible food commodity. Fish products are comparable to meat and dairy products in nutritional quality. These are consumed by about 60% people in many developing countries and contribute above 30% of their animal protein supplies.

Fish is a very good source of protein. It contains all essential amino acids in significant amount. Fish is an excellent source of lysine and sulfur containing amino acids—methionine and cysteine, which are deficient in cereal diets. Thus, fish protein can complement and supplement the amino acid profile of mixed diets.

Fish fat is a very good source of essential amino acids such as linoleic and linolenic acid which cannot be synthesized in human body. Fish oil is particularly rich in polyunsaturated Omega-3 fatty acids (first double bond in third position) which has several neurological benefits in growing children and also plays a role in decreasing the risk of arteriosclerosis and cardiovascular diseases.

Fish meat is a good source of B-complex group of vitamins. Fatty fish also contain adequate A and D vitamins. Some fresh water fish like carp possess high thiaminase activity resulting in low thiamine in such species. Fish meat is particularly valuable with respect to mineral profile. It is a good source of calcium, phosphorus, iron, etc. Marine fish have a high content of iodine. Thus fish products are comparable to meat and dairy products in nutritional quality. These products have very good sensory properties which can enhance the taste of even otherwise bland diets.

## HANDLING OF FISH

Fish is a highly perishable food commodity which requires proper handling and preservation to enhance its shelf life and retain its quality as well as nutritional value. These days, it is a common practice to keep the fish alive for eventual consumption. It requires fish to be first conditioned in a container with clean water. The damaged, sick or dead fish are removed while doing so. The fish are usually kept alive in holding basins at lowered water temperature to reduce the metabolic rate and activity. Low metabolic rate decreases the fouling of water with ammonia, nitrite and carbon dioxide which are toxic to the fish. Holding basins can also be equipped with water filter.

Handling of dead fish involves transfer of catch from gear to vessel, holding of catch, sorting/grading/bleeding/gutting/washing, chilling, chilled storage and unloading. These operations can be performed by manual, semi-automatic and automatic methods. Icing is the oldest method of preserving fish freshness. Ice has the advantage of being low cost, readily available and safe medium which keeps the fish moist and can provide large cooling capacity. In artisanal fisheries also, use of ice is cost effective on small boats and the handling operations remain the same.

The harvested fish should be cleaned and cooled as soon as possible. Due to their strong digestive juices, fish spoil very soon and if not gutted and cleaned promptly, it may develop off flavor and color. A sharp knife, clean cloth or paper towels, plastic bags and crushed ice in an ice chest must be kept ready for gutting and cleaning the fish. With the help of a clean fillet knife the fish should be cleaned and bled. Throat should be cut and gills and entrails are removed. The surface of fish should be wiped with a clean cloth or paper towel. Cleaned fish be first put in plastic bags and then in ice. To prevent contamination during handling of the fish, the hands, working area, cutting boards, knives and other utensils should be properly cleaned with hot water and soap after each use.

For preparing the fillet, fish is washed in clean cold water to remove blood, microbes and enzymes. Filleting is done with a sharp knife with flexible blade. The fish is cut behind the pectoral fin straight down to the backbone and cut is angled towards the top of the head. Knife is run along one side of the backbone, scraping the rib bones without cutting them. The knife is pushed through the flesh near the vent just behind the rib bones and fillet is cut free at the tail. Flesh is cut carefully away from the rib cage. The first boneless fillet is removed by cutting through the stomach skin. Same method is used to get the second fillet. These fillets should then be stored properly at low temperature.

## TRANSPORTATION OF FISH

Fish is a traded live, fresh or frozen. Transportation of live fish requires oxygen for respiration and removal of toxic gases as well as byproducts. Fish is also starved or conditional before transportation to decrease its metabolic rate and increase the packing density.

Fish is transported by land, sea or air. It is very important to maintain the cold chain throughout for fresh, chilled or frozen fish which requires the use of insulated containers or transport vehicles. Air cargo is also used to transport about 5% of the total world catch. It requires special care in handling and excellent communication among the shipper, carrier and consignee. Any leakage can harm cause damage to the aircraft by corrosion or interference to the control mechanisms.

## PRESERVATION OF FISH

Fish is an aquatic creature. As it is removed from its natural habitat, the postmortem reactions set in and the process of spoilage starts. It is a pity that nearly 25% of India's total fish production becomes inedible due to lack of proper preservative techniques. Modern fish handling and preservation techniques are being developed to salvage this precious source of protein and their application is proving to be very useful. India has tropical and subtropical climate which increases the possibility of fish spoilage because of high temperature and humidity. Preservation of fish is as important as its production.

After harvest, fish undergoes three main type of changes—bacterial, enzymatic and oxidative. Initially bacterial growth is slow but afterwards proceeds very fast and cause spoilage. Chemical reactions breakdown protein and other nitrogenous constituents into hydrogen sulfide and indole which emanate strong odor. Besides, marine fish also produce some amount of trimethylamine oxide which is finally converted to trimethylamine.

All these undesirable factors could be reduced or eliminated to preserve the fish quality and enhance shelf life with the help of techniques.

### Temperature Control

These techniques decrease the fish temperature to levels where the activities of microbes or enzymes are reduced or stopped. This is made possible by fish icing refrigeration or freezing (–18°C). Some times chilled sea water (CSW) or refrigerated sea water (RSW) are also used to lower the temperature of small fish caught in large quantities.

Refrigeration is a suitable method for short-term storage of fish. It not only retards spoilage but also retains the natural attributes and nutritive value of fish. Commercially, cold or chilling rooms are used to store bulk harvest. Washed and cleaned fish can be packed and put in ice to transport it to the market. It can preserve the fish for about 48 hours.

Preservation of fish for more than 2 days is accomplished in deep freezer cabinets. Quick freezing of packaged fish is more suitable for retaining the quality attributes of fish for a long time. In India, this facility is available in Mumbai, Mangalore, Cochin, Calicut and Trivandrum. Quick freezing allows the formation of very small ice crystals in fish meat. At about –40°C, the size of these ice crystals is barely 1 mm and the fish appears to be chalky white.

In glazing, frozen fish is sprinkled with a layer of ice or dipped in cold water maintained at 0 to 3°C to effect glazing. This process is repeated until an ice coating of at least 2 mm thickness is made on the fish. This ice cover stops freeze dehydration in fish. It is suitable for whole fish or large cuts. Glazed fish require less freezer space. Glazing of fish should be checked at intervals and if required, a glaze layer may again be applied.

## Control of Water Activity ($a_w$)

Water is essential for microbial and enzymatic reactions and several techniques have been evolved to tie up or remove this water and make it unavailable for these reactions and thus reduce $a_w$. These techniques include salting, salting and smoking, drying, etc.

## Physical Control of Microbial Fish Load

These techniques use heat (blanching, cooking, pasteurization, sterilization), irradiation or microwave heating. Blanching and pasteurization do not completely inactivate microorganisms and often required to be combined with refrigeration to preserve fish products. Sterilized products are stable at room temperature because of complete inactivation of micro-organisms in canning or retortable pouches.

## Chemical Control of Microbial Fish Load

These techniques involve adding chemical agents or decreasing muscle pH to levels that inhibit the microbial growth. Microbial growth in inhibited by decreasing the pH to less than 4.5 by adding organic acids or through marinades, fermentation, etc. Fish fermenting lactic acid bacteria also produce antimicrobial compounds such as nisin bringing about biopreservation.

## Control of O-R Potential

Reduction of oxygen around fish checks the growth of some spoilage bacteria as well as lipid oxidation and this enhances the shelf life.

Vacuum packaging and modified atmosphere packaging (MAP) of fish and fish products brings about this effect. Refrigerated storage of packaged products further enhances the effect.

### Hurdle Technology

A balanced combination of two or more techniques improves the efficacy of preservation while reducing the undesirable effect of severe treatment of any single technique. Salting-drying, salting-smoking etc., along with vacuum or MAP and refrigeration can bring about multiple hurdle effect.

Before preservation, fish is washed with potable water to remove slime, blood, sand and mud. Smaller and larger fish are segregated on the basis of their size, larger fish are cut to remove their viscera as well as other internal organs and cleaned properly.

We can salvage a large quantity of fish by applying the above preservation methods. Besides, fish byproducts can also be utilized in various ways to recover protein and valuable oil to serve the mankind.

## FISHERY PRODUCTS

### Cured and Dried Fish

Salting or curing of fish is popular in India since ages. Salting reduces the water activity and checks the enzymatic reaction and bacterial growth. Salting is done in two ways.

#### *Dry Salting*

Fish fillets are rubbed with table salt and stored in tub or cement tanks. Dry salt is sprinkled on all the body surfaces. Salt to fish ratio varies from 1:4 to 1:8 depending on the fish variety, climate and local practices. Comparatively more salt is applied on fatty fish. After 10–12 hours, fish are washed in their own brine and dried in sun for 2–3 days to bring down the water activity **(Fig. 26.1)**.

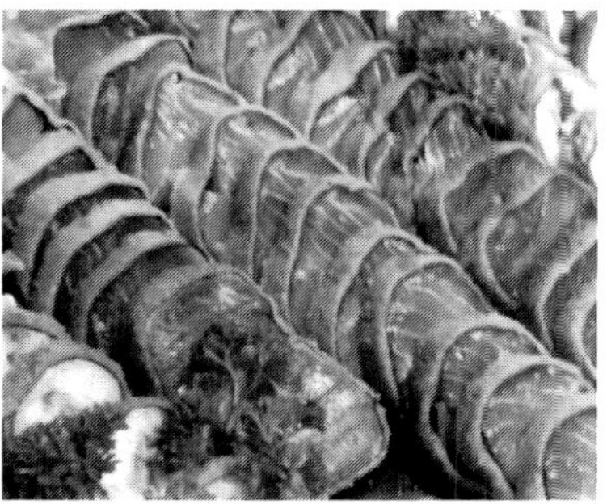

**Fig. 26.1:** Salted fish.

### *Wet Salting*

Use of wet salt is in wide use in Konkan coast of India. Washed fish fillets are kept in concentrated salt solution or brine. Larger fish like salmon, seerfish, black pomfret, etc., are cleaned of their internal organs and split longitudinally. Salt to fish ratio is maintained at 1:3. On first day, the fish are rubbed with dry salt and put on cement surface for partial dehydration. Then these are transferred to brine tanks for 7–10 days period. Such fish keep well for 3–4 months.

Drying is an age old technique of preservation. The objective of fish drying is to reduce moisture and check bacterial and enzymatic degradation. In India, around 35% of the total marine fish is dried in sun. Small sea fish like ribbon fish, silver valley fish, Bombay duck, etc., are spread on the sandy sea shores. Some times mats and larger tree leaves make up the bed for sun drying. Very often, Bombay duck variety of fish is dried on hangers made up of bamboo or rope. In larger fish, internal organs are removed first which are then salted and then subjected to drying.

In ideal process, the fish is washed thoroughly in 10 ppm chlorinated water to remove slime, adhering dirt, etc. Then visceral contents are removed in mackerel. Scales are also removed in sardines. Guffing is not done in small fish like anchovies. After washing and draining, the fish is salted in salt-to-fish ratio of 1:4 on a salting table. Then fish is spread for drying over the clean surface till the moisture contents are reduced to 20%. Dried fish has a shelf life of 2-3 months.

Cured mackerel, a traditional product of India is brine pickled after gutting, dressing and washing. In Colombo curing, a small quantity of Malabar tamarind (Garcinia cambogia) is put in the body cavity of fish for pickling. If saturated brine is fortified with 0.5% propionic acid, then pickled mackerel can keep well up to one year.

Bombay duck, a small high moisture fish is dried whole and unsalted by interlocking the jaws of two fish. There are dried on horizontal wooden pole for 2–3 days to reduce the moisture to 18%. Silver belly fish are also salted by brine pickling for 18–24 hours and then sun dried and packed.

## Cured and Smoked Fish

Smoked fish is not so popular in India because Indian consumers do not prefer smoked flavor in fish. Smoke preservation is done at a very lower scale in some parts of Tamil Nadu and Orissa. However, it is very popular in Norway and Sweden, where sardine, mackerel, hilsa, etc., are subjected to smoking. This treatment is done after cleaning and salting by dry or wet method. Fish are hanged on hooks above smoke surface or in some chambers. Smoke acts as a preservative mainly because of the presence of phenolic compounds.

Smoked fish is a delicacy these days because of the typical pleasant flavor. Such fish are only highly salted, before smoking **(Figs. 26.2 to 26.4)**. These are shelf stable for 5-7 days at ambient temperature but keep well for 3 weeks in cold storage.

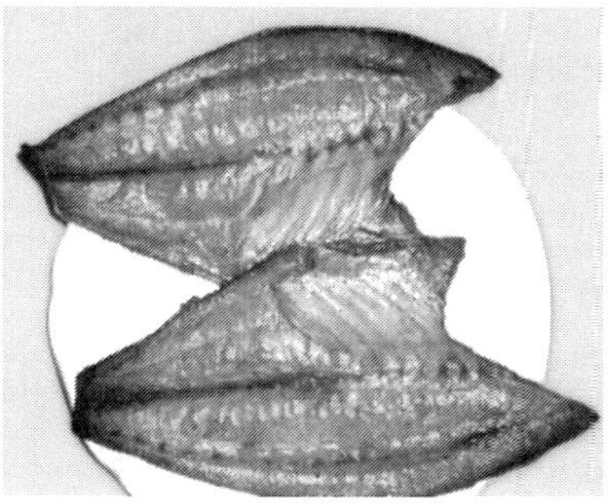

**Fig. 26.2:** Brined and smoked fish.

Smoking may be hot or cold. In hot smoking, cooking is also accomplished in the smoke chamber maintained at 80°C. Fish like trout, eels, sardines, sprats, etc., are hot smoked. In cold smoking, the temperature of kiln should not exceed 30°C. Typical cold smoked fish are cod fillet, salmon, haddock, etc. These are shelf stable for 7 days at 25°C and 6 months at –30°C. The processing of smoked fish is depicted in **Flowchart 26.1**.

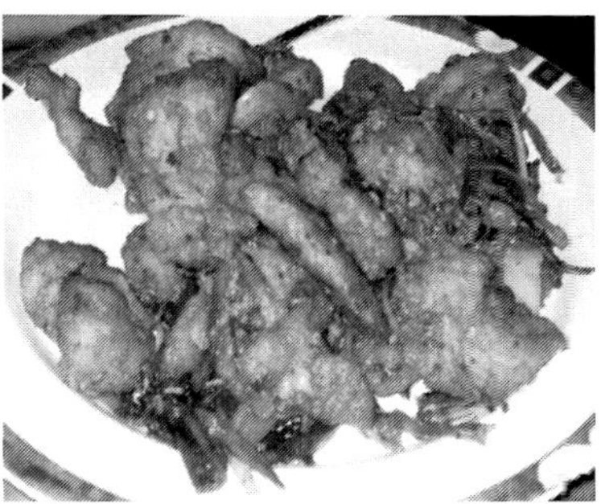

**Fig. 26.3:** Fried fish.

## Canned Fish

Canning of fish started from Europe and then spread to other countries. The method of preservation has the advantage of retaining the natural flavor and other attributes of fish. Large quantities of sardine, mackerel, tuna fish, maniga, etc., are canned at Cochin, Chennai, Calicut, Goa and Mumbai mainly for export.

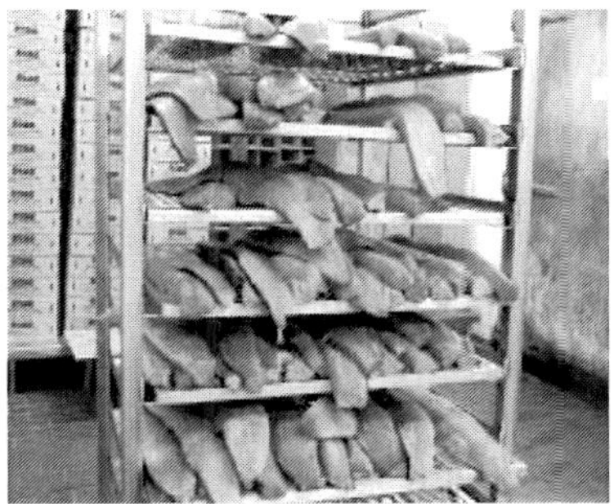

**Fig. 26.4:** Smoked fish.

**Flowchart 26.1:** Processing of smoked fish.

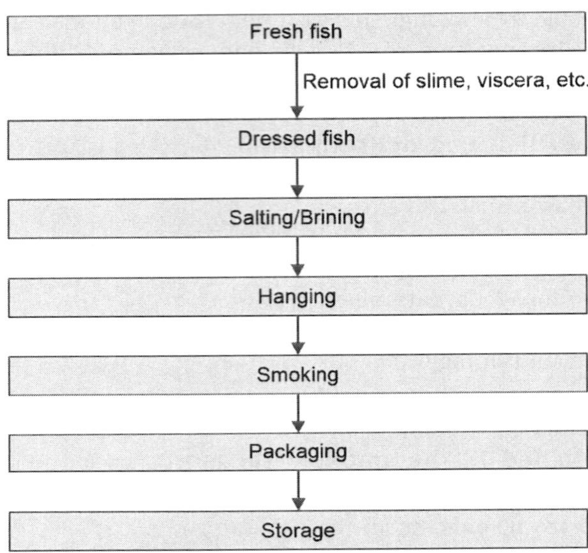


*Note:* It is a general practice to use liquid smoke in modern processing plants.

Canning of fish **(Flowchart 26.2)** involves the following steps:

*Selection and Handling of Raw Material*

The raw material for canning should be of very good quality. It should be temporarily preserved in ice or sprinkled salt or chilled or refrigerated sea water and should be processed as quickly as possible. It is very important to maintain cold chain.

*Salting, Blanching and Precooking*

Generally, fish is salted before canning. It is usually done by immersion in brine at elevated temperature incorporating blanching. In some cases, the temperature may be further increased for precooking. It reduces the bacterial load and fish flesh. It causes sufficient shrinkage (15–30%) of fish enabling easy filling of can.

*Filling in Cans*

It can be done manually or mechanically. A headspace of 1–1.5 cm is usually left. Too little or too much head space can create problems of can bulging or loss of vacuum respectively. It is very common to add brine, refined vegetable oil or tomato soup in canned fish.

**Flowchart 26.2:** Processing of canned fish.

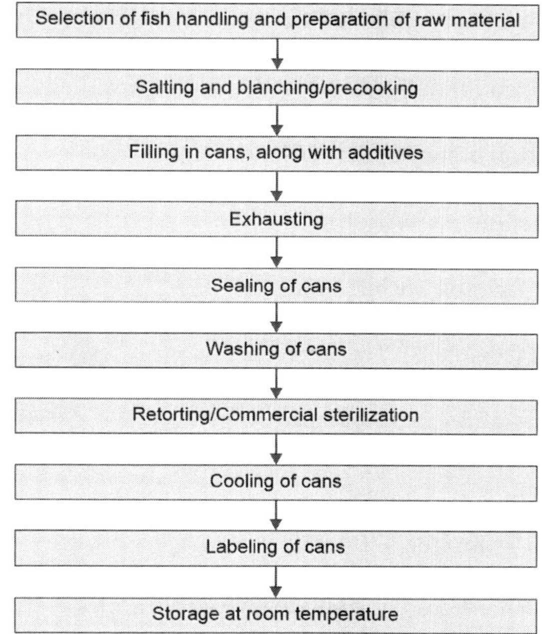


### *Exhausting*

It is the process in which air from the headspace and contents of a filled can is removed before sealing. It is due to exhausting that the can is not strained during heat processing. Besides, during cooling of can, it leads, to the creation of vacuum.

### *Sealing of Cans*

A hermetic sealing between the cover and body of the can is done to check the entry of microorganisms. A good quality tin plate with double seam is desired for efficient can-closing. Code stamping is usually done before sealing.

### *Washing of Cans*

It removes the fish pieces, brine, oil, sauce, etc., adhering on the can surface. A hot detergent such as 1% sodium polyphosphate at 80°C is generally used for washing.

*Retorting or Thermal Processing*

The sealed can are subjected to steam heating at predetermined temperature and pressure for pre-determined time. The time-temperature combination is derived is such a way that it is sufficient to kill or inhibit the microorganisms. An important consideration is the elimination of the spores of Cl. botulinum.

Retorting does not bring about complete *sterility* but a commercial *sterility* in which some spare farming bacteria can be present in dormant state in canned fish **(Fig. 26.5)**. The heat application is enough to kill all viable forms of bacteria having public health significance.

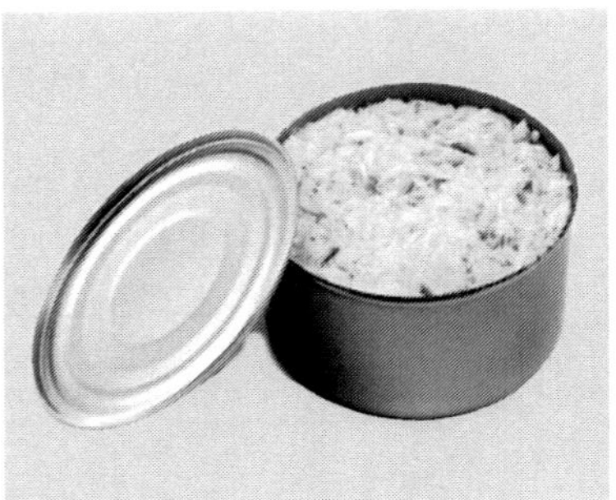

**Fig. 26.5:** Canned fish.

*Cooling of Cans*

After retorting, the cans are immediately cooled to a temperature of about 35°C to eliminate the chances of overcooking and to give a cold shock to the surviving microorganisms, if any.

*Labeling of Cans*

After surface drying, the cans are affixed with labels which provide the approved statutory information including the gross contents.

*Storage*

The cans are packed in bulk containers and stored under cool and dry conditions. The canned fish has a shelf life of 2 years at ambient temperature.

## Fish Protein Concentrate

It is a protein rich flour prepared from ground fish and used as nutritional supplement for humans, being excellent source of highly digestible amino acids. Fish protein concentrate contains as much as 65 to 90% protein, 4 to 8% moisture and very less fat. It is stable at 5°C for 6 months.

**Flowchart 26.3:** Processing of fish protein concentrate.

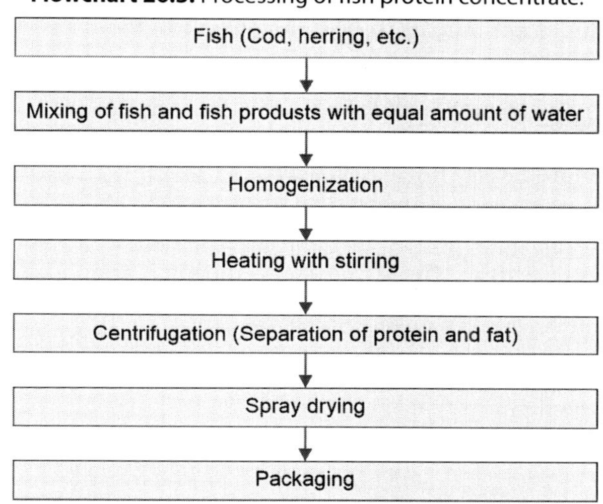


The material is produced hygienically and meets sensory requirement of taste and odor **(Flowchart 26.3)**.

## Surimi

Surimi refers to refined minced fish meat which has been water washed and added with antidenaturant. Thus, surimi is a concentrate of myofibrillar proteins of the fish muscle. It has very good tensile strength and elasticity. This uncooked product is generally frozen stored and serves as a starting material for a variety of processed fish products like fish sticks, fish sausages, kamaboko (a popular fish product of Japan), fish ham, etc. Surimi can be salted or salt free depending on the ultimate use. It cuts down the processing time and ensures uniform quality of several fish products.

After harvesting, the fish is handled in ample amount of ice to retain freshness. The head as well as internal organs are removed. The washed dressed fish or fillets is coarse minced. It is washed in chilled water 4–5 times its volume to remove water soluble proteins. The process is repeated 2–3 times. The material is strained to remove excess water, pigments and fat particles. The process is repeated 2–3 times. Now, additives like sugar, polyphosphate and/or table salt are mixed with the meat, which is filled in polyethylene bags by filling machine and packed in pan. The surimi is quick frozen initially at –35°C and then stored at –30°C.

Quality evaluation and grading of frozen surimi is usually carried out. It should contain 75 to 80% moisture for good texture in the finished product.

## Fish Sausages

These are prepared either from surimi or fish fillets. Surimi based sausages are very much liked in Japan. Comparatively higher content of myofibrillar proteins in the product provides very good gelling capacity and texture. The temperature during cutting and mincing should not exceed 10°C. Use of polyphosphates along with salt gives better results. Casings could be natural without pin holes or synthetic from cellulosic material. The product is cooked at 80°C for 20 minutes and then cooled.

## Fish Balls

Fish mince is mixed with various ingredients which differ from country to country. The material is shaped in the form of balls either manually or through forming machines. Surimi is used as a starting material in Japan. The fish balls are either heat processed or stored frozen. In Philippines, baking power is added to the mince before shaping into balls. The balls are thermo-processed in two stages to enhance binding and imparting crispiness **(Fig. 26.6)**.

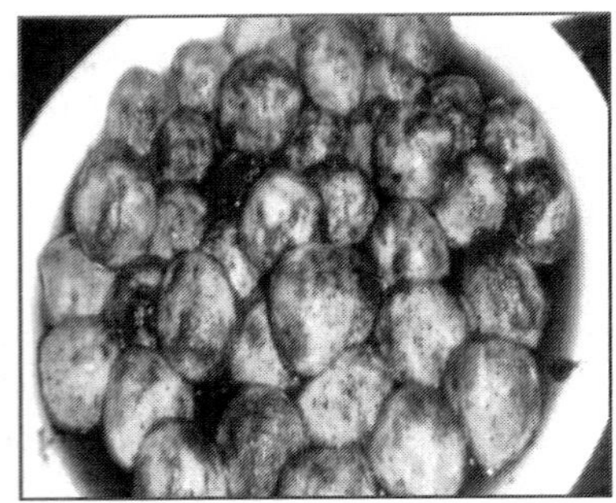

**Fig. 26.6:** Surimi fish balls.

## Fish Curry

It is an important food item in several south-east Asian countries like India, Bangladesh, Sri Lanka, Myanmar, Thailand, etc. A variety of ingredients are added and fish curry is prepared much the same way as meat curry. It is high nutritious and usually consumed along with rice. It has very good consumer acceptability and a properly cooked fish curry is shelf stable only for 2 days at refrigerated temperature.

## Fish Pickle

Usually low value fish like mackerel, threadfin bream, sciaenids, perches, etc., are used for this purpose. These are filleted, washed and applied with salt. The method remains much the same as for meat pickle. This pickle is very popular in coastal regions of South India and is exported in large quantities to the Middle East and other parts of the world to cater to the needs of the people of Indian origin. It is packed in glass or plastic bottles of 500 g capacity for export **(Fig. 26.7)**.

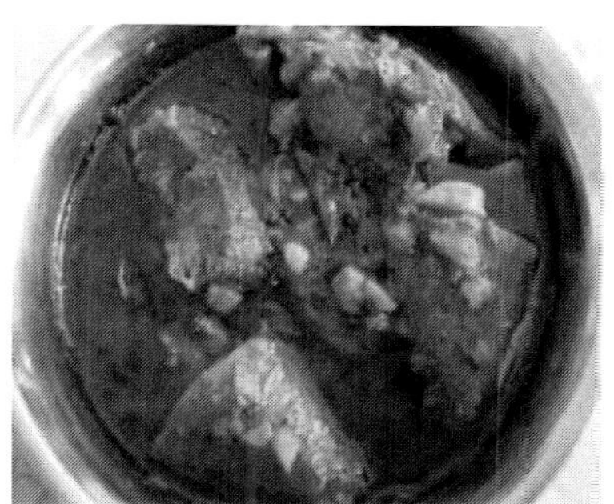

**Fig. 26.7:** Pickled fish.

## Fish Paste

In Malabar coastal areas of India, fish chunks are partially dehydrated and then converted into paste after mixing some dry spices and condiments **(Fig. 26.8)**.

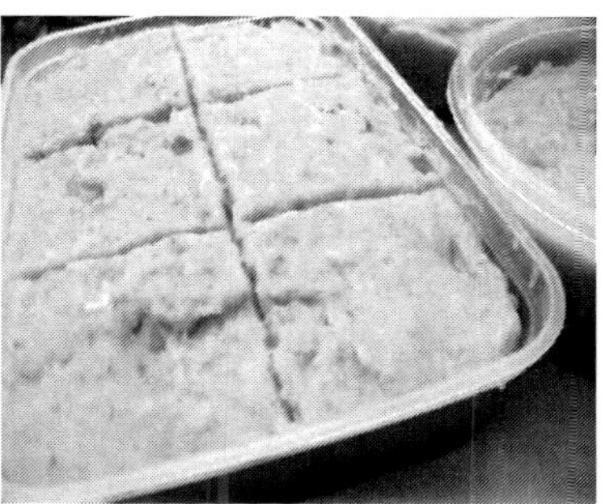

**Fig. 26.8:** Fish paste.

27

CHAPTER

# Organic Meat Food Products

Organic farming is a holistic production management system that dominates the use of synthetic inputs such as synthetic fertilizer and pesticides, veterinary drugs, genetically modified seeds or breeds, preservatives, additives, irradiation, etc. It is a system that promotes and enhances ecosystem health including biodiversity, biological cycles and soil biological activity.

Organic farming has been one of the important priorities right from Tenth Five Year Plan. Agricultural and processed food products export development authority (APEDA) under Ministry of Commerce is making concerted efforts to boost organic production in India. One of the major steps has been the launching of National Programme for Organic Production (NPOP) in 2001 and development of Indian standards for organic production.

Organic foods have gained importance with the increasing awareness of harmful effects of residual pesticides and insecticides in the foods of animal origin. Increasing awareness and knowledge of quality conscious people will pave the way for willing people to pay more for organic products. It is thus essential to increase the availability of organic foods for internal consumption and export.

The demand for organic food is growing nationally as well as globally. It has created new export opportunities for the developing world. Since, organic farming is labor intensive, developing nations can have better chance to boost their export of organic food products, provided international quality standards are achieved.

## NATIONAL STANDARDS FOR ORGANIC ANIMAL HUSBANDRY

### Animal Management

Management techniques in animal husbandry should be governed by the physiological and ethological needs of the farm animals in question. This includes that animals should be allowed to live by their basic behavioral habits and that all management techniques, including those where production levels and speed of growth are concerned, should be directed for the good health and welfare of the animals.

*Standards*

- The accredited certification production program shall ensure that the management of the animal environment takes into account the behavioral needs of the animals and provides for:
  - Sufficient free movement
  - Sufficient fresh air and natural daylight according to the needs of the animals.
  - Protection against excessive sunlight, temperatures, rain and wind according to the withstanding capacity of the animals.
  - Enough lying and/or resting area according to the needs of the animal. For all animals requiring bedding, natural materials shall be provided.
  - Ample access to fresh water and feed according to the needs of the animals.
  - Adequate facilities for expressing behavior in accordance with the biological and ethological needs of the species.
- All animals shall have access to open air and/or grazing appropriate to the type of animal and season taking into account the age and condition, to be specified by the accredited certification program.
- Poultry and rabbits shall not be kept in cages.
- When the natural day length is prolonged by artificial lighting, the accredited certification program shall prescribe maximum hours respective to species, geographical considerations and general health of animals. Herd animals shall not be kept individually.
- The accredited certification program may allow exceptions, e.g., male animals, small holdings, sick animals and those about to give birth.

## Length of Conversion Period

The establishment of organic animal husbandry requires an interim period, termed as conversion period.

*Standards*

- Animal products may be sold as "product of organic agriculture" only after the farm or relevant part of it has been under conversion for at least twelve months and providing the organic animal production standards have been met for the appropriate time.

- The accredited certification program shall specify the length of time for which the animal production standards shall have been met. With regard to dairy and egg production this period shall not be less than 30 days.
- Animals present on the farm at the time of conversion may be sold for organic meat when the organic standards have been met for 12 months.

## Brought-in-Animals

When organic livestock is not available, the accredited certification program shall allow brought-in conventional animals according to the following age limits:

- 2 days old chickens for meat production
- 18 weeks old hens for egg production
- 2 weeks old for any other poultry
- Piglets up to six weeks and after weaning
- Calves up to 4 weeks old that have received colostrums and are fed a diet consisting mainly of full milk.

Accredited certification programs shall set time limits (not exceeding 5 years) for implementation of certified organic animals from conception of each type of animal.

## Breeds and Breeding

- Breeds should be chosen which are adapted to local conditions.
- Breeding goals should not be in opposition to animal's natural behavior and should be directed towards good health.
- Artificial insemination is allowed only upon veterinary necessity.
- Embryo transfer techniques are not allowed.
- Hormonal heat treatment and induced birth are not allowed unless applied to individual animals for medical reasons and under veterinary advice.
- The use of genetically engineered species or breeds are not allowed.

## Mutilations

The accredited certification program shall allow the following exceptions:

- Castrations
- Tail docking of lambs

- Dehorning
- Ringing
- Mulesing

  Suffering shall be minimized and anesthetics used where appropriate.

## Animal Nutrition

- The livestock should be fed 100% organically grown feed of good quality.
- All feed shall come from the farm itself or be produced within the region.
- The diet shall be offered to the animals in a form allowing them to execute their natural feeding behavior and digestive needs.
- The prevailing part (at least more than 50%) of the feed shall come from the farm unit itself or shall be produced in cooperation with other organic farms in the region.
- The following products shall not be included nor added to the feed given to farm animals:
  - Synthetic growth promoters or stimulants
  - Synthetic appetizers
  - Dropping, dung or other manure (all types of excreta) even if technologically processed
- Vitamins, trace elements and supplements shall be used from natural origin when available in appropriate quantity and quality.
- All ruminants shall have daily access to roughage.
- The following fodder preservatives shall be used:
  - Bacteria, fungal and enzymes
  - By-products of food industry (e.g., molasses)
  - Plant based products

## Veterinary Medicine

- The well-being of the animals is the primary consideration, in the choice of illness treatment. The use of conventional veterinary medicines are allowed when no other justifiable alternative is available.
- Where conventional veterinary medicines are used, the withholding period shall be twice the legal period.
- Use of the following substances is prohibited:
  - Synthetic growth promoters
  - Substances of synthetic origin for production stimulation or suppression of natural growth

- ♦ Hormones for heat induction and heat synchronization unless used for an individual animal against reproductive disorders, justified by veterinary indications

## Transport and Slaughter

*General Principles*

- Transport and slaughter should minimize stress to the animal. Transport distance and frequency should be minimized.
- The transport medium should be appropriate for each animal.
- Animals should be inspected regularly during transport.
- Animals should be watered and fed during transport depending on weather conditions and duration of the transport.
- Stress to the animal shall be minimized, especially taking into consideration:
  - Contact (by eye, ear or smell) of each animal with dead animals or animals in the killing process
  - Existing group ties
  - Resting time to release stress
- Each animal shall be stunned before being bled to death. The equipment used for stunning should be in good working order. Exceptions can be made according to cultural practice. Where animals are bled with prior stunning this should take place in a calm environment.

*Standards*

- Throughout the different steps of the process, there shall be a person responsible for the well-being of the animal.
- Handling during transport and slaughter shall be calm and gentle. The use of electric sticks and such instruments are prohibited.
- The accredited certification program shall set slaughter and transportation standards that will take into consideration:
  - Stress caused to the animal and person in charge
  - Fitness of the animal
  - Loading and unloading
  - Mixing different groups of animals or animals of different sex
  - Quality and suitability of mode of transport and handling equipment
  - Temperatures and relative humidity
  - Hunger and thirst
  - Specific needs of each animal

- No chemical synthesized tranquilizers or stimulants shall be given prior to or during transport.
- Each animal or group of animals shall be identifiable during all steps.
- Where the transport is by road, the journey time to the slaughter house shall not exceed eight hours.

## ORGANIC CERTIFICATION

There are several organic food certifying bodies at international regional and national levels.

- Codex alimentarius commission
- International federation of organic agriculture movement (IFOAM)
- UK register of organic food standards (UKROFS)
- SKAL—Netherland
- USDA'S National Organic Programme (NOP): It has four classifications:
    1. *100% organic:* Meat and poultry leveled 100% organic come for animals fed only 100% organic feed
    2. *Organic:* Feed ingredients have to be at least 95% organic
    3. *Made with organic ingredient:* Between 70 and 75% organic ingredients
    4. *Less than 70% organic ingredients*

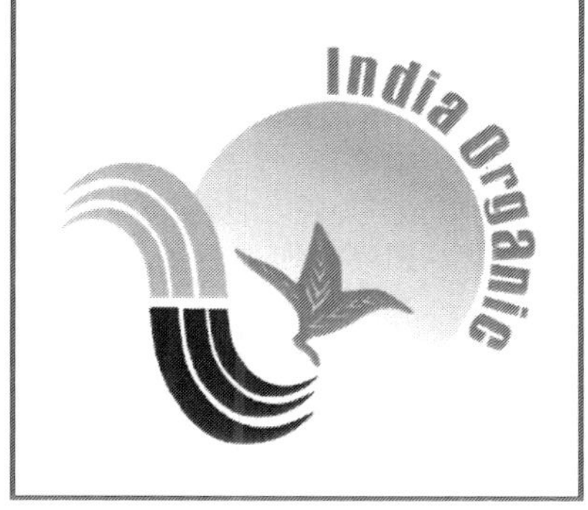


Indian certification has been prepared by APEDA and released as national standards for the organic produce by the Ministry of Commerce. The logo for this certificate has been reproduced here.

Besides, international agencies are also active in India to offer certification services. The standards for organic production are not static. These are being revised periodically at international level and needs to be revised at regional and country level.

## GLOBAL ORGANIC MEAT MARKET

Demand for organic food has become more widely accepted. Markets reflecting this trend includes the USA and EU, and to a lesser extent Argentina and Brazil. The key feature of USA and EU markets is that these are fast growing organic, although even now only a fraction of the total food retail trade is organic. Meat, poultry and eggs have registered 64% growth, followed by dairy with 40% growth. USA is leading followed by Germany, UK and other European countries. Western Europe is currently the largest market for organic food in the world. In USA organic meat and meat products including poultry are the sixth fastest growing commodity group. Organic meat products are expected to capture 5% of total domestic organic food sales by 2003 (USDA, 2001). Organic meat and cheese are the main exported organic products of Austria.

French sales of the organic meat accounted for 3% of total organic production in France. Latin American countries, like Argentina, Brazil and Uruguay produce substantial amounts of organic meat and are seeking to develop export of organically produced meat. In Argentina, more than one million hectares of land are dedicated to organic livestock production, the majority of which produce organic beef cattle and 80% of the produce is exported to the EU. Though little organic beef is produced in Brazil, organic poultry, egg and milk production are growing day by day. New Zealand also exports organic meat to UK and Germany. Japan is the third largest market for organic foods after USA and EU and account for the bulk of Asian market revenues. Organic food is likely to dominate the global niche markets. The quality consciousness and willingness of people to pay more for organically produced products would go up in coming years.

## SCENARIO FOR DEVELOPING COUNTRIES

In developing countries, food security is the prime goal rather than food safety. In this situation, some development has already taken place in the organic crop sector and now the Asian countries are exporting a substantial quantity of organic tea, fresh and dried fruits, vegetables, nuts, rice dried legumes, coffee, sugar, herbs and spices, but the export as well as production of organic meat in most of the developing Asian countries is still an utopia. Though these countries have some excellent breeds of livestock, which are well suited in these climatic conditions, are more resistant to disease, and thrive well on crop residues. Most of the animal husbandry practices with a close resemblance to prescribed organic practices but we failed significantly to convert our advantages into fruitful gains. Small land holding, low level of literacy, lack of information, high stocking density, inadequate production of feed and fodder, high cost of certification, absence of marketing facilities are some hindrances in the way of conversion from traditional to organic. In developing countries, Argentina and Brazil have the most advanced organic livestock sector.

In India, some pockets where the conditions are favorable for organic production need to be developed as organic production zones in the beginning. Ideally, the plan of action for Indian Animal Husbandry with an eye on organic animal products should be drawn on the following lines:

- Promotion of indigenous breeds with improved selection and breeding.
- Construction of animal sheds with space for sufficient movement of animals.
- Emphasizing the importance of grazing and forage feeding.
- Promotion of mixed farming system integrating dairy or poultry as important components, instead of high tech specialized versions of the developed world.
- Promotion of cow milk as a brand to market it for young children, old persons, patients with terminal diseases, etc., and organic cow ghee for religious ceremonies.
- Re-emphasizing backyard poultry for low capital and high nutritive food products.
- Promotion of free range poultry system for egg and meat.
- Strict management of slaughter practice to make them humane and observing all animal welfare measures.
- Promotion of mechanical or at least semi-modern slaughterhouses for small and large animals to produce wholesome meat.
- Making full use of Ayurvedic and Homeopathic products in animal husbandry; authentic products and practices can even be exported to the west.

Some potential areas of the countries (hilly areas, forest areas, rain fed areas), where agriculture is not so well developed, should be identified and some nodal agencies should be established. These agencies will provide the technical support to the farmers, make arrangement for certification and help in marketing. The success of these areas will be a model to the rest of the countries.

28

CHAPTER

# Genetically Modified Animal and Marine Products

Genetically modified (GM) animal and marine products are under development in many parts of the world. The genetic modification of animals and fish is a set of rapidly developing technologies which have a number of interesting and promising applications. It can be used to obtain or improve the desired features of livestock and fish such as disease resistance and food production. The technology can be used for the development of proteins or other substances for therapeutic purposes. Besides, it can also generate an alternative source of cell tissues as well as organs for xenotransplantation and to make models of human diseases.

## GENETIC MODIFICATION

Modern biotechnology utilizes in vitro nucleic acid techniques including recombinant DNA and direct injection of nucleic acid into cells or organelles; or fusion of cells beyond the taxonomic family that overcome natural physiological reproductive or recombination barriers beyond traditional selection and breeding. In fact, GM animals and transgenic animals are synonymous terms to mean recombinant DNA animals. Transgene refers to the recombinant DNA that has been integrated in the genome of the GM animal.

## TECHNIQUES

Several techniques can be utilized for transferring genes into animals depending on their suitability for different species, efficiency of transformation and risk involved. Identification of a gene encoding a desired product trait is the first step in the utilization of gene transfer approach. This gene is incorporated into an expression vector which is carefully selected for different species of animals. Biotechnologists may purposely transfer into the host:

- **Fusion gene**—referring a gene encoding or desired product with an element which will regulate its expression into the host.
- **Transposon**—referring a DNA element capable of breaking itself from one location of the genome and inserting itself into another location to contain fusion gene.
- **Retrovirus**—referring a virus that can integrate itself into a genome and become expressed through the host cells replication process and that has been modified to contain the fusion gene.

Several expression vectors contain marker genes. One type of marker gene only report successful gene transfer while the other type encode gene products so that transgenic animals can be selected for specific purposes.

There are several methods by which the expression vector can be introduced into the host. Some important methods are:

- Direct injection of the expression vector into fertilized eggs or host cells with a very fine glass needle (microinjection).
- Introduction of expression vector into host cells through transient pores in their membrane with the help of electric impulses (electroporation).
- Coating the expression vector on the gold particles which are introduced in host cells by bombardment (particle bombardment).
- Directly adding or knocking out genes in cultured cells and implanting in surrogate dams to generate somatic cell cloned animals which are also transgenic (cell transformation).
- Genes can be introduced into oocytes or spermatocytes and their transformed gametes used for fertilization, generating a whole animal (transformation of gametes).

Use of any of the above method will bring about successful transformation in only small percentage of animals so produced. The transgenic animals can then be identified and bred to develop a transgenic line.

## APPLICATIONS AND THEIR POTENTIAL BENEFITS

GM animals pose a range of possible benefits to food production or human health. Such animals are at various stages of development. Early applications for approval of transgenic animals for food production being several species of fishes expression introduced growth hormone genes. Production of GM livestock is challenging and expensive because of their low productive rate, internal fertilization and slow development. Many transgenic founder animals are mosaic for transgene, i.e., they have it in some but not in all cells. Some examples of application of GM animals could be:

- **Improved animal production:**
  - Increased yield by accelerated growth rate or improved feed conversion rate
  - Improved disease resistance
  - Increased tolerance of environmental conditions such as low temperate
  - Improved digestibility of feed ingredients, e.g., phytase gene in pig
  - Approach could also be to adapt carnivorous fishes to plant based diet
- **Improved product quality:**
  - Change in nutritional profiles
  - Removal of allergens from food
  - Novel ornamental animals such as fluorescent protein genes expressed in zebrafish
  - Novel products including pharmaceuticals for human and veterinary use
  - Bioindicators/sensors for pollution
  - Cells, tissues and organs for xenotransplantation

## LABELING OF GM PRODUCTS

Food labels must be designed to clearly convey accurate information about the product in simple language. This may be the greatest challenge faced by a new food labeling policy which could educate and inform the public without damaging the public trust and causing alarm or fear of GM food products. Consumer interest groups are demanding mandatory labeling. People have the right to know what they are eating.

The FDA's current position on food labeling is governed by the Food, Drug and Cosmetic Act which is only concerned with food additives, not whole foods or food products that are considered GRAS (generally recognized as safe). The FDA contends that GM foods are substantially equivalent to non-GM foods, and therefore not subject to more stringent labeling. The new Food Safety and Standards Authority of India has to prepare adequate guidelines in this matter.

## FOOD-RELATED HAZARDS ASSOCIATED WITH PRODUCING GM ANIMALS

It is very important to consider the hazards or degree of harm that may be posed by GM animals and marine products. The full range of benefits from use of GM animals will depend on advances of technical aspects of their production.

- Introduction of a transgene into an animal is not a precisely controlled process and can result in a variety of outcomes with respect to integration, expression and stability of the transgene in the host.
- The development of pigs for Xenotransplantation raises the possibility that pigs might become more susceptible to human viruses. This could provide an alternative host for spread of human diseases.
- The potential entry of GM animals or their transgenes can affect food safety. The current status of development calls food safety managers to deal first with GM fish and shell fish and somewhat later for some kinds of GM poultry such as ducks and quails.

## APPROACHES TO SAFETY ASSESSMENT OF GM ANIMAL AND MARINE PRODUCTS

The food safety assessment of GM animal products can largely be performed on the lines that have been established for evaluation of GM plants and derived products for the consumer (Codex Alimentarius Commission, 2003). The traditional animal products may serve as a baseline for comparison for assessment of safety. The basic idea is that GM derived food products should be at least as safe as the traditional products.

- In terms of classical risk assessment (CSA), the approach should be to do both hazard identification and characterization. It will involve:
  - Safety assessment of gene product which should be done case-by-case. It will require limited evaluation process of the available data on protein. In theory, production of GM animals may lead to the introduction of many new proteins without a history of safe use into human diet. In the case of unknown proteins, a classic toxicological assessment procedure should form part of the evaluation. A clear distinction should be made between GM animals developed for food purposes and GM animals developed for pharmaceutical or industrial purposes.

- Allergenicity of the newly expressed proteins in the GM animal should be assessed. There is no single parameter that can predict the allergenic potential of a substance. Animal models for allergenicity testing may be useful.
- Unintended effect could be an other concern in GM animal products. Hence, compositional analysis leased on validated scientific method for macro- and micronutrients should be done and compared with the traditional or conventional product.

- Food intake assessment is must on such complex foods to determine the amount of food or food ingredients that can be consumed by an individual or population group. The effect of GM animal products on the vulnerable consumers such as pregnant or lactating woman or specific patent groups should be studied.
- Risk characterization involves integrating the outcome of the full toxicological and nutritional evaluation in order to reach an overall conclusion. If the safety standards are not at par with conventional counterpart, GM animal product should not be approved for marketing.
- Post-market surveillance is an appropriate risk management measure. It may require the establishment of an adequate product tracing system. The use of post-market surveillance should also be done to gain information on the potential long-term or unexpected adverse and beneficial effects of GM animal products.

## ECONOMIC CONCERNS

- Bringing a GM food to market is a lengthy and costly process.
- Many new genetic engineering technologies have been patented, and consumer are worried that patenting these new GM technologies will raise the price of the products so high that third world countries will not be able to afford these products, thus widening the gap between the rich and poor.

Governments around the world are working hard to establish a regulatory process to monitor the effects and approval of new varieties of GM animal and marine products. However, different governments are responding in different ways depending on the political, social and economic climate within a region or country. Government of India is yet to announce a definite policy on GM foods although the matter is being discussed at various platforms.

Lastly, the production of GM animals and derived products raise a variety of ethical and animal welfare issues. It may serve the interest of producer or consumer but it will disturb the natural genetic make up of animals and may derive them to unintended deformities. A proper set of ethical principles need to be established for dignity, fairness and welfare considerations comprising the elimination of genetic welfare and increasing the positive welfare.

# 29 CHAPTER

# Packaging Materials for Livestock and Poultry Products

Food packaging materials can be divided into the following two broad categories:

I. Flexible packing materials
II. Rigid packaging materials

## FLEXIBLE PACKAGING MATERIALS

### Aluminum Foil

Plain aluminum foil in the thickness of 0.025 mm to 0.15 mm is used in packaging food products requiring protection against light, water vapor and gases. Alu foil in gauges less than 0.025 mm have pin holes increasing with the decrease in thickness. These low gauges Alu foils of poor mechanical strengthen are generally laminated to paper or heat sealable films or paper board with suitable bonding agents which markedly brings down their permeability to water vapor and gases.

Flexible pouches of these laminates are used for packaging dehydrated cooked meat. Alu foil provides colorful and decorative printing base in package labeling. Steel foil in gauges from 0.025 mm to 0.1125 mm has also been made available for packaging applications. It is extremely strong, puncture resistant and can be laminated to paper, paper board and other packaging materials.

### Plastics

Plastic films are quite popular in food packaging due to their unique properties. Some physico-chemical properties of plastic films are shown in **Table 29.1**.

#### *Polyethylene (PE)*

It is obtained by polymerization of ethylene. Low density polyethylene (LDPE) is prepared by exposing ethylene to a very high pressure of

**Table 29.1:** Some physico-chemical properties of packaging films.

| *Film* | *Density/ specific gravity* | *Clarity* | *Tensile strength (kg/cm²)* | *Elongation* | *Tear resistance (g/100 gauge)* | *Heat seal range (°C)* | *WVTR (g/m²/ 24 hr at 38°C and 90% RH)* | *GTR (O²) (cc/100 gauge/ m² hr at NTP)* |
|---|---|---|---|---|---|---|---|---|
| Polyethylene (low density) | 0.910–0.925 | Transparent to Translucent | 80–240 | 220–600 | 100–400 | 120–175 | 20 | 4000–12500 |
| Polyethylene (high density) | 0.941–0.965 | Translucent to opaque | 200–350 | 50–400 | 50–300 | 138–155 | 5–10 | 500–4000 |
| Polypropylene | 0.88–0.90 | Transparent | 300–400 | 200–500 | 40–300 | 160–200 | 7–10 | 1200–6500 |
| PVDC/Saran | 1.65–1.70 | Transparent | 500–800 | 40–80 | 10–20 | 135–150 | 2–5 | 10–25 |
| Polyamide (nylon) | 1.13–1.14 | Transparent to Translucent | 700–1000 | 250–500 | 50–150 | 175–250 | Very high | 25–100 |
| Polyester | 1.15–1.39 | Transparent | 750–1500 | 70–120 | 15–75 | 135–200 | 15 | 50–125 |
| polystyrene | 1.05 | Transparent | 350–500 | 10–50 | 5–20 | 120–160 | >100 | 2500–7500 |
| Cellulose acetate | 1.25–1.35 | Transparent | – | 15–50 | 2–10 | 175–230 | Very high | 1500–3000 |
| Cellophane (polycoated) | 1.25 | Transparent to Translucent | – | 15.15 | 2–10 | 100–150 | >20 | 5–10 |

about 1200 atmospheres at temperatures between 150–200°C in the presence of traces of oxygen. High density polyethylene (HDPE) is prepared at 40 atmospheric pressure at temperature between 60–150°C in the presence of metal catalysts. Medium density polyethylene (MDPE) can also be produced.

Their density ranges are as follows:

| | | |
|---|---|---|
| LDPE | : | 0.910–0.925 g/cu cm |
| MDPE | : | 0.926–0.940 g/cu cm |
| HDPE | : | 0.941–0.965 g/cu cm |

Different density grades of this polymer do not differ chemically but their physical properties vary to some extent. Polyethylene is inert chemically and insoluble in all organic solvents upto 60°C. It is tasteless, odorless and non-toxic in nature.

It has a softening point of about 99°C for film grades and the melting point range between 110 to 115°C. So, it can be conveniently used up to a temperature of about 70°C. One of the most advantageous features of the polyethylene is its heat-sealability to itself to give liquid tight seals. It is due to this reason that LDPE is extensively used in coating and laminating composite packaging materials, where it forms the inner-most layer requiring good heat sealability **(Fig. 29.1)**. The film is capable of elongation from 400 to 600% before being ruptured.

Low density polyethylene (LDPE) provides the benefit of maximum flexibility and very low cost. It retains flexibility even at low temperatures (–60°C). It has very low permeability to water-vapors, but it is fairly permeable to oxygen or carbon dioxide or odors. HDPE film is about three times less permeable to water vapor than LDPE. The permeability rate increases by two to five-fold with every 10°C rise in storage temperature. Thus, LDPE meets the requirement of being a fairly tough water-vapor proof film at low temperature. LDPE begins to swell on prolonged contact with oil and grease and offers little resistance to them against grease resistance property of HDPE, which has very high thermal stability as well and offers excellent protection against moisture loss. It is used in film form as well as rigid plastic containers including milk bottles.

*Polypropylene*

Polypropylene is produced by polymerization of propylene at low pressure in the presence of catalysts. It has very high flex strength, resistance and a good gloss surface. It softens at about 150°C and melts at 170°. It is readily heat sealable. The film has low water vapor permeability and a good resistance to oil and grease.

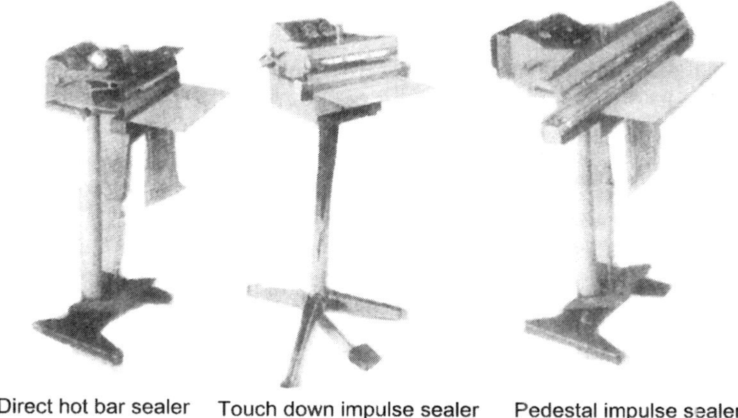

Direct hot bar sealer  Touch down impulse sealer  Pedestal impulse sealer

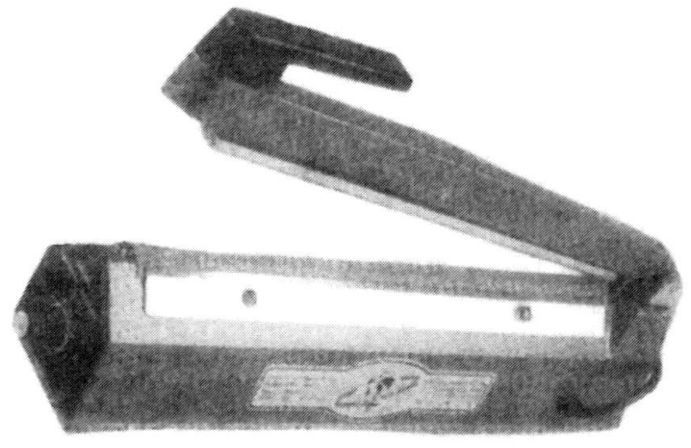

Imulse sealer

**Fig. 29.1:** Different types of sealing machines.

The unoriented film is stable at low temperature and is a poor gas barrier, making it suitable for wrap packaging. Mono and biaxially oriented films are used for shrink packaging whereas heat-set biaxially oriented films are used for laminations. It can be co-extruded with polyethylene to impart desired sealing and barrier characteristics. Polypropylene lamination with other films is utilized for vacuum and gas packaging of processed meats. In dairy industry, it may be suitably put to use in packaging of cheese.

*Polyamides (Nylons)*

Polyamides, usually called Nylons in trade, are condensation polymers of diamines with diacids. They are inert, heat resistant due to high softening and melting point and have excellent mechanical strength. They are grease resistant and have low permeability gases but are fairly permeable to water vapors. They are usually coated or used in combination with other materials to produce packaging materials of good inertness as well as low permeability. Nylon-6, Nylon-11, Nylon-12, etc., have found use in packaging of foods. Nylon-6 films are tasteless and odorless making them ideal for packaging of processed foods. It can be sterilized by steam/gas or gamma radiation technique. It can also be used for boil-in-bag processing of convenience foods. It offers excellent gas barrier properties. So, a major use of Nylon-6 is in packaging of bacon using automatic vacuum-packaging process. Nylon composites - laminates or co-extruded films with LDPE are used in the packaging of oils and fats.

*Polyester*

Polyester is the condensation produce of a polyalcohol with diacids or its anhydride. The polyester of most importance in food packaging is polyethylene terephthalate (PET), a condensation product of ethylene glycol and terephthalic acid, better known in US trade as Mylar. It is crystalline linear polymer of excellent mechanical strength and inertness. It has moderate water vapor and low gas permeability. It is resistant to high temperature and can be handled in thin gauges. So, it is widely used in lamination with aluminum foil as outer, abrasion-resistance layer for food pouches.

PET bottles and containers can be molded in any shape, size and color to suit specific product requirements. These are extremely clear, virtually unbreakable, very light weighing just about 1/15th the weight of glass, excellent gas barrier and are most hygienic for packaging edible products. These are quite economic due to cut in handling and transportation cost and prevention of breakage loss. The enhanced visual appeal of the product in PET containers leads to higher sales.

*Cellophane*

Although cellophanes have a natural polymer, cellulose as major constituent, these are frequently classified as plastics. Plain cellophane is made from sulphite pulp **(Flowchart 29.1)**.

**Flowchart 29.1:** Manufacture of plain cellophane.

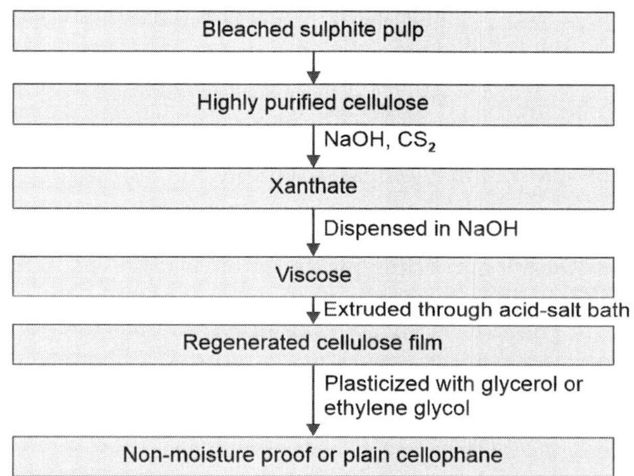


It can be suitable coated on one side or both sides to impact desired functional properties. The usual coatings are nitrocellulose, PVDC, vinyl copolymer and polyethylene. This cellulosic film has assumed importance in flexible packaging due to low cost, heat resistance, good machinability and dimensional stability. It has been customary to letter designate the functional properties of the cellulosic film. The following letter designations are of common use:

A. Anchored
C. Colored
D. Demi (one side) coated
M. Moisture proof
O. Opaque
S. Heat sealing
T. Transparent
XX. Polymer coated

MSADT cellophane is coated only on one side with a special nitrocellulose or polyethylene. At the time of packaging fresh meat uncoated side is kept in direct contact with meat.

*Ethylene-vinyl Acetate (EVA) Copolymers*

EVA film is obtained by copolymerization of LDPE and vinyl acetate (up to 20%). Copolymerization allows package tailoring of polymers to suit specific functional requirements. EVA is far superior to PE in clarity, flexibility and resistance. Its high impact strength offers comparatively thin gauge of this film for similar applications than PE. However, it is unstable at high temperature and has higher water and gas permeability.

EVA coating on bags and industrial sacks improves stackability. Bags can be produced to stretch wrap products like frozen poultry without the use of a shrink tunnel. EVA is also suitable for lamination due to good adhesion and heat sealability.

### *Polystyrene (PS)*

It is a transparent and brittle plastic which is usually copolymerized with acrylonitrile and butadiene to make it flexible. Polystyrene is a multiutility plastic. It can be thermoformed as cups for yoghurt, ice cream, cheese, etc., whereas expanded polystyrene can be thermoformed as meat trays.

### *Rubber Hydrochloride (Pliofilm)*

This film is produced by the action of hydrochloride on natural rubber. It is non-toxic, stretchable, grease resistant and heat sealable. It is a good gas barrier and has found use in the short-term packaging of meat and cheese.

### *Vinyl Films*

Polyvinyl chloride (PVC) films are made by polymerizing vinyl chloride in the presence of catalysts. Since it is a hard brittle material, it has to be plasticized to make it flexible. Food grade plasticizers, catalysts and stabilizers are used to obtain PVC of food grade. PVC bottles are used for packing edible oil, pickles, etc.

Vinylidene chloride copolymer (Saran, Cryovac) is produced within 13–20% vinyl chloride. It contains very little plasticizers, stabilizers and slip agents. This film is clear, nontoxic and its permeability to water vapor and gases is very low. It is almost impervious to odor transmission. This film is used for packaging of meat, sausages and cheese.

Polyvinyl acetate copolymer is used for packaging meat and cheese as a seamless coating. It is also used as a coating on paper. Polyvinyl alcohols are insoluble in many organic solvents but readily soluble in water. Hence, they are used as lining on paper for oil and fat packaging.

### *Ionomer*

Ionomer is a unique thermoplastic with ionic bonds. In Surlyn-A, an ionomer of LDPE, ionic bonds serve to increase overall bond strength, melt strength and yield superior oil, grease and solvent resistance. It has a very good clarity. An ionomer usually serves as an ideal bonding agent between two films and has better seal strength.

## Specific Films

### *Shrink Films*

Many thermoplastic films such as polyethylene, polypropylene, polyvinylidene chloride, polyester and polystyrene can be mono- or biaxially oriented to stay stretched at ambient temperature. This property is built into the plastic film during manufacture by stretching it under controlled temperature and tension to create molecular orientation and then locking the film in this stretched condition by cooling **(Fig. 29.2)**.

Shrink films are used for wrapping comparatively large and uneven cuts of fresh meat. These are also frequently recommended for storage

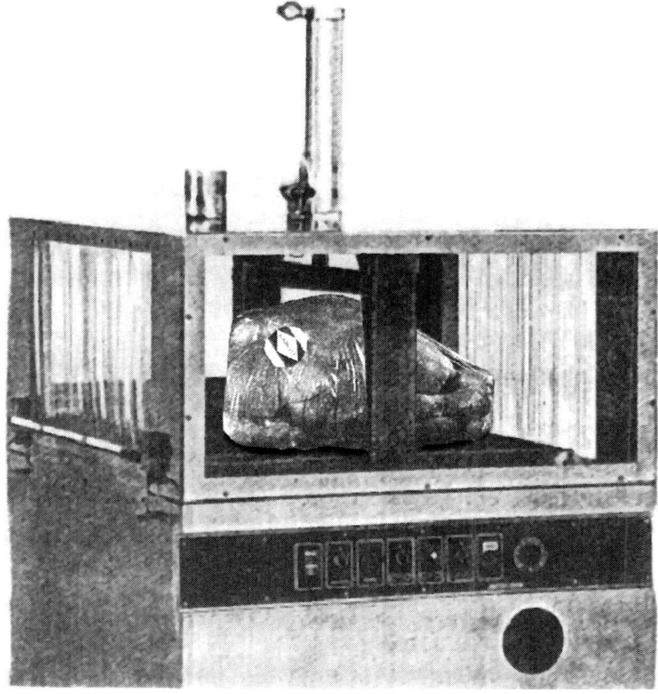

**Fig. 29.2:** Shrink pack and shrinkage tank to effect the same.

of carcass quarters and dressed poultry under frozen conditions. Uneven meat cuts or dressed birds are over-wrapped with such films and passed through hot air tunnel or dipped in water tub maintained at 90°C for few seconds to effect shrinkage of the film. The stretched films shrink almost to their original size.

Shrink films usually have high structural strength and can withstand storage temperature down to –45°C. These packaging films offer neat appearance, contour tight package and are easy to handle.

*Composite Films*

a. **Laminate:** Laminate is a combination of different flexible packaging materials such as paper, plastics or foil bonded together by heat/ adhesive forming a composite structure of uniform thickness and flexibility. Lamination greatly improves the barrier properties, provides required functional properties and heat sealability. Some typical laminates are:
   Polyester/PE
   Nylon/PE
   Paper/Alu foil/PE
   Polyester/Alu foil/PE, etc.
b. **Coextruded film:** It is obtained by simultaneous extrusion of two or more polymers in a molten stage, from a common die to emerge out as a single layer. The advantage of co-extrusion over lamination comes from the ability to produce composite film (consisting of many layers) in one pass. This process reduces the film thickness and cost of the composite structure. Some typical co-extruded films are:
   *LDPE/HDPE/LDPE*
   *LDPE/LDPE*
   *LDPE/HDPE*
   *LPPE/HDPE/Ionomer*
   *LDPE/Nylon/HDPE, etc.*

## Paper

In flexible packaging, the basic papers used may be:

i. Bond paper
ii. Tissue paper
iii. Litho paper
iv. Kraft paper
v. **Glassine paper:** They have high resistance to air and grease. A plasticizer may be added to give the paper softness and machinability for wrapping ice candy.

vi. **Parchment paper:** They have good grease resistance and high wet strength. It is generally used as wrapper for butter.

## RIGID PACKAGING MATERIALS

### Metal Cans

Metal cans are primarily used for heat-sterilized food products. These are made up of tinplate or aluminum or tin-free steel. Tin plate consists of a base sheet of steel with very thin tin coating on either side applied by hot dipping or electrolytic process. Atypical tinplate may be 0.01 inch thick with tin coating contributing only about 0.0006 inch to this thickness. Tin layer is more uniform with electrolytic tin coating process. Differential tin coating may be applied on the internal and external side of cans. The thickness of internal coating should be appropriate for food whereas the external tin coating may be thinner and generally applied to prevent corrosion on long term storage.

To make the can more suitable for specific packaging applications, lacquers are applied to the tin. The composition of the lacquer (enamel), which is applied as a very thin layer depends on the foods stuffs to be packed. Lacquers must be nontoxic and free from odor or taste. It must adhere firmly and should not deteriorate. Sulfur-resistant internal lacquers usually zinc oxide added oleoresins are used for meat products to check the discoloration (sulfur staining) arising as a result of decomposition of meat proteins. Others in use are phenolics, epoxy esters, etc., external lacquers include alkyds, acrylics, vinyl, etc., and are usually pigmented. They are less exposed to food contact but must survive processing and be receptive to decorative printing.

Can bodes are soldered, welded or cemented. Soldering is being replaced these days to avoid contamination of foods by lead from the soldered side seams. Many easy open devices like panels for meat products are available these days. Use of cemented cans are restricted to nonprocessed products because the cement is not capable of standing processing. Aluminum cans have not been used extensively for heat sterilized food products. An interior lacquering is usually necessary. Shallow drawn cans have less space and have been used for packing processed meat and fish products. Deep drawn aluminum cans usually have round shape and are used for processed food products like powdered milk, condensed milk, etc.

The double seaming process is now gaining ground because of its ability to form a hermetic seal. This is necessary to prevent leakage and also to prevent sucking in of bacteria when the contents are being processed. The overlap of cover hook and body hook expressed as a percent of the seam length is called percentage overlap. An overlap of 45% or above should be achieved in double seaming.

Due to shortage of metallic tin and its high cost, tin free steel (TFS) has been developed by replacing tin with chromium metal. Advantages of tin free steel cans are ease of fabrication, strong corrosion resistance against acid and alkali solution, strong resistance to sulfur staining and suitability for attractive printing. Lacquered tin free steel cans can be used for products like meat, fish and vegetables. Advantages of metal cans are excellent strength, excellent machinability and production of products in commercially sterile conditions. The drawbacks are comparatively more weight and problems of reclosure and disposal.

## Glass Containers

Glass containers are one of the most versatile packages used in food packaging. These are universally available and hold a distinct place in the packaging field. The advantages of glass from food packaging point of view are:

- It is chemically inert in nature.
- It allows excellent product visibility.
- It is an excellent barrier to solids, liquids and gases.
- It can be molded into various shapes and sizes.
- Good quality glass containers can withstand sterilization temperature.
- It is refillable.

### *Disadvantages*

- It is fragile. So breakage risk is also there.
- It is comparatively heavy weight.
- It is not so easy to dispose of.

### *Package Forms*

| | | |
|---|---|---|
| Bottle | : | Neck round, much narrower than body. |
| Jars | : | Wide mouthed bottles, no appreciable neck. The opening permits insertion of fingers. |
| Tumbler | : | Like jars but open ended. |
| Jag | : | Large sized bottles with carrying handles. |
| Carboys | : | Heavy shipping containers shaped like a short necked bottle having three gallon or more capacity. Typically they have been used with a wooden crate holder. |

Vials and ampules : Small glass containers used mainly for pharmaceuticals. May be used for food color, flavor, etc.

## Rigid Plastic Packages

**Thermoformed containers** are prepared by exposing the plastic sheet to heat and forming into a female or around a male mold. Vacuum forming, pressure forming and several other techniques are used. Thermoformed trays have many food applications ranging from meat trays to formed polystyrene foam trays for eggs. The plastics used for thermoformed trays are HDPE, PVC, PS and PP, cellulose acetate is also used for this purpose. The specific plastic selected is dependent on the food packaged and storage requirements needed.

**Polystyrene trays** are clear but become brittle at low temperature whereas linear polyethylene trays are somewhat flexible but they give a cloudy appearance. All thermoformed trays are generally covered with a heat sealable plastic film or aluminum foil laminates. Most widely used plastics are polystyrene and polypropylene. One of the major advantages of the use of polystyrene is its excellent clarity. In general, advantages of rigid plastic containers are low cost and ease of fabrication.

## Wooden Boxes and Crates

Wooden boxes are usually solidly walled, rectangular and nailed containers. They vary in size as per the requirement of load. The top, bottom and size of a box provide the structural strength. Wooden crates are lighter in weight and spaces are left between boards. Here frame members carry the load. A sheath made up of corrugated fiber board may be used before the item is put in wooden crate.

## Fiberboard and Cardboard Boxes

Fiberboard or cardboard boxes are used to make shipping cases used exclusively in bulk packaging. They are made by gluing various liner and corrugated plies. Corrugated fiber board and boxes may be made up of 3, 5 or 7 plies. Their main advantages are versatility, light weight, disposability and low cost. Major disadvantage being low wet strength, which can be improved by various coatings.

30

CHAPTER

# Testing and Specifications of Packaging Materials and Packages

## THICKNESS OF PACKAGING FILMS

Thickness can be defined as the perpendicular distance between the inner and outer surfaces of a packaging material. It has a profound influence on the physicochemical and strength properties of the packaging films, e.g., low-density polyethylene films of 100 gauge and 150 gauge thickness have tensile strength of 3.7 and 4 kg/15 mm, elongation value of 300 and 250%, bursting strength of 0.98 and 0.90/ $cm^2$ and testing resistance of 27 and 18 g respectively in machine direction. Water vapor and gas transmission rates of plastic films also decrease with increase in thickness, e.g., high-density polyethylene films of 200 gauge and 300 gauge thickness have water vapor transmission rate (WVTR) of 1.9 and 1.5 g/$m^2$/24 hrs at 38°C and 90% relative humidity (RH).

Thickness of plastic films is measured on dial gauge or micrometer **(Fig. 30.1)**. Usually ten readings are taken at different places in the films and their average is taken as a measure of thickness. High-quality films do not show much variation in thickness measurement at different points.

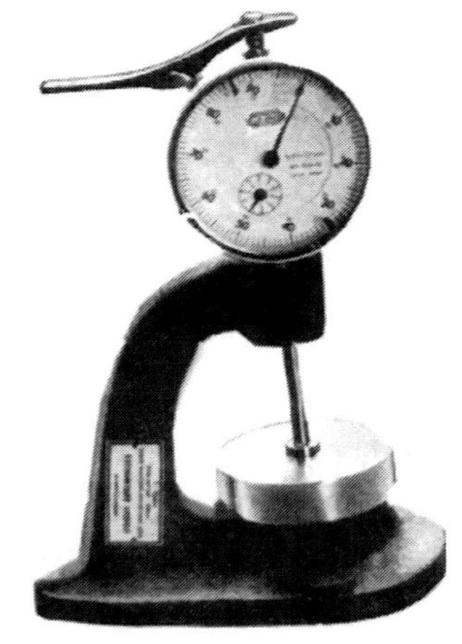

**Fig. 30.1:** Thickness gauge tester.

Thickness of plastic films is measured in gauge in British system, mil in American system, mm in metric system and micron (μm) in continental system. The following factors can be of much help in their inter-conversion:

100 gauge = 1 mil
= 1/1000 inch
= 0.001 inch
= 0.025 mm
= 25 micron (μm)

## STRENGTH PROPERTIES OF PACKAGING FILMS

### Tensile Strength

The strength of a packaging film determines its resistance to rupture when subjected to a pulling force. It is expressed in kg/15 mm width.

High tensile strength is necessary for flexible packaging materials to hold heavy packages and when packages are formed in semi-automatic or automatic pouch forming and filling machines and also in operations such as coating-laminated or printing.

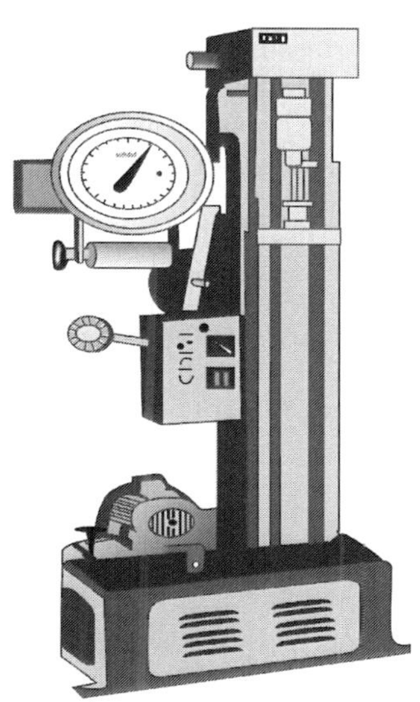

**Fig. 30.2:** Tensile strength tester.

Most of the films and laminates have a tensile strength of 3-6 kg/15 mm width. It is less in transverse direction (TD) than in machine direction (MD). All strength parameters in packaging films are taken in both the directions because the values differ. The molecular orientation of a packaging film in MD and TD are very much different. The tensile strength is more in the MD than in the TD.

Elongation properties of a packaging film are measured on the tensile strength tester itself **(Fig. 30.2)**. It denotes the length to which the film can be stretched by using a pulling force. It is expressed in percentage.

For packages which are likely to experience drop during distribution require material of higher elongation value of 200–500%, whereas some plastic films like low-density polyethylene (LDPE) show an elongation value of 300–500%.

## Bursting Strength

It is a measure of the pressure which a packaging material sheet can resist before bursting. It is expressed in kg/cm$^2$. The bursting strength values can be used as a rough guide to complete the general strength properties of packaging films. Most of the unsupported films and laminates have bursting strength values between 0.7 and 2.0 kg/cm$^2$.

**Tester:** This machine operates on the uniform pressure distribution principles of hydraulics. The fluid expands under uniformly increasing pressure against a distensible rubber diaphragm and simultaneously into a pressure gauge. The material to be tested is clamped securely into the machine and hydraulic pressure is applied. As the material bursts, the pressure drops suddenly, but the indicator remains static to indicate the exact pressure at which the bursting occurred **(Fig. 30.3)**.

## Puncture Resistance

It gives a reliable indication of the protection by the packaging materials and containers against puncture hazards in handling and transit. It is expressed in Oz/tear inch and is measured by puncture resistance tester **(Fig. 30.4)**.

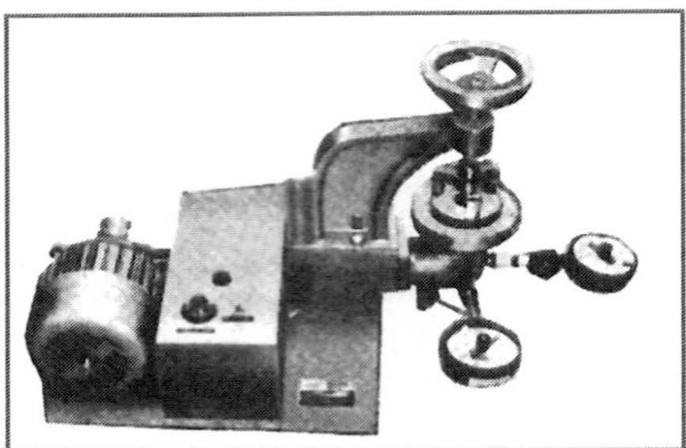

**Fig. 30.3:** Bursting strength tester.

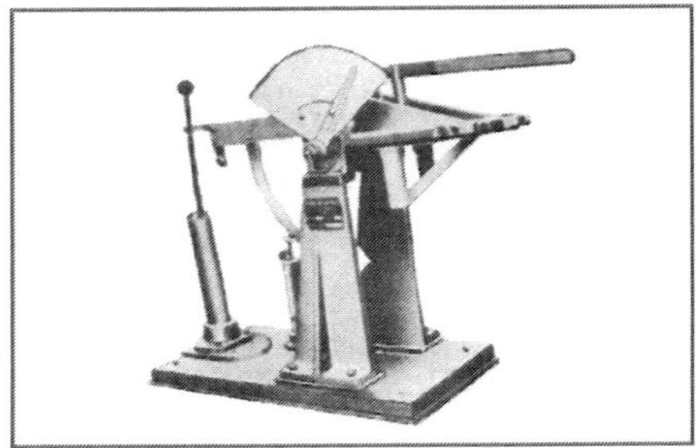

**Fig. 30.4:** Puncture resistance tester.

### Tearing Resistance

This is the measurement of the resistance to the propagation of a slight tear in the flexible packaging material. It is expressed in gm. This property is important for packaging materials which are used to package sharp-edged food products. Tearing strength depends on orientation of molecules in the packaging material. PE has a very high tear resistance values since high elongation is normally associated with high tear resistance.

## CHEMICAL IDENTIFICATION OF DIFFERENT PLASTIC FILMS

To find out the given sample, one square inch samples of known film is cut and placed in a 50 mL round bottom flask together with 15 mL of appropriate solvent. The flask is filled with water cool reflux condenser to prevent solvent loss. Carry out the procedure as shown in the diagram and find out the given sample **(Flowchart 30.1)**:

**Flowchart 30.1:** Procedure.

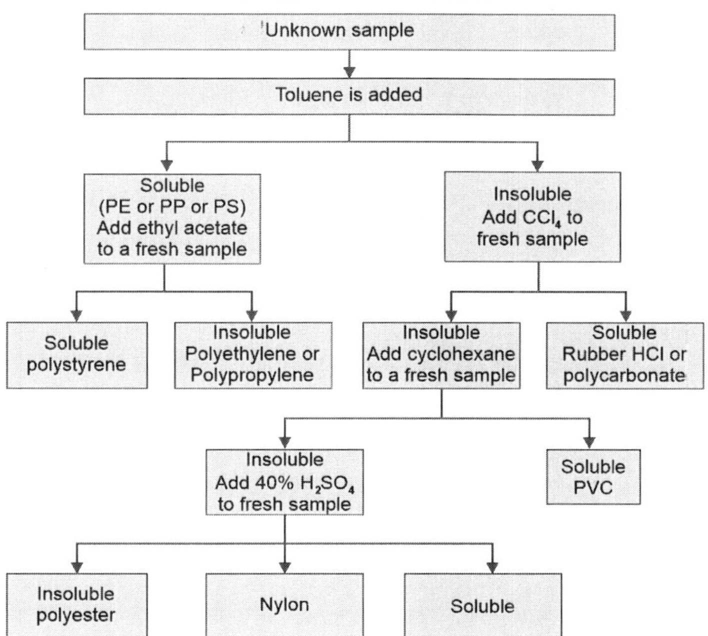

## IDENTIFICATION OF PACKAGING FILMS BY FLAME TEST

Burning behavior of plastic packaging films and the color and other characteristics of flame can guide us to their tentative identification which can be further confirmed on the basis of chemical tests.

The pieces of films are burnt on a Bunsen flame for a short while and the burning characteristics—the flame, film response, smell, etc., are carefully recorded. **Table 30.1** can be of much help in this respect:

**Table 30.1:** Burning characteristics of packaging films.

| *Plastic film* | *Characteristics of the flame* | *Burning behavior of the film* | *Smell* | *Self-extinguishing or not* |
|---|---|---|---|---|
| Polythene | Yellow top with blue bottom | Melts and drips | Burnt paraffin | No |
| Polypropylene | -do- | -do- | Acrid burnt | No |
| Polyvinyl chloride | Orange yellow with green edges | Darkens rapidly, softens and decomposes | Typical chlorine | Yes |
| Polyamide (nylon) | Yellow top with blue bottom | Melts and drips with froths. Drips cannot be crushed | Burning hair | Yes |
| Polyester | Burns steadily with yellow black flame | No drips | Pleasant resin odour | No |
| Polythene | Orange yellow with black sooty smoke | Softens, without drip | Marigold odor | No |
| Cellulose acetate | Yellow top with blue bottom | Melts, burns quickly with irregular charred beads | Burnt vinegar | No |

## WVTR AND GTR OF PACKAGING FILMS

### Water Vapor Transmission Rate (WVTR)

Moisture loss or gain, through the packaging films or package during storage and distribution affects the quality and shelf-life of food. WVTA is measured as the quantity of water vapor in grams which will permeate through one square meter of a film in 24 hours at 38°C and 90% RH. Thus, WVTR determines the efficiency of a packaging film to the transmission of water vapors. Films and laminates of very low WVTR are used for the packaging of hygroscopic foods.

WVTR is measured with the help of specially designed aluminium dish which is filled with finely ground calcium chloride at the bottom. Now accurately weighed plastic film is put over the dish and all the sides are sealed with microcrystalline wax by using a wax applicator. The initial weight of dish is noted.

The dish is put in the humidity cabinet at a temperature of 38°C and 90% RH **(Fig. 30.5)**. The increase in weight of the dish is noted every day for six days. Average gain in weight of aluminium dish in 24 hours gives the quantity of water vapor which could permeate through the film. The same is calculated on the basis of square meter area of the film. The observations are taken in duplicate.

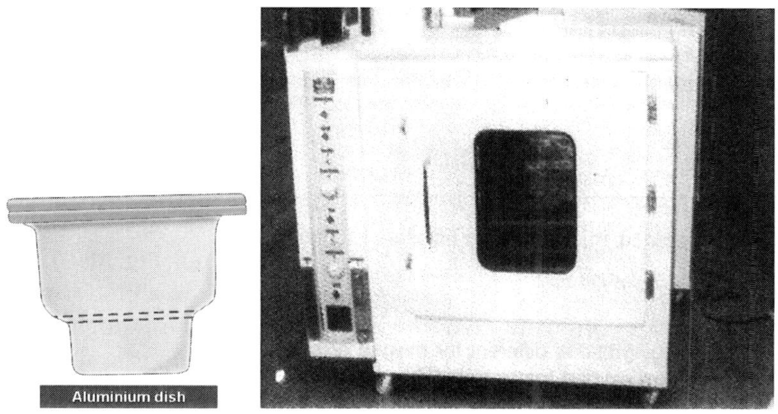


**Fig. 30.5:** Humidity cabinet.

### Gas Transmission Rate (GTR)

Gas transmission rate is measured as the effectiveness of a packaging film in resisting the permeability of a particular gas through a unit area. The measurement is done in terms of change in volume at constant pressure. At normal temperature and pressure (NTP) it is calculated as cc/m$^2$/24 hrs.

GTR of a packaging film is different for oxygen or carbon dioxide of other gases. Films of low oxygen transmission rate (OTR) or oxygen barrier laminates are selected for oxygens sensitive foods to prevent the development of oxidative rancidity.

## PERFORMANCE EVALUATION OF TRANSPORT PACKAGES

### Bulk or Wholesale Packaging

This packaging is done with the aim to transport a product from the point of production or wholesaler to the retainer in sound condition. Bulk packaging should meet all the necessary requirements for a very good transport worthiness.

### Unit or Retail Packaging

It is also called consumer packaging because size of packaging is optimized such that the food contents can suffice the requirement of a family. It does not involve fresh packaging exercise at the retail store. So, there is no chance of pilferage or underweighing at the retail store. However, unit packaging invariable adds to the cost of the product.

The tests are used to evaluate the transport worthiness of bulk packages.

#### *Drop Test*

This is the most important test for testing the performance of package during transport, especially that of bulk packages such as corrugated fibre boxes, wooden shipping containers, etc.

The package is kept on resting table of drop tester **(Fig. 30.6)**. By pressing the lever the container is allowed to fall on a platform at the bottom, by the corner sides and edges. The fall is straight and perfectly vertical. The height and weight relationship is as follows **(Table 30.2)**:

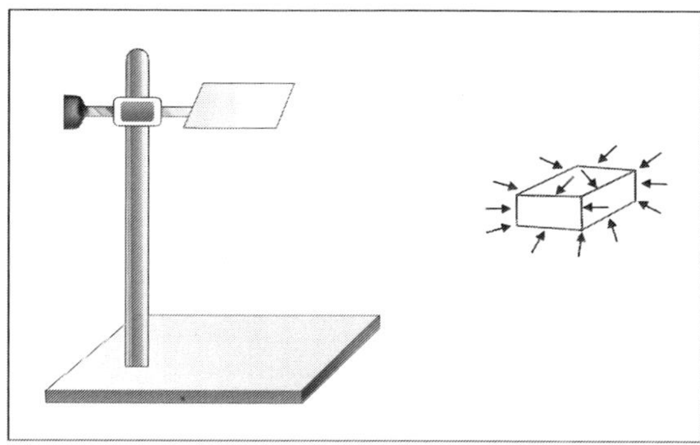

**Fig. 30.6:** Drop tester.

**Table 30.2:** The height and weight relationship is drop test.

| *Weight* | *Height* |
|---|---|
| 0–10 kg | 105 cm |
| >10–25 kg | 90 cm |
| >25–125 kg | 75 cm |
| >125–250 kg | 60 cm |

Height is adjusted as per the weight of filled-in packages and observations are made.

*Inclined Impact Test*

The bulk container is kept on the inclined impact tester which moves with the speed of 8 km/h. Each phase of the container is tested for 6 inclined impacts. A bulk package must be able to bear these impacts for excellent transport worthiness **(Fig. 30.7)**.

*Vibration Test*

It is conducted to test the packages which are to be transported by train. The packages are put on the vibration table which vibrates with the speed of 120 cycles/min. for a known time. An hour of vibration represents 1,000 kms transit by train.

*Stack Load Test*

Bulk containers are tested for the load they can bear. By stacking different weights on the package their stackability during shipment is determined.

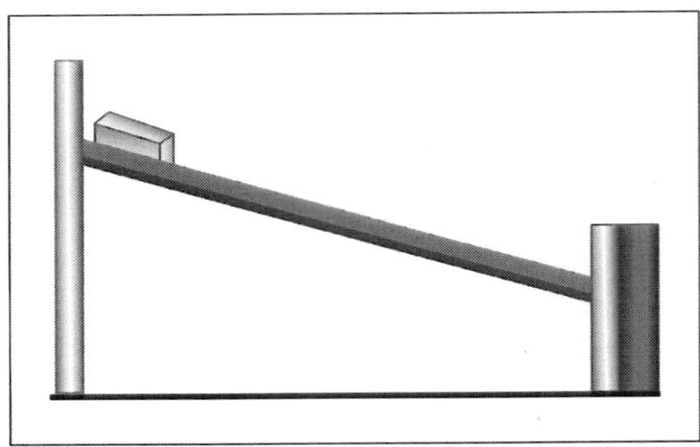

**Fig. 30.7:** Inclined impact tester.

*Rolling Test*

Certain containers may have to be rolled during shipment. So the capacity of a container to withstand rolling is also tested.

All these tests to evaluate transport worthiness are not done on all packages or containers. Various combinations are followed as give hereunder:

- **Combination 1**
    - Drop test
    - Vibration test
    - Rolling test
- **Combination 2**
    - Inclined impact test
    - Vibration test
    - Rolling test
- **Combination 3**
    - Drop test
    - Inclined impact test
    - Rolling test

## PACKAGING SPECIFICATIONS

Meat food products should be packed in such suitable containers as are described in the 'Fourth Schedule' of MFPO (1973).

- All containers shall be securely packed and sealed.
- New sanitary top can made from suitable type of the plate shall be used. The can shall be lacquered internally. They shall be sealed hermetically after filling. The lacquer used shall be sulphur-resistant and shall not be soluble in fat or brine.

- Cans used for filling pork, meat shall be coated internally with edible gelatin, lard or lined with vegetable parchment paper before being filled.
- The exterior of the cans shall be free from major dust, rust perforation and seal distortion. Can shall be free from leaks.
- Bottle and jars used for packing shall be clear and must be capable of being sealed hermetically.
  - Meat food products packed in hermetically sealed containers shall be processed to withstand spoilage under commercial condition of spoilage and transport.
  - Packaging material shall be cleaned and should be stored in clean and sanitary manner to prevent contamination of the final product.
  - No water other than potable water shall be used for cooking or cooling of any hermetically sealed container.
  - After processing, container should be handled in such a way to avoid contamination of product. Both running and other can conveying equipment shall be maintained in clean condition and good repair.
  - Processing food hermetically sealed containers shall be inspected to exclude the defective containers.
  - Every manufacturer shall provide adequate facilities for the random sampling.
  - The manufacturer shall cause an appropriate table to be affixed to each container after packing it with meat food products derived from meat which has been previously inspected and passed.
  - Specimen of all labels shall be first approved by the licensing authority before use.

## LABELING SPECIFICATIONS AS PER MFPO

The following particulars be clearly marked on the label:
- Net weight or volume of the content at the time of packing.
- Name of the product.
- Name of the manufacturers and place of manufacture.
- Where any preservative or any coloring agent other than natural color is added, a statement to the fact that it contains permitted preservatives or coloring agents other than natural color.
- License number and category of manufacture.
- Name of the product shall always be the common name which shall clearly identify the article packed and understood by the

consumer. In case of product prepared by salting, smoking, drying and cooking, etc., the process should be so indicated on the label.

- When any artificial flavoring agent is permitted to be used, this fact shall appear in prominent letter word (a flavored/artificially flavored).
- Every trade name shall have the prior approval of licensing authority. Any statement, word, picture or design that may convey false impression should not appear on the label.

The contents, ingredients should appear on the label in the decreasing order of their weight.

## MICROBIOLOGICAL EVALUATION OF CANNED FOODS

It is a general practice to take 12 cans as samples from each canning line per day or a production lot which refers to the cans produced under essentially same conditions. Association of Food and Drug Officials of US specify the examination of 10 packs per production lot.

Of the twelve cans, one half (6) are incubated at 37°C for 7 days whereas other half are incubated at 55°C for 14 days. These cans are examined daily for swells and bacteriological examination of swelled cans is normally conducted. At the end of incubation period, all the cans are opened and checked for spoilage, odors, discoloration and pH. The equipment required for total plate count include bottles of 99 mL, tubes of 9 mL, a high speed blender if solid food is examined, pipettes of 10, 1 and 0.1 mL and Petri dishes.

The number of bacteria in food is so large that in order to obtain discrete colonies in petri dish, the food must be cultured after dilution. The first dilution of usually 1:10 is prepared by placing 10 mL of food in 90 mL of diluents. In semisolid foods, a 1:10 dilution of food should be made by taking a quantity and adding the required amount of dilution water into sterile blender and blending for 2–3 minutes. Portion of 50 g of food and 450 mL of diluents are often used for this purpose. Further serial dilution is made from this and suitable media re-used for systematic microbiological evaluation as per ICMSF (1978).

MFPO (1973) specifies that canned meat products have to be tested essentially for trace elements like lead, tin, arsenic, copper and zinc which are health hazards beyond a particular limit.

## TAINT PROBLEMS IN PACKAGED FOODS

Taint refers to an undesirable change in the sensory qualities of packaged foods. It may be in form of undesirable taste or odor of a food product with or without adverse effect on color, texture, etc. Besides, food stuff may be rendered unacceptable in a container due to the presence of harmful trace elements, dirt, organic matter, etc.

Plastic packaging materials which come in close contact with foods may contain various additives such as plasticizers, stabilizers, colorants, besides residual monomers, solvents and catalysts. Minute quantities of these substances can, at times, lead to major effect on the acceptability of packaged foods. Traces of harmful elements including tin beyond a certain limit can migrate into canned foods causing taint. Several process deficiencies such as inadequate control of lamination, coating or printing or even heat sealing at excessive temperature may promote degradation of the polymer leading to taint in packaged food products. These are some of the most likely causes, although tainting can occur because of any of the following several reasons:

- Migration of normal constituents of a packaged material into the food product.
- Migration of food constituents into the packaging material.
- Migration of harmful trace elements of container into the foodstuff.
- Improper processing.
- Contamination of packaging material.
- Storage of packaged foods in the proximity of highly odorous substances.
- Penetration of printing ink or adhesive or inadequately dried varnish into the food product.

## Precautions to Check Taint Problems

- It is utmost important to use only food grade packaging materials.
- Paper-based packaging material should be stored in cool and dry places.
- In plastic packaging, processing conditions specified by the manufacturer should be strictly followed.
- Tin plate cans should be uniformly lacquered and chances of any solvent residue be eliminated.
- Coating, bonding and printing of laminates should be done under the direct supervision of qualified and experienced professionals.
- Plastic films for use in contact with livestock products should conform to Global Migration Tests especially with water, acetic acid and n-Haptane.
- Metal containers should be subjected to Blend test, Lacquer coating test, Porosity test, etc., to eliminate the main causes of taint in canned foods.

31

CHAPTER

# Sensory Evaluation of Meat Products in Practice

Demand for ready-to-eat products is increasing everyday and development of products and processes is regarded as a major thrust area. Therefore, it is the responsibility of meat technologists to cater to the culinary requirements and sensory quality of meat and meat products.

Sensory threshold of human senses is far ahead of the known instrumental techniques. Meat is one of the most palatable food items for non-vegetarians. Meat technologists, students and technicians involved in quality control of fresh and processed meats, new products development, storage studies and investigation of various palatability related problems require a thorough knowledge of Sensory Evaluation Techniques.

Sensory evaluation of foods including meat refers to their scientific evaluation through the application of human senses. Even though highly sensitive measuring instruments are now available, the importance of sensory analysis has grown over the years instead of doing down. The reason being that our senses which are biological detectors can perceive odor, taste, etc., even below the lowest limit of instrumental sensitivity. Instruments usually analyze only a single component at a time whereas the overall impression and taste of a food product can be properly assessed only by human sensory perception.

Specialized or product-oriented panel testing uses small number of trained panelists who function as testing instruments. Such panelists can easily identify differences among similar meat products or intensities of flavor, texture, appearance, etc., because they are selected on the basis of their sensory ability and specially trained for such a task.

## SELECTION AND TRAINING OF PANELISTS

The criteria identified for selection of panelists include willingness, availability, capability, sensitivity, selectivity, dependability and general health. The potential panelist should be asked to fill up questionnaire indicating their food likes or dislikes and food restrictions/allergies if any. For institutional sensory evaluation exercises, it is always useful to maintain a file regarding all potential panelists.

These panelists are invited to an orientation session where the panel leader explains the importance of sensory evaluation, shows the testing facilities and satisfies their curiosity. To screen the sensitivity of the panelists, recognition test (qualitative determination) and threshold test (quantitative determination) are employed. The recruited panelists are subjected to training for improving their individual sensitivity and memory, which enable them to arrive at precise and consistent sensory judgments. They are also familiarized with the important sensory qualities of meat products and commonly used test procedures. Training is the best accomplished by personal interviews, group discussion and improving their sensitivity further by serial dilution tests so as to enable them to use their senses as biological receptors **(Fig. 31.1)**.

A group of workers utilized five, 30 minutes training sessions to train the panelists for sensory evaluation of sausages. They concluded the training sessions when the sensory scores did not vary more than +1 from the mean scores (on 8-point hedonic scale). In contrast another group utilized only four preliminary sessions to train the panelists for sensory evaluation of bacon. In general, training to be given to selected individuals, till they become familiar with the attributes of the meat and meat products and attain a very good performance on hedonic or rating scale. In any particular study or test, substitution of panel members should be avoided.

On the basis of the training provided/required the sensory panels are categorized either trained or semi-trained. The trained panelists are able to establish the intensity of sensory character or overall quality of meat and meat products. They are usually involved in all developmental and processing studies.

Semi-trained panelists are persons normally familiar with the quality of different classes of meat and are in a position to discriminate differences and communicate their reactions. In a semi-trained panel, individual variations are generally balanced by involving greater number of panelists.

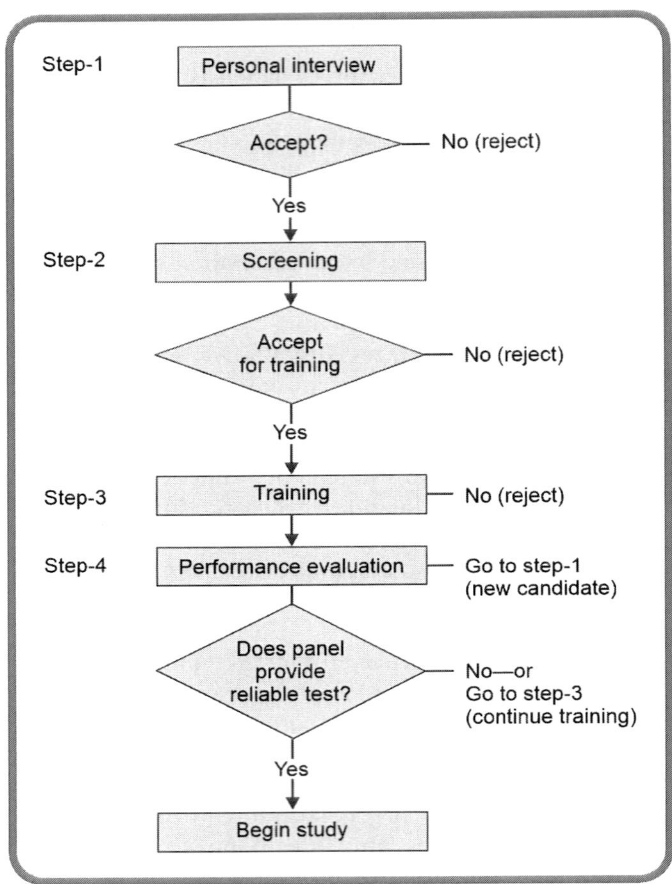


**Fig. 31.1:** Steps in selection and training of panelists. (Adapted from Cross et al., 1978)

## PREPARATION AND PRESENTATION OF SAMPLES

### Testing Environment

The sensory evaluation laboratory should be separate from the sample preparation room. The only connection allowed may be 45 × 30 cm pass-through. The laboratory should have independent air conditioning with exhaust for positive pressure to eliminate external odors. It should have separate booth for each panelist having wash basin, water for oral rinsing, thermostatically controlled heating device, writing table, chair, water beakers and arrangements for colored as well as neutral white lights. Besides, the sensory laboratory should have provision for white plastic serving trays, paper napkins, forks, knives and group discussion area equipped with a large table and stools to sit 12–15 persons. A relative humidity of 70–75% and a temperature of 20 ± 2°C have been reported as ideal laboratory conditions **(Fig. 31.2)**.

## Preparation of Sample

The sampling for sensory evaluation should be done in such a way that the sample taken represents the total batch. However, it should be ensured that all meat samples to be presented for evaluation are safe for consumption. Panelists should never be asked to taste or eat nay meat that has become moldy. In case, meat has been presented or treated in such a way that might make it unsafe microbiologically or chemically, then only the appearance and odor attributes may be evaluated.

Cross et al. (1978) reported considerable variation amongst meat scientists in the size and amount of sample presented for sensory evaluation. In view of this, AMSA (1978) recommended samples with 1.32 to 2.5 diameter cubes or slices of 1.3 × 1.3 × 1.9 cm of hot meat. However, Ennis (1990) used cubes of 1.1 × 1.1 cm for Canadian style bacon and boneless hams. As a thumb rule, the amount of sample should be enough for the panelists to have at least two bites in case of solids and 15 mL for liquids.

## Number and Presentation of Samples

At least two pieces (cubes or slices) from steaks, roasts or chops or nay other meat products should be presented to each panelist in a random order unless the statistical design calls for evaluation of position effects within the muscle. The samples should be assigned suitable codes in such a way that they should not give the panelists any hind of the treatments, preferably a 3-digit random numbers (Watt et al., 1989). In this context, recommended use of 3 digits selected from a table of random numbers ideally or more than two sessions per day or ten sessions per week. When the number of attributes is more, the sample number per session may be decreased. Generally six attributes and six samples are considered as absolute maximum for trained panelists because the sensory receptors become fatigued. Bohneukamp and Berry (1987) studied the effect of sample number

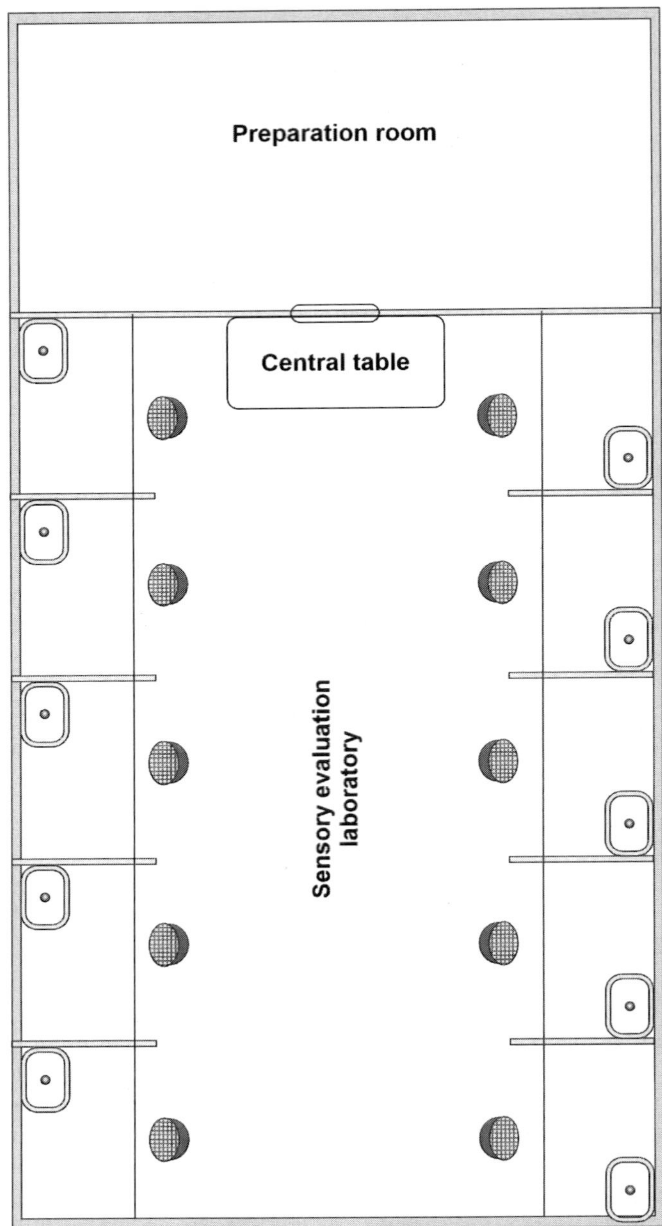


**Fig. 31.2:** Outline of a sensory evaluation laboratory.

on the sensory perception of panelists and reported discrimination between formulations in first six samples distinctively as compared to the later samples. In paired difference test, a maximum of three pairs may be allowed whereas in consumer panel not more than two samples should be presented at a time. Meat samples should be prepared as uniformly as possible and presented as quickly as possible to prevent changes that occur during holding.

## Reference/Control Sample

Reference sample is many a times either used in sensory testing, which can be designated reference/control sample against which all other samples are to be compared or it can be hidden control coded and served to the panelist with the experimental samples. The hidden control must be sufficiently similar to the sample being tested so that it is not immediately identified. It should be coded in the same way as experimental samples using a different code number each time it is presented to the panel. While conducting a storage study, control sample must be stored under same storage conditions for comparative study or it may be a fresh sample to see the storage effects. If the purpose of study is to produce a product which is an improvement on existing one, then the existing sample can serve as a control. If the scores assigned by the panelists for hidden control vary considerably, then the concerned panelists should be given further training and their scores may have to be excluded from the data set.

## Temperature of Sample

Meat and meat products are generally taken warm, so they should be judged at those temperatures. Most of the comminuted meat products should be evaluated at 40–60°C although steaks, chops and roasted may be evaluated at 70°C. however, ham and luncheon meat should be judged at room temperature. The samples may be warmed to the temperature of presentation by spacing the time interval. This can be accomplished by placing them in a double boiler. It has been suggested to avoid placing cut samples in an oven or a heating device which has a drying effect. Increased holding time before sensory evaluation lowers the sensory ratings.

### Time of Conducting Panel

The optimal testing time is of utmost importance in the sensory evaluation. In general, panelists are more sensitive when slightly hungry. The ideal testing time for conducting the sensory evaluation of meat and meat products is late morning/late afternoon or at least one and half hours after lunch. Eating highly spiced food, smoking, taking drinks with lingering after-taste and sucking candies or chewing gum have to be avoided before the test. After such activities a gap of 30 minutes may be allowed prior to conducting sensory evaluation.

### Conducting of Sensory Evaluation

The panel leader must be knowledgeable enough about the basic principles of sensory evaluation, testing procedure, statistical design and interpretation of results. He should guide the panelists on which attributes they should concentrate and make their opinion on the test sheet. Expectation errors can occur when panelists are given too much information about the nature of the experiment or the types of samples before tests are conducted. Panelists should be given only that information which they need to satisfactorily perform their task. When the evaluation is underway, they should be discouraged from discussing their judgments with each other. Before having the first bite, the panelists should rinse their mouth with the neutral or demineralized water. Oral rinsing in between the samples is also essential. Glass distilled water is not suitable for this purpose as it may cause a cardboard like flavor. Panelists may be directed to fill up the test sheets on the spot correctly as per the instructions.

## DISCRIMINATORY SENSORY EVALUATION TESTS

Modern sensory evaluation requires trained sensitivity along with reliable, precise and reproducible ratings of small differences in sensory perception. This work can be accomplished by specialized or analytical panelists with ability to determine the difference in treatments and magnitude of differences in perception. The specialized panel consists of small number of trained persons usually 5–20. The differences can be known by various discriminatory and descriptive tests. To predict the future market performance of meat and meat products for a given geographical area, consumer panel can be used. These panelists do not require trained sensitivity and may consist of laboratory workers, plant employees or general public, usually 100 or more in number. However, they should be able to follow the instructions on the use of scoring chart. The consumer preferences may be influenced by eating habits, education, sex, age group and income, etc., in spite of these drawbacks, consumer panels provide actionable and reliable guidance for the product development.

The specialized panels need to be properly selected, trained and then involved in the analytical sensory testing. It will enable them to use their senses as analytical biological detectors without any personal likes or dislikes. At present following tests are used for sensory evaluation of meat and meat products.

## Recognition Test

Recognition test is a qualitative determination for the identification of four basic tastes. This is a pre-requisite before the prospective panelists are selected. It allows to identify the taste blind persons who may be rejected at the initial stage itself. Very dilute aqueous solutions of sucrose, sodium chloride, citric acid and caffeine are prepared and presented in random order to the candidates. They submit their test sheets containing taste identity of different samples to the panel leader who verifies them and accept or rejects them. Similarly, odor recognition and aroma recognition tests are also conducted.

## Threshold Test

Threshold test is a quantitative determination which is conducted to measure the sensitivity of the prospective sensory panelists with respect to four basic tastes. A concentration series of aqueous solutions of sucrose, sodium chloride, citric acid and caffeine is presented to the panelists. Each series is arranged in order to increasing concentration and needs to be tested in the same sequence. Retasting is not allowed. The lowest concentration or concentration threshold of each panelists is determined which is further improved during training.

## Difference Tests

Recognition and threshold tests are basic exercises and more attention is paid to conduct test with food as we do not consume only aqueous solutions in our day to day life. Difference tests are analytical exercises for the recognition of small and minute variations. The trained panelists act as instruments to detect difference between any two samples. These tests are based on difference threshold which is defined as the concentration at which the difference is recognized. It has been reported that beginners receive the sample with 30% difference but with training and concentration of the panelists, a difference threshold of 10% is reached. The three main difference tests are paired difference test, triangle test and duo-trio test.

*Paired Difference Test*

Paired difference test is applied in product testing, as well as panel training and selection. In this test there is a direct comparison of two samples for a single attribute. Several paired samples are presented to panel members. Each pair consist of a control sample and an analytical sample. The panelists have to state whether the two samples can be differentiated. It is essential to present the samples in complete randomness so that the panelists respond to each trial-set independently. There are limitations to this sensory test but it can be used to generate useful information. Poste et al. (1991) have outlined several samples of this test in various foods.

**Test Sheet**

Name of the Panelists..........................................Date....................

Product......................................................................................

Samples Numbers

| | |
|---|---|
| A | B |
| C | D |
| E | F |
| G | H |

Panelist must mark the sample pairs in which he or she is able to differentiate between the samples.

*Triangle Test*

This is the most widely used difference test specially for panel selection, training and meat product testing. In this test three samples are presented in a row randomly, two being alike and one different. The odd sample is required to be identified. Retasting is now allowed. Triangle test has been conducted successfully for product development and testing in beef, pork turkey, meat batters and products. Usually it is not sufficient to note a difference between samples. The kind of difference must be characterized. This additional task is accomplished with the help of extended triangle test especially helpful in product development.

**Test Sheet**

Name of the Panelists............................................Date.................

Product.......................................................................................

Samples Numbers

| | | |
|---|---|---|
| A | B | C |
| E | F | G |
| H | I | J |
| K | L | M |

Encircle the odd sample.

*Due-trio Test*

Due-trio test is intermediate between the paired difference and triangle test. The panelists receive one sample marked control along with one or several pairs of samples. The panel members are required to identify the sample which matches the control. This method is particularly advantageous for identification of off notes and products having lingering after taste. Paired difference and duo-trio tests have been compared by Mahony et al. (1986). They have highlighted the difficulties encountered in their adoption. Brook and Pearson (1989) used duo-trio test for detection of odor threshold of the androstenone responsible for boar taint in pork. The statistical analysis of data obtained from these difference tests can be done by binominal distribution.

**Test Sheet**

Name of the Panelists..............................................Date...............

Product.......................................................................................

Samples Numbers

| | | |
|---|---|---|
| K | K | A |
| K | A | K |
| K | A | K |
| K | A | K |

Panelists must mark the sample which resembles the control (K). Retesting may be allowed once.

## DESCRIPTIVE SENSORY EVALUATION TESTS

### Ranking Test

Ranking is a process of arranging three or more samples for increasing or decreasing degree of a specified attribute, overall quality or response. In this test coded samples are presented simultaneously in sufficient amount enabling the panelists to check their first impression. They are just assigned to rank the samples according to their preference. Hence, the samples are evaluated in relation to each other. Ranking tests are useful in storage life evaluation to each other. Ranking tests are useful in storage life evaluation of meats, product development, consumer preference, training of panelists and studies on meat tenderness. Ranking data can be statistically analyzed by rank analysis and ANOVA. The major limitations of this test are that the degree of difference can not be known and the individual likings or dislikes badly influence the results.

*Example*

The rank sum of four samples A, B, C and D are 44, 21, 42 and 63, respectively in a ranking test. Interpret the findings (least significance difference = 20).

*Interpretation*

Rank sum of sample A = 44bc
B = 21a
C = 42b
D = 63c

The rank sum indicates that B is the most liked sample whereas D is the least liked sample. Sample C is liked more than sample A but less than sample B. Thus, ranking in descending order will be:

B > C > A > D

Statistically, most liked sample B has significantly higher ranking than all others. The difference in the ranking of samples A and C is not significant. Sample D has significantly lower ranking than sample C, whereas difference in the ranking of A and D is not significant.

*Hedonic Scoring or Rating Test*

This test is used to measure the degree of preference or acceptance for a particular product which can be easily inferred from the hedonic scaling or rating. This method relies on panelists capacity to report directly and precisely their feelings of likes and dislikes. Several variations of the traditional 9-point hedonic scale have been used effectively. These include reduced number of rating categories (not less than five), greater number of like rating categories, omission of neutral rating categories, etc., the product samples may be tested singly for determining the acceptability of a new and unusual food product where there are no similar products for comparison. This test can also be used in multiple sample comparisons for preference screening.

In paired or multiple sample comparisons, the samples may be presented simultaneously or successively in a balanced order. The panelists may be asked to evaluate various attributes in each sample and mark the scales or ratings accordingly. It is emphasized that the instructions by the panel leader should not give any idea about the treatments, otherwise it may influence the panel ratings.

The hedonic scale rating test can yield both absolute and relative information about the test sample. The numerical scores obtained in the test can be subjected to ranking analysis and ANOVA to determine difference in degree of liking between or among the samples. This hedonic scale rating test can be used for new product development, product matching, product improvement, process changes, cost reduction exercises, storage stability and consumer preference. An 8-point hedonic scale was followed by Keeton (1983) for different attributes like tenderness, flavor, etc., in pork patties where scale 8=extremely desirable and 1=extremely poor. The same hedonic scale after suitable modification has been adopted by the scientists of the Division of Livestock Products Technology, Indian Veterinary Research Institute, Izatnagar, UP, India to evaluate different attributes like general appearance, flavor, texture, juiciness, mouth coating and overall acceptability, etc.

In fresh meat storage experiments, especially pertaining to microbiological studies, a 7-point hedonic scale can be adopted for evaluation of appearance and odor attributes, wherein score 7 denotes a fresh and score 1 a putrid sample.

## SCORE CARD FOR APPEARANCE AND ODOR PANEL

Name.............................................................Date..........................

Kind of meat ...........................................................................

Scoring guide:

7 = Fresh
6 = Fairly fresh
5 = Just acceptable

4 = Just spoiled
3 = Well spoiled
2 = Nearly putrid
1 = Putrid

| Sample no. | Appearance | Odor |
|---|---|---|
| A | | |
| B | | |
| C | | |
| D | | |

Remarks

Signatures

## SPECIALIZED SENSORY EVALUATION TESTS

### Flavor Profile Test

It is a descriptive method of sensory analysis which provides a written record of the products perceptible aroma, flavor components (notes), feeling factors and after taste. The panelists characterize the individual components of odor and flavor in the sequence of their perception. Then using a constant rating scale, the intensity of each component is assigned the numerical value followed by the subjective judgment of total quality or else the amplitude of flavor harmony is scored. A properly screened and trained panel consisting of four or five members is used. The panelists first independently examine the product, record their impressions and report feelings to the panel leader for an open discussion. Once the consensus is reached on the components and their order of perception, the panel leader summarizes the report form.

The selection and training of panelists is of paramount importance in the flavor profile method, because the accessors are not to express their likes or dislikes. Their main task is to (a) recognize the fine nuances or odour, taste and feel, (b) assess these nuances qualitatively and (c) apply scaling system in such a way that there is no major disagreement among the judges on the score level to be applied for a particular degree of intensity. Flavor profile method is designed to achieve the concordance among panelists and reach agreement on the odor of perception. They are also required to subjectively assess the amplitude of the product. ASTM (1968) defines amplitude as "the initial overall intensity impressions including both the separately identifiable factors and underlying unidentifiable part of the flavor complex". The product is judged as to whether it is weak in overall character, or some notes are so strong as to imbalance the flavor harmony of the product. High scores are given when the specific flavor components of the particular meat product are of high intensity **(Table 31.1)**.

The flavor profile is applied in the monitoring of the competitive meat products quality, storage life, development of newer products, quality control, effects of ingredient substitution, processing change or packaging and correlation of sensory with instrumental measurements. The method has considerable appeal because the results could be obtained rapidly. It has been possible to successfully profile the chicken flavor to twelve different terms.

In many food products, the flavor harmony is so inbuilt that it is very difficult to make analysis of individual components. In these cases, the flavor harmony is imbalanced by dilution with water or preparing an aqueous profile extract. This method is referred to as dilution flavor profile test. This test has been successfully applied in the investigation of smoked fish, smoked ham, etc.

It has been suggested that flavor profile testing does not require statistical analysis, and relies on the collective judgement of the

**Table 31.1:** Flavor descriptors for various species of meat.

| *Beef* | *Lamb* | *Pork* | *Poultry* | *Fish* |
|---|---|---|---|---|
| Beefy | Gamey/ muttony | Porky | Chickeny poultry | Boiled Chicken/ buttery |
| Broth/meaty | Fatty | Sex taint/ boar odor | Meaty | Nutty/pecan |
| Cooked beef fat | Bloody/ serum | Fatty | Brothy | Grainy/ corn green vegetable |
| Serum/ bloody browned | Browned/ Caramel Liver/organ meaty | Bloody Browned | Browned Liver/organy | Shellfish Briny |
| Grainy/cowy | Meaty | | | |
| Livery/organ meat | | | | |

trained panelists. However, numerical values of intensity rating can be statistically analyzed by principal component analysis and multivariate analysis of variance.

## Texture Profile Test

It is a descriptive method and provides a systematic approach to the measurement of textural dimensions of a food in terms of its mechanical, geometrical, fat and moisture characteristics along with the degree to which each is present in order to enhance their perception **(Table 31.2)**. A panel consisting of 6 to 9 properly screened and trained members is used to identify the textural attributes and establish the evaluation procedure; first individually and then in a group discussion. The panel leader moderates the discussion and records the panel findings. The sequence for assessment of textural attributes has been discussed in three stages. The initial perception on first bite includes both mechanical characteristics such as hardness, viscosity, brittleness, etc., and geometrical characteristics depending on the product structure. The second stage of masticatory perception during chewing also includes mechanical characteristics like gumminess, chewiness, adhesion, etc., and geometrical characteristics depending upon the product structure. The third stage involves residual changes that occur during mastication which includes rate of breakdown, type of breakdown, moisture absorption, mouth coating, etc.

**Table 31.2:** Texture descriptors for some species of meat.

| *Stage* | *Chicken breast* | *Lamb* | *Frankfurters* |
|---|---|---|---|
| Surface | None | Smoothness<br>Surface moisture<br>Fat type<br>Fat amount<br>Amount of particles | Surface moisture<br>Type of moisture<br>Surface<br>Smoothness |
| Partial Compression | Springiness | Elasticity (Springiness) | Elasticity (Springiness) |

*Contd...*

*Contd...*

| *Stage* | *Chicken breast* | *Lamb* | *Frankfurters* |
|---|---|---|---|
| First bite | Initial cohesiveness<br>Hardness Initial juiciness<br>(Moisture release) | Compressibility (Cohesiveness)<br>Moisture release<br>Amount of fat<br>Type of fat<br>Cohesiveness (Disintegration) | Hardness<br>Cohesiveness<br>Uniformity<br>Amount of fat<br>Type of fat<br>Cohesiveness (Disintegration)<br>Graininess |
| Mastication | Hardness<br>Cohesiveness of mass<br>Saliva produced<br>Particle size and shape<br>Fibrousness<br>Chew count<br>Bolus size<br>Bolus wetness | Chewiness<br>Number of chews<br>Stringiness (Fibrousness)<br>Moisture release<br>Moisture Absorption<br>Cohesiveness (of mass)<br>Fat type<br>Fat amount<br>Rate of breakdown<br>Uniformity<br>Density<br>Connective tissue amount | Chewiness<br>Moisture release<br>Oiliness<br>Moisture absorption<br>Cohesiveness of mast<br>Lumpy<br>Grainy<br>Skin<br>Description of breakdown |
| Residue | Ease of swallowing<br>Residual particle<br>Tooth pack<br>Mouth coating | Ease of swallowing<br>Mouth coating type<br>Mouth coating amount<br>Particle type<br>Particle amount<br>Tooth packing | Ease of swallowing<br>Mouth coating<br>Oiliness<br>Particles |

The textural profile test can be applied in new product development, product matching, product improvement, process changes, storage stability and quality control of various meat products. This test has been successfully used in canned meat sauces, beef patties, chicken breast, cooked beef, restructured beef steaks, Australian sausages and rabbit meat. A modified textural profile scheme to assess the textural characteristics of cooked bacon has been used by involving four stages namely physical visual test, incisor bite, mastication and overall acceptability. Unstructured scale labeled with terms at two or three points were used to quantify the observation made at each stage. The statistical analysis of the data can be conducted by graphic representation, principal component analysis and multivariate analysis of variance.

# 32 CHAPTER

# Meat Eating and Animal Welfare

Meat is a highly nutritious food. It is almost fully digestible. It is appealing to the senses of taste and olfaction. The nutritive value of meat is attributed to its abundant high quality proteins, essential fatty acids, some important minerals and vitamins.

Meat is a concentrated source of superb quality proteins with very high biological value. It is rich in essential amino acids. Meat fat contains ample amount of essential fatty acids. In general, meat is a good source of all important minerals except calcium. It is rich in iron. Lean meat is an excellent source of B-complex group of vitamins. It has only traces of fat-soluble vitamins.

It is a paradox that most of the principal meat species themselves are plant eaters. They are living reservoirs of human food. By any ethics, they are required to be treated well. Since we are exploiting their potential for our benefit, we must look after their comfort and well-being during their limited lifespan. In fact, our interests are inter-related.

Animal welfare relates to the physical fitness and mental well being of the animals. In good welfare conditions, the animal is able to cope up with its environment with ease. In stress conditions, the animal gets alarmed, heart rate is increased and normal behavior is also changed. Good management practices and enough housing space provide good animal welfare. In a herd high mortality rate indicates poor welfare. Removal of the animals from the acclimatized environment also evokes a stress response. Besides, transportation to long distances in crowded space and sudden jerks may result in physical injury, bruising or broken bones causing lot of pain to the animals. Prevalence of bruises is also an indicator of poor welfare.

Here it will be pertinent to note that cruelty against animals is punishable under PCA Act (1960). The main provisions of the Act are reproduced hereunder:

## THE PREVENTION OF CRUELTY TO ANIMALS ACT, 1960

### Short Title

1. This act may be called the Prevention of Cruelty to Animal Act 1960.
2. Definitions: In this act, unless the context otherwise requires:
   a. “Animal” means any living creature other than a human being.
   b. “Board” means the animal welfare board established under section 4.
   c. “Captive” animal means any animal (not being a domestic animal) which is in captivity or confinement.
   d. “Domestic” animal means any animal which is tamed.
   e. “Local authority” means a municipal committee, district board or other authority.
   f. “Phooka or Doom De” includes any process of introducing air or any substance into the female organ of a milch animal.

## ANIMAL WELFARE BOARD

1. Constitution of the board consists of:
   a. The inspector general of forest, government of India, ex. officio.
   b. The animal husbandry commissioner to the government of India, ex. officio.
   c. One person to represent such association of veterinary practitioners.
   d. Two persons to represent practitioners of modern and indigenous system of medicine.
   e. One person to represent each of such three societies dealing with the prevention of cruelty to animals.
2. Term of office and conditions of service of the members of the board are three years.

## CRUELTY TO ANIMALS

1. Treating animals cruelly. If any person:
   a. Beats, kicks, overrides, overdrives, overloads, or otherwise treats any animals so as to subject it to unnecessary pain.
   b. Promotes or takes part in any shooting or competition wherein animals are released from captivity for the purpose of such shooting, he shall be punishable with fines which may extend to fifty or one hundred rupees or with 3 months imprisonment or with both.

2. Penalty for practicing of "Phooka or Doom De" he shall be punishable with fine which may extend to one thousand rupees or with imprisonment for 2 years or with both.

## Experimentation on Animals

Penalties—if any Person:

a. Contravenes any order made by the committee under section 19 or Institutional Animal Ethics Committee set up under Breeding and Experiments on Animals (Control and Supervision) Rules, 1998 of the Act require location of animal houses in a quiet atmosphere and premises to be kept tidy, hygienic and animal protected from drought and extremes of weather. Animal cages for small animals and stables for large animal shall be such that animals can live in comfort and overcrowding is avoided. It requires animal attendants to be suitably trained. It also stipulates that if an animal is suffering from abnormally severe pain at any stage of experiment, it shall be painlessly destroyed. Institutional Animal Ethics Committee is also required to maintain a record of the animals under its control and custody in the specified format.
b. Commits a breach of any conditions he shall be punishable with fines which may extend to two hundred rupees.

## Performing Animals

Restriction on exhibition and training of performing animals applied to be registered under this Act which when not entitled to be so registered, he shall be punishable on conviction with fine which may be extended to five hundred rupees.

# TIPS FOR GOOD ANIMAL WELFARE

1. Animals should be housed in such a space that these are able to perform their normal behavior patterns. European Union has specified the space requirement for pigs as 0.65 $m^2$ per animal and for caged hens as 550 $cm^2$ per bird to live in.
2. At the farm, animals should be handled in a humane way. Husbandry practices should be adopted keeping in view the overall comfort of the animal in mind. The flooring and fence design should reduce the injuries to the animals.
3. Design of the restraint system should be evolved keeping in mind the highest considerations for animal welfare.

4. During transport, care should be taken to avoid any unnecessary suffering of the animals. The loading and unloading should be made smooth with the help of low slope wooden ramps. Proper mode of transport, overhead protection, provision of enough space and ventilation should be taken care of.
5. In the lairage, it is advisable not to mix strange animals, especially males. If possible, animals from the same herd should be kept together with adequate straw bedding. There should be provision of ample drinking water.
6. In the slaughter house, an animal awaiting slaughter should not be allowed to view the sticking of the other animal. Fear triggered by strange movements, noises and smell leads to severe physiological stress. It is further enhanced by the separation from fellow animals.
7. A suitable stunning procedure that can keep the animal in unconscious state for about a minute, should be followed. The sticking should be completed well before the animal is expected to regain the consciousness. The techniques should conform the socio-religious needs, least painful slaughter and good meat quality at the same time.

Meat is a highly nutritious human diet. The debates on animal welfare should not be allowed to come in the way of its popularity. In fact, it will be appropriate to direct the efforts to improve the well being of food animals and the conditions at the slaughter house simultaneously in order to popularize meat in the human diet. It should be borne in mind that excited, stressed, fatigued, suffocated, bruised and injured animals can never yield wholesome meat. So, human welfare is also linked to animal welfare.

# 33 CHAPTER

# Biotechnological Approaches in Processing and Packaging of Poultry Products

Indian meat and poultry industry represents a major success story in the present era. Among various reasons for increased consumption are relatively low costs of production, the rapid growth rate, high nutritional value and introduction of many innovative processed meat products. Chicken meat can make many positive contributions to the diet of those with low income. Maintaining this appreciable position will require innovations, new ideas and strategies in the ever-increasing competitive food market. Poultry products processing makes use of various unit operations and technologies to convert relatively bulky, perishable and typical raw materials into more useful, shelf-stable and palatable products. Processing contributes to food security by minimizing waste and losses in the food chain and by increasing food availability and marketability. Poultry products are also processed in order to improve their quality and safety.

Biotechnology is the use of living systems and organisms to develop or make useful products, or any technological application that uses biological systems, living organisms or derivatives thereof, to make or modify products or processes for specific use. It is a more extreme scientific method that offers the potential to improve the quality, yield, and safety of animal products by direct genetic manipulation of livestock. In essence, biotechnology is a new approach to the methods of genetic selection, crossbreeding, administration of growth hormones, processing of products and packaging and labeling. However, progress in this area is very slow and has a long way to go before having an impact at the commercial usage level.

Biotechnology in the meat and poultry processing sector makes use of microorganisms for the preservation of meat and for the production of a range of value-added products such as enzymes, flavor compounds, vitamins, microbial cultures and food ingredients.

Biotechnology applications in the meat-processing sector, therefore, target the selection and manipulation of microorganisms with the objective of improving process control, product quality, safety, consistency and yield, while increasing process efficiency. The main uses of biotechnology in the poultry processing sector can be summarized as follows:

## BIOTECHNOLOGICAL APPROACH IN POULTRY MEAT PROCESSING

### Meat Fermentation

Meat fermentation is a low energy, biological acidulation as well as preservation method which results in unique and distinctive meat properties such as flavor and palatability, color, microbiological safety, tenderness, and a host of other desirable attributes of this specialized meat item. Changes from raw meat to the fermented product are caused by cultured or wild microorganisms which lower the pH. Since this is a biological system, it is influenced by many environmental factors that need to be controlled to produce a consistent product.

Beef, lamb, and pork have more saturated fat and less moisture than chicken, turkey, and mechanically de-boned poultry and therefore the former species produce a firmer texture and are less susceptible to rancidity and off flavors than poultry products when used in fermented sausages. Mechanically de-boned poultry is usually limited to 10% (although some use 100%) due to the softer texture. Meat intended for fermentation should have a pH of 6.8 and below. Higher levels of glucose should be used in sausages that initially have a higher pH such as poultry. Also, if poultry is used, the product should be heated to at least greater than 68.9°C or other temperature/time combinations to destroy *Salmonella* spp.

The fermentation bioprocess is the major biotechnological application in food processing. Fermentation processes have been developed to upgrade plant and animal materials, to yield a more acceptable food, to add flavor, to prevent the growth of pathogenic and spoilage microorganisms, and to preserve food without refrigeration. Fermentation bioprocessing makes use of microbial inoculants for enhancing properties such as the taste, aroma, shelf-life, safety, texture and nutritional value of meat. Most of the commercially available meat starter cultures contain mixtures Lactic Acid Bacteria (LAB), Gram-positive Catalase-positive Cocci (GCC+, mostly *Staphylococcus* and *Kocuria* species) and less importantly yeasts and molds. These bacterial groups are responsible for the basic microbial reactions that occur simultaneously during fermentation; the decrease of pH values via glycolysis by LAB, the reduction of nitrate, and the development of aroma by GCC+. They are, by definition, used to drive the fermentation process in the desired direction, reducing the variability in the quality of the product, limiting the growth of spoilage bacteria by accelerating fermentation, and improving the sensory properties of fermented meat products.

The meat starter cultures are divided into two categories. The first generation of starter bacteria, generally derived from cultures for vegetable fermentation, such as L. plantarum and pediococci, were mainly selected for their acidification properties. A second generation developed isolating strains of meat origin, such as *L. sakei* and coagulase-negative staphylococci (CNS) that harbored phenotypic traits of technological relevance. This second generation is now widely used in the industrial processes of fermented meat production.

Development of a third generation of functional starter cultures with increased diversity, stability, and industrial performance is underway. Using comparative genomics, microarray analysis, transcriptomics, proteomics, and metabolomics, the natural diversity of wild strains that occur in traditional artisan foods is being explored.

Nitrate is added to fermented chicken sausages for its capacity to fix and obtain the typical color of cured products, rather than for its antimicrobial properties. To be effective, the added nitrate must be reduced to nitrite. Besides contributing to flavor, *Staphylocuccus* and *Kocuria* also have a role for their nitrate reductase and antioxidant activities. These microorganisms reduce nitrate to nitrite, which is important for the formation of nitrosylmyoglobin, the compound responsible for the characteristic red color of fermented chicken. The flavor and aroma of fermented meats is a combination of several elements. The bacterial community contributes to flavor development through carbohydrate dissimilation, peptide metabolism, and lipolysis. To ensure the sensory quality of fermented sausages, the contribution of the proteolytic and lipolytic activities of staphylococci is fundamental.

## Genetically Modified Organisms as Additives and Processing Aids in Poultry Products

Genetically modified microorganisms are now not only used to produce pharmaceuticals, vaccines, specialty chemicals, and feed additives, but they also produce vitamins, additives, and processing agents for the food industry and even for processing of poultry meat. The use of microorganisms for production of food additives and other valuable substances is not new. Genetic engineering, however, has made it possible to modify bacteria and fungi to make them produce substances at a more economic advantage than conventional, industrial methods. In many ways, these biotechnological methods have replaced chemical, synthetic production. The advantages are obvious: microorganisms grow rapidly and in most cases are easy to cultivate. Unlike conventional production methods, they do not need high temperatures, pressures, or harsh chemicals. Using microorganisms is much more environmental-friendly than conventional chemical-synthetic methods; they use less energy and mostly renewable resources. Production leftovers are easily biodegradable and have minimal impact on waste water. In order to biotechnologically produce a certain substance, microorganisms must be identified that produce the substance naturally. There are many known bacteria and fungi that produce valuable substances.

Genetically modified microorganisms are now not only used to produce pharmaceuticals, vaccines, specialty chemicals, and feed additives, they also produce vitamins, additives, and processing agents for the food industry and even for processing of poultry meat. Examples:

- Vitamin $B_2$ (coloring, riboflavin E 101)
- Vitamin C (preservative, ascorbic acid E 300)
- Thickener, xanthan (E 415), acidity regulator, citric acid (E 330)
- Preservative, natamycin (E 235), nisin (E 234), lysozyme (E 1105)
- Various amino acids, e.g., the flavor enhancer glutamate (E 621) the sweetener aspartame (E 951) or the flour treating agent cysteine (E 921)
- Enzymes (proteases) make meat more tender and improve aroma.

## Enzymatic Chicken Meat Protein Extraction

Meat and bone is to a large extent separated from each other by cutting at the slaughterhouse before the meat is sold to the consumers. Four to five percent of the meat remains, however, with the bones after the cutting process and is often wasted with the bones because it is difficult to remove. The remaining meat can, however, easily be extracted from the bones with the help of enzymes and the "meat protein extracts" can be injected into meat cuts or used in processed foods such as chicken soups and sausages as an alternative to meat or soy-protein. Animal production is responsible for considerable greenhouse gas emissions and using enzymes to increase the yield of protein from slaughtered animal could help reducing pressure on the climate. Enzymatic meat protein extraction was introduced in full scale production in the 1990 but spreading has so far only been limited. The amount of greenhouse gasses could also be limited if enzymes are applied in poultry meat processing to reduce waste.

## Processed Chicken Preservation and Added Functionality

In recent years, there has been a considerable increase in studies of natural antimicrobial compounds on and in the food produced by LAB, referred to as bioprotective cultures, it may act as starter cultures in food fermentation processes, such as dry chicken sausage manufacturing, or they may protect foods from any detrimental organoleptic changes. The ability to produce different antimicrobial compounds, such as bacteriocins and/or low-molecular mass antimicrobial compounds may be one of the critical characteristics for effective competitive exclusion. The production of bacteriocins, one of the most promising technological features of starter cultures. Foods which have health benefits beyond their nutritional content (functional foods), and particularly foods containing probiotics, are products that are growing in popularity. Probiotics are available as dietary supplements or they may be incorporated directly into foods. They are live microorganisms that when administered in adequate amounts confer a health benefit on the host. Commercial probiotic cultures, such as strains *L. rhamnosus* GG, *L. rhamnosus* LC-705, *L. rhamnosus* E-97800, and *L. plantarum* E-98098, have been tested as functional starter culture strains for fermented chicken products in northern Europe without negatively affecting the technological or sensory properties of the finished products.

## Meat-based Bioactive Compounds and their Utilization

Since chicken contains an abundance of proteins with high biological value, also a fundamental source of essential amino acids and some valuable minerals and vitamins. Some of these nutrients are either not present or have inferior bioavailability in other foods. In addition to these basic nutrients, much attention has recently been paid to meat-based bioactive compounds such as conjugated linoleic acid L-carnitine detected in the skeletal muscle of chicken assists the human body in producing energy and in lowering the levels of cholesterol, also, it helps the body to absorb calcium to improve skeletal strength and chromium picolinate to help build lean muscle mass. Glutathione present in chicken is an important antioxidative compound providing cellular defense against toxicological and pathological processes. Accumulation of bioactive peptides in meat products by fermentation is another good strategy for developing functional meat products. Bioactive peptides could be generated in fermented meat products, since meat proteins are hydrolyzed by proteolytic enzymes during fermentation and storage. Rediscovery of traditional fermented meats as functional foods is also an interesting direction. Numerous physiologically active components including bioactive peptides have been discovered in these traditional fermented foods. Thus, traditionally fermented meats are attractive targets for finding new functional meat products. Although bioactive peptides are yet been utilized in the meat industry, such peptides are promising candidates for ingredients of functional foods. Several food products containing ACE (Angiotensin I-converting enzyme) inhibitory peptides have been successfully marketed for hypertensive persons.

## BIOTECHNOLOGICAL APPROACH TO PROCESSING OF EGG PRODUCTS

### Desugaring Albumen for Egg Powder Preparation

Desugaring albumen is necessary to prevent Maillard reaction (initially a bonding of glucosidic hydroxyl groups and amine groups of peptides) which causes brownish discoloration of dried albumen. Besides albumen also loses solubility and acquires metallic off-flavor. Glucose can be removed by:

- Yeast fermentation: 3-hour fermentation at 37°C with strains of Saccharomyces, e.g., S. cerevisiae.
- Controlled bacterial fermentation (the most commonly used method) of the many organisms studied, a strain of *Klebsiella pneumoniae* has been generally adopted by the industry.
- "Enzyme" fermentation: Glucose oxidase is used to convert glucose in albumen to gluconate and catalase to break down $H_2O_2$.

Whole egg and egg yolk for powder preparation also requires desugaring to prevent Maillard reactions and additionally, reaction of glucose with phospholipids,especially cephalin causes discoloration of dried whole egg or yolk powder. Glucose oxidase and catalase system have been used almost exclusively to remove glucose with incubation at 100°C in order to deter growth of undesirable microorganisms.

### Yolk Cholesterol Removal

Microbial and enzymatic treatment of yolk cholesterol provides an alternative way to reduce yolk cholesterol economically and efficiently. Successful attempts have been made to degrade over 60% yolk cholesterol by Rhodococcus equi No. 23 without steroid intermediate accumulation. A 40% bioconversion was reached in a 60 min period by Rhodococcus equi. A bioconversion of 93% over 3-day incubation with cholesterol oxidase (COD) from *Pseudomonas fluorescens* and *Nocardia erythropolis* has also been reported. Previously, quantitative work has been done on the properties of both rough and purified COD from a mutant, ODG-007, of *Brevibacterium* sp., the only steroid-like bioconversion product of cholesterol was cholest-4-en-3-one. So it can be deduced that the bioconversion product of yolk cholesterol, by cholesterol oxidase from the same enzyme source,might be cholestenone alone. The converted choelstenone was characterized as a major component of oviductus ranae, a traditional Chinese medicine, and is reported to have an antiobesity effect without any detectable clinical or necropsy anomaly. The process of yolk cholesterol conversion, catalyzed by COD from a mutant ODG-007 of *Brevibacterium* sp. was thoroughly studied to obtain detailed information, and also optimum conditions, for the bioconversion of yolk cholesterol in a cost-efficient way which might be applicable in the food industry.

## BIOTECHNOLOGICAL APPROACH TO PACKAGING OF POULTRY PRODUCTS

These are appropriately covered under intelligent packaging systems that include a sensor or indicator to provide information about the quality of packaged food.

### Biosensors in Packaging System

The recently developed biosensor technologies represent an additional area with potential for application in intelligent meat packaging systems. Biosensors are compact analytical devices which detect record and transmit information pertaining to biological reactions. They consist of a bioreceptor specific to a target analyte and a transducer to convert biological signals to a quantifiable electrical response. Bioreceptors are organic materials such as enzymes, antigens, microbes, hormones and nucleic acids. Transducers may be electrochemical, optical, or calorimetric and are system dependent. Intelligent packaging systems incorporating biosensors have the potential for exceptional specificity and reliability. Market analysis of pathogen detection and safety systems for the food packaging industry suggests that biosensors offer considerable promise for future growth. Some commercially available biosensor, incorporating antibodies printed on polyethylene-based plastic packaging capable of detecting target pathogens such as *Salmonella* sp., *Campylobacter* sp., *Escherichia coli* 0517 and *Listeria* sp.

Some multinational companies have developed a system based on a biosensor for temperature monitoring. The system monitors the accumulated effect of temperature on products over time. The system consists of a chipless RF circuit with a built-in biosensor which can be read with a handheld scanner at various points in the supply chain. Information is stored in a database and can be used to analyze the cold chain and validate that the agreed temperature has been maintained.

## Indicators in Packaging System

Indicators may be defined as substances which indicate the presence, absence or concentration of another substance, or the degree of reaction between two or more substances by means of a characteristic change, especially in color. A number of commercially available indicators are available for use with packaged chicken and meat products.

A time-temperature indicator (or integrator, TTI) is defined as a device (small tag or label) used to show a measurable, time-temperature dependent change that reflects the full or partial temperature history of a food product to which it is attached. Operation of TTIs is based on mechanical, chemical, electrochemical, enzymatic or microbiological change, usually expressed as a visible response in the form of a mechanical deformation, color development or color movement. Therefore, the visible response gives a cumulative indication of the storage temperature to which the TTI has been exposed. TTIs are classified as either partial history or full history indicators, depending on their response mechanism.

## Bioactive Edible Coating

The incorporation of antimicrobial compounds into an edible coating is being explored by dipping or spraying onto the meat. Selection of the incorporated active agents is limited to edible compounds, because they have to be consumed with the coating layers and meat together. The aforesaid chitosan-based films associated with other bioactive compounds (bacteriocins, organic acids, etc.) may also be included in these packaging concepts. The effectiveness of bacteriocin-protective cultures has mainly been studied in meats. The potential association of a chitosan-based packaging with bacteriocin could be interesting against strains, which are common meat product contaminants. Although this system was only studied as a preservative agent using a chitosan-carnosine based combination and a chitosan-sulfate combination, the results have shown potential applications for edible films.

Utilization of biotechnological tool to achieve the goal of food security in the form of processing and packaging is todays demand to mitigate the requirement of huge consumer population. Since meat and meat products are important in the diet in most developed countries, healthier meat and meat products would contribute to human health. In the field of meat processing, proper application of favored microbe-based fermentation process is one of the keys for development of innovative and healthy chicken products, as it not only improves the products quality and acceptability but also the storability and economic viability of the products. Utilizing meat-based bioactive compounds including bioactive peptides generated from meat is a promising means for developing attractive functional meat products. The biosensors and quality indicators offer potential advantages with respect to product safety and distribution besides brand differentiation for meat products.

# 34
CHAPTER

# Pesticide Residues in Meat: A Public Health Concern

The substances intended for preventing, destroying, repelling or mitigating any pests are commonly called as pesticides. Pests include certain insects, plant pathogens, weeds, mollusks, birds, mammals, fish, nematodes (roundworms), and microbes that are detrimental to agriculture, livestock, spread disease or cause nuisance. Food and Agriculture Organization (FAO) has defined the term of *pesticide* as *"Any substance or mixture of substances intended for preventing, destroying or controlling any pests, including vectors of human or animal disease, unwanted species of plants or animals causing harm during or otherwise interfering with the production, processing, storage, transport or marketing of food, agricultural commodities, wood and wood products or animal feedstuffs, or substances which may be administered to animals for the control of insects, arachnids or other pests in or on their bodies."* The term includes substances intended for use as a plant growth regulator, defoliant, desiccant or agent for thinning fruit or preventing the premature fall of fruit. It also encompasses substances applied to crops either before or after harvest to protect the commodity from deterioration during storage and transport. The use of pesticides has been in practice in the public health sector for disease vector control and in agriculture to control and eradicate crop pests for the past several decades. The positive side of the use of pesticides include enhancement of economic potential in terms of increased production of food and fiber as well as prevention of vector-borne diseases, whereas on the negative front it has resulted in serious health implications to man and his environment in the form of variety of known and unknown toxic symptoms.

Pesticides may be used in variety of different ways during the production of food. Small amounts of pesticides used in these ways can be found in or on foods and are called residues. These pesticide residues are undesirable substances in foods and may be either chemical or biological in nature. Many of the modern agricultural practices intended for enhanced production are responsible for objectionable residues in the products to be consumed by human beings. Although, it has become almost inevitable to follow these practices, 60,000 species of invertebrate pests and plant diseases in the field and storage, and 8,000 species of weeds compete with man to incur substantial loss of production. Besides use in intensive agricultural production, pesticide application is being done globally to check the losses during harvesting and storage. This has resulted in potential risk of various life-threatening diseases such as cancer, leukemia, reproductive disorders besides disruption of body's immune, endocrine and nervous system.

Keeping in view the hazards involved in the use of pesticides World Health Organization (WHO) has referred the pesticide residue as any substance or mixture of substances in food for man or animals resulting from the use of a pesticide and included any specified derivatives, such as degradation and conversion products, metabolites, reaction products and impurities that are considered to be of toxicological significance. Meat is one of the such food commodities which is quiet vulnerable to residues either from pesticides or drugs because of their unwarranted and indiscriminate use. Surveillance and monitoring of the pesticide's residue in meat and their products were relatively a neglected area until last decade. But now a days, consumers are very much concerned about impact of pesticide residues in food. International trade in food commodities is also at risk because of essential certificate with respect to pesticide residue. The present article aims to focus on some of the pertinent issues such as entry of pesticides to meat or meat products and its status in India, their effects on human health, monitoring and regulation of pesticide residues in meat and meat products and available alternatives for pesticides.

## ENTRY OF PESTICIDES IN MEAT/MEAT PRODUCTS AND STATUS IN INDIA

Pesticides are not a modern invention. Elemental sulphur dust was used by ancient Sumerians to protect their crops from insects. Medieval farmers experimented with various substances and chemicals for use on common crops. In 1939, Dichlorodiphenyltrichloroethane (DDT) was discovered to be extremely effective and became most widely used insecticide in the world. It was also extensively used in the malaria control program in India. Today use of several pesticides is quiet regular in the entire food chain. The principal sources of pesticide residues in crops, food animals, soil, water and almost all food commodities might be due to carry-over from insecticide application to soil or to growing crops, leaching of herbicides or insecticides into groundwater, disposal of pesticides in streams and rivers or effluents of pesticide industry in water bodies and into soil which could be finally translocated in crops. Extra label use of pesticides directly on animal body or their surroundings have been also found to be associated with residues in products such as milk or meat. The animal ingests these pesticides through their feed and fodder or water, which later on gets accumulated in tissues and finally reaches to table meat.

The pesticides of class organochlorine such as DDT, Lindane or hexachlorobenzene, heptachlor, heptachlor epoxide, aldrin/dieldrin are most persistent in environment and therefore major cause of health hazard. As compared to food grains, very little information is available from India on the pesticides in meat and meat products because of their indirect entry pathway. Studies on meat contamination in the 1970s indicated relatively low residues, at <1 mcg/g of DDT and HCH **(Table 34.1)**, compared to agricultural products. The goat, sheep buffalo, pig, chicken and fish tissue were found to contain <1 mcg/g of DDT and HCH. Among several meat products, greatest contamination was reported in chicken muscle followed by goat and beef collected in Lucknow, India.

The occurrence pattern of organochlorine pesticide residues in adipose tissue, liver and kidney samples of goats, sheep and oxen collected from the local slaughterhouse in Bangalore was studied by Nath et al. (1998). DDT was found to be in higher concentration in most of the tissues analyzed. The mean concentrations (mcg/g) of HCH, HCH, p,p'-DDE and DDT residues were 0.021, 0.057, 0.056 and 0.17 in adipose tissue; 0.006, 0.013, 0.005 and 0.110 in liver and 0.002, 0.004, 0.001 and 0.003 in kidney tissue respectively. Endosulfan was not detected in any of the sample. In a similar study Aulakh et al. (2005) investigated occurrence pesticides in muscles of poultry in Punjab and found mean concentration of HCH, DDT, endosulfan sulfate and heptachlor epoxide residues to be 0.11, 0.24, 0.10 and 0.07 mcg/g respectively but none of the muscle samples exceeded maximum residue limits (MRL) for these organochlorine pesticides. Biswas et al. (2005) screened a total of 122 buffalo meat samples comprising 92 *longissimus dorsi* (LD) and 30 *silver side* (SS) for pesticides (cypermethrin, deltamethrin and Carbaryl). Residue concentrations were far below the MRL and carbaryl residues were present in 3 LD samples and 2 SS samples.

**Table 34.1:** Mean concentration of DDT and HCH (mcg/g wet wt) in meat collected from various locations in India.

| *Year* | *Location* | *DDT* | *HCH* | *References* |
|---|---|---|---|---|
| 1975–76 | Calcutta | 1.5 | 1.2 | Mukharjee et al., 1980 |
| 1979 | Delhi | 1.0 | NA | Sharma et al., 1979 |
| 1979 | Bombay | NA | 0.6 | Banerjee, 1979 |
| 1980–1981 | Punjab | 0.25 | 0.19 | Singh and Chawla, 1988 |
| 1981–83 | Uttar Pradesh | 0.24 | 0.20 | Kaphalia et al., 1985 |
| 1989 | Various states | 0.1 | 0.48 | Kannan et al., 1992 |

*Source:* Jadhav and Waskar (2011)

## EFFECTS OF PESTICIDE RESIDUES ON HUMAN HEALTH

The World Health Organization and the UN Environment Programme estimate that about 3 million workers in agriculture in the developing world experience severe poisoning from pesticides every year while as many as 25 million workers in developing countries may suffer mild pesticide poisoning yearly. The fate of pesticides inside the body depends on category of pesticides. Pesticides can be classified by target organism, chemical structure, and physical state. They can also be classed as inorganic, synthetic, biologicals or based upon their biological mechanism, function or application method. The persistence and ultimate fate of pesticides in the food, soil, water, and air of human environment is affected by such interrelated factors as volatility, solubility, ultraviolet irradiation, surface adsorption, systemic action, hydrolysis, chemical rearrangement, etc. Within the body, the pesticides may be metabolized or it may be stored in the adipose tissue or excreted unchanged. In order to facilitate the clearance of poorly excretable lipophilic pesticides, there is a group of enzymes that are specialized for the conversion of lipophilic materials to hydrophilic metabolites which can readily be eliminated by excretion in body wastes. Metabolism will probably make the pesticide more water soluble and thus more easily excreted. The toxicity of pesticide residues may be influenced by number of factors such as health status of individuals (more toxicity in nutritionally deficient people), the interaction among the pesticides themselves if there is exposure to more than one (as is usually the case) and various environmental factors. The rate of elimination is a major factor governing the severity and duration of any toxic effects in human beings.

Pesticides are a public health concern and have been associated with a range of disorders and diseases. Exposure to pesticides may cause acute and delayed health effects. It may lead to a variety of adverse health effects. Along with certain environmental chemicals, pesticides are known to cause endocrine disruption by mimicking or antagonizing natural hormones in the body and it has been postulated that their long-term low-dose exposure are increasingly linked to human health effects such as immunosuppression, hormone disruption, diminished intelligence, reproductive abnormalities and cancer. Many studies have examined the effects of pesticide exposure on the risk of cancer. It has been found to have associations with: leukemia, lymphoma, brain, kidney, breast, prostate, pancreas, liver, lung, and skin cancers. Neurotoxicity of pesticides has been explained by Dale et al. (1962), who reported that adipose tissue acts as a protective reservoir. They reported that p,p'-DDT residues in the adipose tissue can be mobilized during starvation, reach tissues such as brain and produce symptoms of neurotoxicity. Thus, pesticide residues are known to cause nerve damage. The risk of developing Parkinson's disease is 70% greater in those exposed to even low levels of pesticides whereas long term exposures may increase the risk of dementia. Strong evidence also exists for other negative outcomes from pesticide exposure such as birth defects, fetal death and neurodevelopmental disorders.

## MONITORING OF PESTICIDE RESIDUES AND RELATED REGULATIONS

There is a growing concern about pesticide in foods. The government agencies are trying to regulate their use in almost all countries. Pesticide regulations differ from country to country. In Europe, recent EU legislation has been approved banning the use of highly toxic pesticides including those that are carcinogenic, mutagenic or toxic to reproduction, those that are endocrine-disrupting, and those that are persistent, bioaccumulative and toxic (PBT) or very persistent and very bioaccumulative (vPvB). In the United States, the Environmental Protection Agency (EPA) is responsible for regulating pesticides under the Federal Insecticide, Fungicide, and Rodenticide Act (FIFRA) and the Food Quality Protection Act (FQPA). The EPA regulates pesticides to ensure that these products do not pose adverse effects to humans or the environment. Pesticides produced before November 1984 continues to be reassessed in order to meet the current scientific and regulatory standards. All registered pesticides are reviewed every 15 years to ensure they meet the proper standards. During the registration process, a label is created. The label contains directions for proper use of the material. Based on acute toxicity, pesticides are assigned to a Toxicity Class.

With the passage of WTO sanitary and phytosanitary measures, strict regulations on their use are being enforced. Codex *Alimentarius Commission* has formulated standards using the term like Maximum Residual Limits (MRL) and Acceptable Daily Intake (ADI) to create uniform standards for maximum levels of pesticide residues among countries participating in international trade. Acceptable daily intake or ADI is a measure of the amount of a specific substance (residue in the present context) in food or drinking water that can be ingested (orally) on a daily basis over a lifetime without an appreciable health risk. It is usually expressed in mg/kg of body weight per day. An ADI value is based on long term studies on animals and observation of humans. The ADI does not take into account allergic reactions that are individual responses rather than dose-dependent phenomena. The "Joint FAO/WHO Meeting on Pesticide Residues (JMPR)" is an expert body for harmonizing the requirement and risk assessment of the pesticide residues. The body meets annually to conduct scientific evaluations of pesticide residues in foods. It provides advice on acceptable levels of pesticide in food moving in international trade. The ADI estimates of JMPR forms the essential basis for Codex maximum residue limits (MRL) for food and agricultural commodities circulating in international trade for the benefit of the governments of member countries and regions.

Codex maximum residue limits for pesticides (MRL) is the maximum concentration of a pesticide residue (expressed in mg/kg) recommended by Codex Alimentarius to be permitted in or on food commodities and animal feeds. MRLs are based on GAP data and foods derived from JMPR following toxicological assessment of pesticides and its residue and review of residue data from supervised trials. In fact, MRL is not a safety standard. It is a legal limit that is allowed on the food. Safety is defined by ADI. Thus, MRLs of all foods taken in a day must be within ADI.

In India, the Insecticide Act, promulgated in 1968 and enforced on 1st August, 1971 envisages to regulate the import, manufacture, sale, transport, distribution, and use of insecticides, with a view to prevent risks to human beings or animals, and for matters connected therewith. More than 200 pesticides are registered under section 9(3) of this act. Almost three dozen of pesticide/pesticide formulations have been banned for use to date and another 10 have been under restricted use. According to Prevention of Food Adulteration Act and Rules, Maximum Residue Limits for about 19 pesticides residues in meat and poultry have been defined. The Food Safety and Standards Authority of India have been established under the Food Safety and Standards Act, 2006. Tolerance limit of pesticides, veterinary drugs residues, etc., under section 21 have been incorporated in the law. In coordination with different research organization toxicological evaluation of pesticides is being carried out in the country regularly. Presently, MRLs are on a higher side in India **(Tables 34.2 and 34.3)**. Therefore, even if legal MRL standards are met in India, our exposure is not safe. We have to revise our standards to make sure that ADI is not exceeded **(Table 34.4)**.

**Table 34.2:** PFA Maximum Residue Limits for pesticide residues in meat and poultry.

| *S. No.* | *Pesticides* | *Tolerance (ppm or mg/kg)* | *S. No.* | *Pesticides* | *Tolerance (ppm or mg/kg)* |
|---|---|---|---|---|---|
| 1. | Aldrin, dieldrin | 0.20 | 11. | Carbendazim | – |
| 2. | DDT | 7.00 | 12. | Benomyl | 0.10 |
| 3. | Fenitrothion | 0.03 | 13. | Carbofuran | 0.10 |
| 4. | Lindane | 2.00 | 14. | Cypermethrin | 0.20 |
| 5. | Chlorfenvinphos | 0.20 | 15. | Edifenphos | 0.02 |
| 6. | Chlorpyrifos | 0.10 | 16. | Fenthion | 2.00 |
| 7. | 2,4D | 0.05 | 17. | Fenvalerate | 1.00 |
| 8. | Ethion | 0.20 | 18. | Phenthoate | 0.05 |
| 9. | Monocrotophos | 0.02 | 19. | Pirimiphos-methyl | 0.05 |
| 10. | Trichlorfon | 0.10 | | | |

**Table 34.3:** Maximum Residual Limits (MRL) of pesticides in cattle meat (Codex Standard).

| *Pesticides* | *MRL (ppm)* | *Pesticides* | *MRL (ppm)* |
|---|---|---|---|
| Aldrin/Dieldrin | 0.2 | Endosulfan | 0.1 |
| Chlordane | 0.05 | Fenvalerate | 1.5 |
| Aldicarb | 0.1 | Heptachlor | 0.2 |
| Carbaryl | 0.1 | Hexachlorobenzene | 0.2 |
| Chlorpyrifos | 2.0 | Lindane | 1.0 |
| Cypermethrin | 0.02 | Monocrotophos | 0.02 |
| DDT and Its metabolite | 5.0 (Fat) | Propoxur | 0.05 |
| Decamethrin/ Deltamethrin | 0.03 | | |

**Table 34.4:** Acceptable Daily Intake (ADI) for Indian Pesticides.

| *Name of pesticide* | *JMPR-ADI (mg/kg bw)* | *Year of review* |
|---|---|---|
| D.D.T. | 0.005 (Conditional) | 1983 |
| Malathion | 0.3 | 1997 |
| Methyl Parathion | 0.003 | 1995 |
| Dichlorvos—D.D.V.P. | 0.004 | 1993 |
| Monocrotophos | 0.0006 | 1995 |
| Phorate | 0.0005 | 1996 |
| Ethion | 0.002 | 1990 |
| Endosulfan | 0.006 | 1998 |
| Cypermethrin | 0.05 | 1996 |
| Acephate | 0.01 | 2002 |
| Chlorpyrifos | 0.01 | 1999 |
| Lindane | 0.005 | 2002 |
| Endrin | 0.0002 (PTDI) | 1994 |
| Dieldrin | 0.0001 (PTDI) | 1994 |
| Carbaryl | 0.008 | 2001 |

*Source:* CSE (2004)

## ALTERNATIVES TO REDUCE THE RISK OF PESTICIDES IN MEAT AND MEAT PRODUCTS

It has been explained above that animal tissue gets the residue of pesticides in their tissue mainly through the contaminated feed, fodder or water. Therefore, the strategies to reduce the pesticides residue in meat and meat products should directly through the reduction of their use in agriculture. Undoubtedly pesticides reducing the losses are enhancing efficiency of agricultural production system but some alternates have also been suggested considering the health hazard associated with their use. Some evidence shows that alternatives to pesticides can be equally effective as the use of chemicals. Alternatives to pesticides include methods of cultivation, use of biological pest controls (such as pheromones, neem-based pesticides and microbial pesticides), genetic engineering, and methods of interfering with insect breeding. Application of composted yard waste has also been used as a way of controlling pests. Cultivation practices include polyculture (growing multiple types of plants), crop rotation, planting crops in areas where the pests that damage them do not live, timing planting according to when pests will be least problematic, and use of trap crops that attract pests away from the real crop. Release of other organisms that fight the pest such as natural predators or parasites entomopathogenic fungi, bacteria and viruses of the pests are other example of alternatives to pesticide use. Thermal treatment of soil through steam, interfering with insects' reproduction, using traditional *Panchagavya*, the "mixture of five products are some proven alternates. Under Integrated pest management (IPM), mixture of behavior-modifying stimuli to manipulate the distribution and abundance of insects was also suggested to reduce the pesticides uses. Even some of the food processing technologies are being investigated as probable means for reduction of pesticides in consumable products. Removal of residues in food by processing is affected by type of food, insecticide type and nature and severity of processing procedure used. Food processing treatments such as washing, peeling, canning or cooking have been reported to lead a significant reduction of pesticide residues, although these findings in meat processing are yet to be investigated.

# 35 CHAPTER

# Healthier Meat and Meat Products and their Role as Functional Foods

Diet is one of the important factors influencing the health and well-being of the people. Meat consumption is increasing in India as it is being attached with the quality of life. Meat and meat products are important sources of proteins, vitamins and minerals and also contribute to the intake of fat, saturated fatty acids, cholesterol, table salt, etc., Presence of inappropriate proportions of these elements and their association with obesity, coronary heart diseases, atherosclerosis, etc., is influencing the image of meat products. Various international health organizations including WHO have recommended lowering of daily intake of dietary fat between 15 and 30% of total calories, limiting saturated fat to less than 10% of the total calories and cholesterol content to less than 300 mg per day as a means of reducing the risk of such health problems. Meat and meat products inherently lack in dietary fiber, which is again not conducive for a good health. In order to uphold the consumption of this highly nutritious food item and reduce the risk of diet-related diseases in consumers, strategies have to be evolved to provide them healthier meat products. The concept of healthier foods encompasses the basis of functional foods which typically denote processed foods having disease-preventing and/or health-promoting benefits in addition to their normal nutritive value. Such foods should be derived from naturally occurring ingredients, consumed as a part of daily diet and involved in regulating specific processes for humans including preventing the risk of disease, delaying aging process and improving immunological ability.

## STRATEGIES FOR ACHIEVING HEALTHIER MEAT AND MEAT PRODUCTS

The meat industry is coming under heavy pressure to come up with meat products in which undesired constituents are either eliminated or reduced within appropriate limits, while beneficial constituents are enriched or incorporated. This will require a detailed planning from animal production, handling of raw meat as well as other ingredients and then product reformulation. Various strategies in the development of healthier meat products are briefly described below:

## Modification of Carcass Composition

The composition of animal carcass differs depending on the species, breed, age, sex, type of feed, etc. Various techniques have been worked out to induce desirable changes in various meat constituents by employing genetic selection, manipulation of feed type and feeding schedule, using growth promoters and nutrition partitioning agents and immunization of animals against target hormones.

Significant changes could be achieved in carcass composition through selection of genetic lines resulting in reduction of fat and increase in unsaturated fatty acid percentage. In pigs, restriction of energy intake will reduce carcass fat, whereas provision of excess protein will increase the lean fat ratio. Desirable fatty acid profile can be achieved in pig and poultry (monogastric) by manipulating dietary fatty acid composition. Feed supplementation with vitamin E in these two species resulted in meat with comparatively higher vitamin E, better lipid stability and sensory quality. It has been possible to produce eggs, chicken and beef with several fold increase in Omega 3, DHA and vitamin E contents through feeding strategies. Several studies have shown that feeding conditions of animals influence the contents of bioactive components, such as L-carnitine and CLA in meat.

Partitioning agents like growth hormones, anabolizers, etc., and target immunization can alter metabolism and selectively promote protein synthesis and reduce fat deposition. In pigs, somatotropin administration can bring about not only substantial increase in carcass protein but also significant reduction in carcass fat and saturated fatty acids.

## Manipulation of Meat as a Raw Material

Meat composition can be altered to some extent by intervention during the conversion of muscle to meat or handling raw meat before the actual processing commences. Extensive trimming can be undertaken to remove external fat and limit internal fat from the carcass. The process can be further extended to trim the fat from the primal cuts and retail cuts as well. In order to produce emulsion-based or ground meat products with minimum fat, it is possible to reduce particle size and then separate or extract fat through physicochemical techniques such as cryofiltration, centrifugation, decantation, etc. However, such an extreme limitation of fat is bound to have some impact on the sensory quality of the resultant product which will need to be addressed.

## Reformulation of Meat Products

Formulation of a meat product is the appropriate time to bring about the desired characteristics in the final product. It could be accomplished by limiting certain undesirable components and incorporation of some health-enhancing ingredients. The newly developed product should have tailored functional characteristics with good sensory quality, safety, convenience and shelf-life. We can approach the reformulation of the meat products on the following lines:

### *Reduction of Fat Content and Calories*

Generally, meat products contain 15–25% of fat, which need to be lowered to 10% or even less. It can be partially achieved by reformulating the product with lean meat. However, it results in technological problems because juiciness of meat product is immediately affected followed by texture. Lot of research work is being conducted to evolve low-fat meat products. These have been categorized as lean and extra lean on the basis of fat percentage in the finished meat products. Several fat replacers have been identified. Fat replacers have been defined as ingredients that contribute minimum calories to formulated meat products and do not drastically change the flavor, juiciness, mouth feel, viscosity or other organoleptic and processing properties. These include added water to some extent. Carbohydrate-based fat replacers such as carrageenan, alginate, potato starch, tapioca starch, oat fiber, soy flour, barley flour, etc., alone or in combination have been shown to have good potential.

Milk protein derivatives like skim milk powder, sodium caseinate, milk coprecipitate, whey protein concentrate, etc., have also proved to be good fat mimetic as well as texture modifying agents. Among vegetable proteins, soy proteins are widely used in the formulation of low-fat meat products. Others like corn gluten meal, texturized peanut protein could also be used. A zein-based fat replacer has been commercially marketed, which simulates the sensory and physical characteristics of emulsion-based products. All these ingredients possess the unique property of binding water which helps in preventing the sensory feeling of dryness in emulsion-based patties, sausages, nuggets, etc. Lowering of fat level will improve the nutritional quality by reducing calorific value and cholesterol content. This condition will minimize the chances of obesity, hypertension and cardiovascular diseases.

*Modification of Fatty Acid Profile and Reduction of Cholesterol*

It is not only the fat but the fatty acid profile and level of cholesterol which needs to be attended. Animal fat contains lot of saturated fatty acids and good amount of cholesterol. So instead of using animal fat in meat products, a shift should be made to use vegetable oils such as sunflower oil, soybean oil, safflower oil, linseed oil, olive oil, canola oil, etc. These oils are high in mono and polyunsaturated fatty acids and free from cholesterol. Sunflower oil and soybean oil are rich in health-promoting omega-6 fatty acids, whereas linseed oil is rich in omega-3 fatty acids. Use of unsaturated fatty acids will lower serum triglycerides, thereby reducing the chances of thrombosis and atherosclerosis. Still another advantage of using vegetable oils is that they contain a wide range of phytosterols which have been found to reduce the LDL cholesterol. Vegetable oils like sunflower oil, palm oil and cotton seed oil are also good sources of antioxidant vitamin, tocopherol.

*Reduction of Table Salt/Sodium Content*

Sodium chloride or common table salt is an essential part of human diet. Considerable concerns are now being expressed about the amount of sodium chloride in the diet. On population basis, it has been established that consumption of more than 6 g sodium chloride per person in a day was associated with an age-increase blood pressure and the total dietary salt be maintained at about 5-6 g per day. Sodium constitutes 40% of sodium chloride and excess of sodium has been implicated in arterial hypertension. Hence, it is desired that ways and means should be devised to reduce sodium chloride content of these products to make them healthier without much effect on the sensory acceptability of these products.

Meat as such is relatively poor in sodium, containing only 50–90 mg of sodium per 100 g. However, the sodium in meat products is much higher because of table salt content, which can be 2% in emulsion-based or ground meat products to as much as 4–6% in cured meat products. The technologists should endeavor to substitute 50% of the sodium chloride normally present in meat products to make them healthier. Salt reduction leads to loss of functionality, increased cooking losses and lower acceptability due to decrease in textural properties and flavor. Finding a suitable sodium chloride substitute is a big challenge because of its unique, pure salty taste and flavor enhancing properties. Sodium chloride can be partially substituted by other compounds that have somewhat matching properties. A combination of chlorides of sodium, potassium and magnesium has been advocated for satisfactory results. A number of sodium chloride substitutes are presently being tried for partial replacement. These include chloride, lactate, phosphate and sorbate of potassium; lactate and ascorbate of calcium, glutamic acid, glutamate and recently transglutaminase.

Seasoning with herbs, spices and vinegar is a healthy way to enjoy great flavor with less sodium. Different herbs have their own flavor strength. Strong flavor herbs include bay, cardamom, curry, ginger, mustard, black pepper, rosemary and sage. Medium flavor herbs required in moderate amount include basil, celery seed and leaves, cumin, fennel, garlic, marjoram, oregano, mint, savory, thyme and turmeric. Delicate flavor herbs may be used in large quantities and combine well with most other herbs and spices. This group includes chervil, chives and parsley also.

#### *Incorporation of Dietary Fiber*

Dietary fibers consists of plant polysaccharides, oligosaccharides, lignin and associated plant substances, which are resistant to digestive enzymes of human beings. These can be classified as soluble or insoluble fibers. Soluble fibers dissolve in the water of food and form a viscous gel which can trap certain food components and make them less available for absorption. Insoluble fibers remain metabolically inert and provide bulking or can be prebiotic and ferment in the large intestine. Both the types of fibers have numerous health benefits including maintaining bowel integrity and gut health, lowering blood cholesterol levels, controlling blood sugar levels and providing a non-caloric bulking agent that can help in weight loss by replacing caloric food components such as fat. Increased proportions of fibers in foods are known to reduce the risk of cardiovascular diseases, diverticulitis, constipation, irritable colon, colon cancer, diabetes, etc. In addition to health benefits, dietary fibers in meat also have other advantages such as fat replacement, increased water-holding capacity, fat-binding properties, cooking yield and improved oxidative stability when fiber source is associated with phenolic antioxidants.

Incorporation of dietary fiber has been successful in various meat products from different plant food sources: grains (oatmeal/bran, barley flour, wheat bran, rice bran, etc.), legumes (black bean, kidney bean, lentil flour, gram flour, pea hull flour, etc.), vegetables (sweet potato, carrot, bottle gourd, cabbage, capsicum, turnip, broccoli, etc.) or fruits (apricot, orange pulp, apple pulp, peach, raw banana, etc.). Besides, chicory root powder (inulin), flaxseed, etc. have also been used in meat products. Dietary fibers, especially from vegetable and fruit origin, are carrier of bioactive compounds. It is interesting to note that incorporation of most of the dietary fibers not only imparts one or more health-enhancing effects but also technological benefits as well.

*Enrichment with Meat-based Bioactive Compounds*

The Foundation for Innovation in Medicine in 1991 defined bioactives as "any substance that may be considered a food or part of a food that provides medical or health benefits including the prevention and treatment of a disease." Bioactive compounds have been shown to exhibit physiological benefits upon ingestion. Most bioactives are naturally occurring compounds that can be extracted from the plant or animal sources. A prerequisite for physiological action of many bio-actives is that (a) sufficient quantities of components are present in the food system, (b) compounds remain physically and chemically active during production, storage and consumption and (c) upon consumption pass through the human digestive system in the form that allows the compounds to be optimally absorbed in the intestinal tract. Some of the important ones are:

**Conjugated linoleic acid (CLA)**

Conjugated linoleic acid have been shown to exert anticarcinogenic, antioxidative and immunomodulative properties. CLA might also play a role in the prevention/control of obesity, diabetes and modulation of bone metabolism. Conjugated linoleic acid was initially identified as anticancer compound from ground beef extract. It is a group of positional and geometric isomers of octadecadienoic acid. It is most abundant in fat and muscle of ruminant animals because rumen bacteria convert lenoleic acid to CLA by their isomerase. Even though ruminant meat and milk products are rich sources of CLA, further enrichment of these products are required to obtain potential health benefits of CLA in human population. CLA is also available as a food additive for incorporation in other foods.

## BIOACTIVE PEPTIDES

Naturally occurring angiotensin I-converting enzyme (ACE) inhibitory activity has been identified from the proteolytic degradation products of native proteins including those from meat, dairy, fish, eggs, etc. Bioactive peptides recovered from the hydrolysis of skeletal muscle proteins including myosin, tropomyosin, troponin, actin and collagen have been shown to vary in size and ACE inhibitory activity. These fractions could be generated using enzyme technology, concentrated and incorporated into functional meat products at the acceptable level (being mostly bitter). Preformed bioactive peptides would be promising ingredients in emulsion-based meat products, where they can remain active in lipophilic matrix. Upon digestion of lipid in intestine, the peptides would be absorbed into the blood and reduce blood pressure. Generation of bioactive peptides, being practiced in some fermented dairy products, can also improve the functionality of fermented meat products.

**Histidyl dipeptides**

Carnosine and anserine are antioxidative histidyl dipeptides that are found in significant amount in meat. Carnosine is a dipeptide from amino acids: β-alanine and L-histidine. Anserine is N-methylated derivative of carnosine. The concentration of carnosine ranges from 500 mg/kg in chicken thigh to 2,700 mg/kg in pork shoulder, whereas anserine is particularly rich in chicken muscles. Both are absent in foods of plant origin. Carnosine and anserine play a major role in muscle tissue as pH buffer and show antioxidative properties. Carnosine exert antioxidative effect as free radical scavenger, metal chelator and a hydrogen donor and thus also bring about color stabilization in meats. It has been also reported to promote several biological reactions resulting in improved wound healing, reduce cell damage in Alzheimer disease patients, slow aging and increased muscle strength and endurance.

**L- carnitine**

L-carnitine (hydroxy trimethyl amino butyric acid) plays a key-role in fat metabolism by transporting long chain fatty acids across the mitochondrial membranes to produce energy. Human body can synthesize some L-carnitine in liver and brain but requirement depends on the activity. L-carnitine is frequently recommended as a food supplement for boosting fat combustion in weight reduction diets and to enhance performance in sports. It helps the body to absorb calcium to improve bone strength and has a positive influence on memory and concentration.

Meat is a good source of L-carnitine (20–40 mg/100 g in pork, 40–60 mg/100 g in mutton, 65–88 mg/100 g in beef). A drink product containing L-carnitine is advertized and marketed in USA claiming maintenance of stamina and recovery from fatigue. Similarly a functional product containing L-carnitine and carnosine of beef origin is being marketed in Japan.

**Taurine**

Meat is particularly rich in taurine (110 mg/100 g in lamb and 77 mg/100 g in beef). Despite being an amino acid structure it does not build protein in the body, but plays a role in several physiological conditions such as bile acid conjugation, development of retina and nervous system, modulation of calcium level and a positive ionotropic influence on the cardiac muscle. It is also reported to offer protection in oxidative stress and immune challenge situations. Taurine is added to energy drinks with the claim that it enhances physical and mental capacity.

**Creatine**

Creatine and its phosphorylated derivative creatine phosphate play an important role in muscle energy metabolism. Though, red meats contain approx. 359 mg/100 g of taurine. Still, meat consumption alone cannot enhance sport performance because the lowest dose for enhanced performance is four times the content in 100 g meat. Creatine supplements are given to athletes in order to improve performance.

Besides, several other endogenous compounds like Coenzyme Q10, glutathione, lipoic acid, spermine, etc., have also been identified in skeletal muscle. Coenzyme Q10 (Ubiquinone) has good antioxidant properties and its supplements have shown beneficial effects in some studies. Glutathione is a component of glutathione oxidase enzymes which play a role in immune response and enhancing iron absorption by contributing to the *meat factor*.

Eating a healthful diet is the responsibility of the consumer. Fortunately, consumers are now becoming conscious of the diet-related problems and are anxious to reform their diet to derive health benefits. Meat technologists should accept this challenge and develop a variety of meat products which are not only health-enhancing but palatable and safe as well. Thus, industry will be able to provide functional or designer meat foods reformulated for the specific purposes. The possibilities of enrichment of meat-based bioactive compounds have to be fully explored to stand out against competitive products. The idea of using food for health purposes is opening up a whole new field for meat industry. Our endeavor should be to incorporate several sets of health-enhancing properties in various types of meat products. Consumers have to be offered integrated functional meat products to maximize the advantages of this premium commodity.

# 36 CHAPTER

# Optimizing Shelf-Life of Meat and Meat Products using Innovative Packaging Solutions

Packaging is the scientific method of containing food products against physical damage, chemical changes and further microbial contamination and to display the product in the most attractive manner for consumer preference. It can be described as a coordinated system of preparing goods for transport, warehousing, logistics, sale and end use. Packaging contains, protects, preserves, transports, informs, and sells. In many countries it is fully integrated into government, institutional, industrial, business and personal use. Packaging fresh meat is carried out to avoid contamination, delay spoilage, permit some enzymatic activity to improve tenderness, reduce weight loss and where applicable, to ensure an oxymyoglobin or cherry-red color in red meats at retail or customer level. When considering processed meat products, factors such as dehydration, lipid oxidation, discoloration and loss of aroma must be taken into account. Traditional food packaging was meant for mechanical supporting of otherwise non-solid food and protecting food from external influences. The shelf life of packaged food depends on both the intrinsic nature of food and extrinsic factors. Intrinsic factors include pH, water activity ($a_w$), nutrient content, presence of antimicrobial compounds, redox potential, respiratory rate, and the biological structure, whereas extrinsic factors include storage temperature, relative humidity, and the surrounding gas composition.

Vacuum packaging maintains the product in an oxygen deficient environment to achieve its preservative effect. It has the inherent disadvantage of keeping the meat in mechanical strain which may increase drip loss. An alternative to vacuum packaging, with added cost, is modified atmosphere packaging wherein meat and meat products are stored under various gaseous atmospheres to achieve enhanced shelf life. Active packaging is the deliberate incorporation of certain additives into packaging systems (whether loose within the pack, attached to the inside of packaging material or incorporated within the packaging material itself) with the aim of maintaining or enhancing product quality and shelflife. Principal active packaging systems involve oxygen scavenging, moisture absorption, carbon dioxide and finally antimicrobial systems. These concepts are successfully utilized in the US and Japan but have seen only limited development in Europe. This could be due to legal restrictions, lack of knowledge about both the acceptability of these systems to consumers and their effectiveness in packaging or to their economic and environmental impact. Consumers now look forward to labeling with shelf life dating on the food itself as an assurance of quality, nutrition and safety. Intelligent packaging (sometimes described as smart packaging) is packaging that in some way senses some properties of the food it encloses or indicate history of the environment in which it is kept and is able to inform the manufacturer, retailer and consumer of the state of these properties. Although distinctly different from the concept of active packaging, features of intelligent packaging can be used to check the effectiveness and integrity of active packaging systems.

## VACUUM PACKAGING

Vacuum packaging of meat is meant to retard or completely check the oxidative reactions and inhibit the microbial growth by eliminating oxygen. It is widely used to extend the storage life of fresh chilled meats by maintaining an oxygen deficient environment within the pack. The air within the package must be evacuated effectively to almost anoxic levels (less than 500 ppm) to prevent irreversible browning due to low levels of residual oxygen. The exclusion of oxygen from the meat surface as soon as possible, after the breaking of the carcass into primal and subprimal cuts, retains the potential to reoxygenate meat following retail pack display. The application of a vacuum to 0.8–0.9 atmospheres is generally sufficient to produce satisfactory vacuum, so that most potent pathogenic aerobic bacterial growth is inhibited. The oxygen level should be less than 1 percent and carbon dioxide less than 10 percent in vacuum packaged meat. Lactobacillus and Brochothrix thermosphacta are the dominant bacteria in vacuum packaged meat. However, vacuum packaged meat having pH below 5.8 overcomes the danger of Brochothrix thermosphacta. This is due to the longer lag phase of this bacterium in comparison to competitive bacteria and also due to its sensitivity to low pH and temperature.

Vacuum packages for meat are four basic types. The first one involves use of heat shrinking flexible packaging material around the primal cuts. When exposed to heat it shrinks and increases film thickness, improves mechanical resistance and reduces the drip loss. The second type involves use of preformed plastic bags/pouches made up of polyamide (PA) as the outer layer, while the inner core is polyethylene (PE). Polyamide provides barrier properties and physical strength while polyethylene provides sealing properties. The third type involves use of thermoform trays in line from a base web. Here the product is placed into the tray and then a film web is allowed to cover the tray from a second reel of film followed by pack evacuation and vacuum sealing. The fourth one is called vacuum skin packaging, in which meat is placed in a rigid preformed tray or on the flat surface of a flexible base material followed by heat softening, evacuation and vacuum shrink sealing. This technique is recommended for long term storage of primal and sub primal cuts of buffalo meat. It ensures a shelf life of 8–10 weeks at 00C. Vacuum packaging of lamb and pork is avoided for different reasons. Lamb may have a shelf life of 3 weeks only because of comparatively high pH. However, lambs with ultimate pH less than 5.8 can be vacuum packaged for shipment to distant destinations. Pork starts with a large load of bacteria and pork cuts are reported to have a shelf life of 2 weeks only at 1°C.

Vacuum shrink packaging in Cryovac barrier bags may provide a means of storage and transport of frozen carcasses, sides or quarters to overseas destinations. A suitable film for vacuum packaging must have a good mechanical strength and barrier properties, besides making perfect seals Vacuum packaging is done either in laminates or coextruded films.

**Some of the typical laminates in use are:**

Aluminum foil/Polyethylene
Polyamide/Polyethylene
PVDC/Polyester/Polyethylene
Polyester/Polyethylene
PVDC copolymer film
Copolymer coated cellulose/PE film
Nylon/EVA

Vacuum packaging is recommended for long term storage of dressed whole or halved poultry because it ensures a shelf life of 5–6 weeks at 2°C. Vacuum packaging reduces the volume of air sealed with meat. The residual oxygen, if any, is quickly consumed by meat. Thus, vacuum packaging provides a good avenue for keeping the product at a better level of quality. The advantages of vacuum packaging can be enumerated as follows:

1. There is saving of space and energy during storage, transport and distribution.
2. There is no loss in weight.
3. The natural flavor of the product is preserved.
4. The product has better keeping quality.
5. The display of the product is better which help in better marketing and fetching better price.

Vacuum packaged product is stored in a refrigerator at 0–2°C. Storage of chilled meat in gas impermeable packs restricts the growth of *Pseudomonas* sp., thus extending the shelf life of meat. The most common bacteria on stored vacuum packaged poultry meat are the lactic acid bacteria mainly *Lactobacillus* sp. However, a puncture or slit or loose seal in vacuum pack may result in blue or green discoloration. Interestingly, vacuum packaged buffalo meat has been found to have the lower fiber diameter and higher sarcomere length. Thus, vacuum appears to enhance ageing of meat resulting in comparatively tender meat.

## MODIFIED ATMOSPHERE PACKAGING (MAP)

Modified atmosphere packaging is an important preservation method for fresh and minimally processed foods. Modified atmosphere packaging encloses food products in high gas barrier materials, where gas environment has been changed once to slow the respiration rate, reduce microbiological growth and retard enzyme spoilage with the final aim of prolonging the shelf life. It is also referred as controlled atmosphere packaging with certain conditions. In controlled atmosphere packaging (CAP) system, the package atmosphere is altered initially and then maintained during the entire period of storage. These techniques are used for a wide range of shelf stable and ready-to-eat chilled foods.

Modified atmosphere combined with low temperature delays the deleterious effects and maintains quality of chilled stored meat for extended periods. The atmosphere inside the package is modified in such a way to extend the shelf life of meat while retaining its color, flavor and weight. The package air can be suitably replaced by gases usually nitrogen, oxygen or carbon dioxide alone or in combination. Different meats have varying modified atmosphere requirements. In red meats, oxygen maintains the much-desired bright red pigment-oxymyoglobin associated with freshness while carbon dioxide inhibits the growth of meat borne microorganisms. The most commonly used gas mixture for fresh red meat is high oxygen which is minimum 60–70% and 30–40% carbon dioxide. Buffalo meat and beef need high oxygen content to maintain a bright red color. Pork needs less oxygen due to high fat content. Nitrogen serves as an inert filler to balance a gas mixture. However, its use increases the cost of packaging.

Carbon monoxide is used in very low concentration and gives cherry red color. The sulphur dioxide has inhibitory effect on bacteria in acidic pH and is used in fermented meat products. Argon, an inert noble gas has some antimicrobial activity and is also sometimes utilized in vacuum packaging of meat and meat products. High standards of hygiene and temperature controls are essential prerequisites for the quality and safety of MAP packed meat and meat products. A gaseous atmosphere of 99% carbon dioxide/1% carbon monoxide was found to be best for preserving the desirable pork loin. Pork loins in such MAP obtained the highest consumer acceptance scores after 24 h of storage. Chops from high pH carcasses had comparatively higher color scores and aerobic plate counts and less discoloration. Overall pH was the best indicator of color and microbiological stability.

In general, the ideal MAP gas mix. for various meat and meat products can be summarized as follows:

| | |
|---|---|
| Raw red meat | 70% $O_2$, 20% $CO_2$, 10% $N_2$ |
| Raw pork | 80% $CO_2$, 20% $N_2$ or even 100% $CO_2$ |
| Raw dressed poultry | 40% $CO_2$, 60% $N_2$ or 50% $CO_2$, 50% $N_2$ |
| MDPM | 20–30% $CO_2$, 0–10% $O_2$, 70-75% $N_2$ |
| Cured meats | 10–15% $CO_2$, 85–90 %$N_2$ |
| Raw offal | 80% $O_2$, 20% $CO_2$ |
| Combination products | 30% $CO_2$, 70% $N_2$ |

## ACTIVE PACKAGING

Active packaging has been defined as packaging, which changes the condition of the packaged food to extend shelflife or to improve safety or sensory properties, while maintaining the quality of packaged food. Packaging may be termed as active when it performs some desired role in food preservation other than providing an inert barrier to external conditions. The development of a whole range of active packaging systems, some of which may have applications in both new and existing food products, is fairly new. Active packaging includes additives or freshness enhancers that can participate in a host of packaging applications and by so doing, enhance the preservation function of the primary packaging system. Active packaging is one of the innovative food packaging concepts that have been introduced as a response to the continuous changes in current consumer demands and market trends. Major active packaging techniques are concerned with substances that absorb oxygen, moisture, carbon dioxide, flavors/odors and those which release carbon dioxide, ethylene antimicrobial agents, antioxidants and flavors.

## Oxygen Scavengers

High levels of oxygen present in food packages may facilitate microbial growth, off flavors and off odors development, color changes and nutritional losses, thereby causing significant reduction in the shelf life of foods. Although oxygen sensitive foods can be packaged under MAP or vacuum conditions, such techniques do not always facilitate the complete removal of oxygen. Therefore, control of oxygen levels in food packages is important to limit the rate of such deteriorative and spoilage reactions in foods.

Oxygen absorbing systems provide an alternative to vacuum and gas flushing technologies as a means of improving product quality and shelf life. Using an oxygen scavenger, which absorbs the residual oxygen after packaging, quality changes in oxygen sensitive foods can often be minimized. Oxygen absorbers can also be a complement of vacuum packaging to avoid photo-oxidation phenomena, in particular for sliced delicatessen products. Indeed, presentations in small packages with a transparent cover to show the food product are more and more appreciated. However, if oxygen traces are still present when the package is put on the shelf, the photo-oxidation phenomena start to take effect, leading to a rapid discoloration of the meat. Existing oxygen scavenging technologies utilize one or more of the following concepts: iron powder oxidation, ascorbic acid oxidation, photosensitive dye oxidation, enzymatic oxidation (e.g., glucose oxidase and alcohol oxidase), and unsaturated fatty acids (e.g., oleic or linolenic acid) rice extract or immobilized yeast on a solid substrate. Structurally, the oxygen scavenging component of a package can take the form of a sachet, label, film (incorporation of scavenging agent into the packaging film), card, closure liner or concentrate. Ageless® (Mitsubishi Gas Chemical Co., Japan) is the most common oxygen scavenging system based on iron oxidation. The sachets are designed to reduce oxygen levels to less than 1%. Iron based oxygen scavenger along with catalysts have been successfully used in sliced, cooked and cured meats.

## Carbon Dioxide Scavengers and Emitters

The function of carbon dioxide within a packaging environment is to suppress microbial growth. Therefore, a carbon dioxide generating system can be viewed as a technique complimentary to oxygen scavenging. Since the permeability of carbon dioxide is 3–5 times higher than that of oxygen in most plastic films, it must be continuously produced to maintain the desired concentration within the package. High carbon dioxide levels (10–80%) are desirable for foods such as meat and poultry in order to inhibit surface microbial growth and extend shelf life. The advantages of carbon dioxide are that it acts on all the food inside the packaging and does not require contact between the food and package, whereas the disadvantage is that it changes the color of meat.

$CO_2$ may be used in conjunction with oxygen scavengers to maintain an atmosphere that is favorable for the preservation of certain products. In the case of fishery products, fresh and processed meats, cheeses, and baked goods, a high concentration of carbon dioxide in the atmosphere of the package is advantageous because it maintains the organoleptic properties of the products and exerts a bacteriostatic effect. Collapse of the package or development of a partial vacuum may also be a problem for food packed with oxygen absorbers. To overcome this problem, the dual action of oxygen absorber/emitter of carbon dioxide absorbs oxygen and generates an equivalent volume of carbon dioxide. Ageless® G and FreshPax exert dual effects as they have the ability to absorb oxygen and emit carbon dioxide. Freshilizer® is another $CO_2$-releasing product used to extend the shelflife of fresh meat. This innovative package consists of a tray with a perforated false bottom in which a porous sachet containing sodium bicarbonate/ascorbate is deposited. When exudates from meat come in contact with the sachet, it releases carbon dioxide, so that the carbon dioxide absorbed by the meat is replaced continuously. Carbon dioxide absorbers (sachets), consisting of either calcium hydroxide and sodium hydroxide, or potassium hydroxide, calcium oxide and silica gel, may be used to remove carbon dioxide during storage in order to prevent bursting of the package. Food applications include their use in packs of fresh meat, dehydrated poultry products and beef jerky.

## Moisture Absorbers

The main purpose of liquid water control is to lower the water activity of the product, thereby suppressing microbial growth. Several companies manufacture drip absorbent sheets or pads such as Cryovac® Dri-Loc® (Sealed Air Corporation, USA), Thermarite® or Peaksorb® (Australia), Toppan (Japan) and Fresh-R-Paxe (Maxwell Chase Technologies, LLC, USA) for liquid control in high water activity foods such as meat and poultry. These systems consist of a super absorbent polymer located between two layers of a microporous or nonwoven polymer like polyvinyl acetate blanket. Such sheets are used as drip-absorbing pads placed under whole chickens or chicken cuts.

## Chlorine Dioxide Generators

Chlorine dioxide can exist in gaseous, liquid or solid state. Its efficiency against bacteria, fungi and viruses can be delivered from a solid state, called Microspheres (Bernard Technologies, USA), through the interaction of moisture to produce a controlled and sustained release of chlorine dioxide in gaseous form. According to the company, no residue is left, nor is the food product contained in the packaging tainted in any way. Sustained and controlled release of chlorine dioxide is related to exposure to humidity greater than 80% and light. The result is a high activity against a broad spectrum of microorganisms including actively growing vegetative cells and spores. Microsphere powder can be delivered from sachets previously incorporated in the packaging. The sustained and controlled release of chlorine dioxide from the Microspheres can be varied from peak delivery of 1 ppm–100 ppm for periods of days to 6 weeks. Applications for this technology are just beginning to unfold in the food industry to reduce food safety risks for meat, poultry, fish and dairy products.

## Preservative Releasers/Antimicrobial Packaging

Microbial contamination and subsequent growth reduces the shelf life of foods and increases the risk of food borne illness. Traditional methods of preserving foods from the effect of microbial growth include thermal processing, drying, freezing, refrigeration, irradiation, MAP and addition of antimicrobial agents or salts. However, some of these techniques cannot be applied to food products such as fresh meats. Antimicrobial packaging is a promising form of active packaging especially for meat products. Incorporation of bactericidal agents into meat formulations may result in partial inactivation of the active compounds by meat constituents and therefore exert a limited effect on surface microflora. Antimicrobial food packaging materials have to extend the lag phase and reduce the growth phase of microorganisms in order to extend shelf life and to maintain product quality and safety.

The classes of antimicrobials listed range from acid anhydride, alcohol, bacteriocins, chelators, enzymes, organic acids and polysaccharides. Antimicrobial packages have had relatively few commercial successes except in Japan where Ag-substituted zeolite is the most common antimicrobial agent incorporated into plastics. Ag-ions inhibit a range of metabolic enzymes and have strong antimicrobial activity. Antimicrobial films can be classified into two types: those that contain an antimicrobial agent which migrates to the surface of the food and, those which are effective against surface growth of microorganisms without migration. Besides these flavor/odor absorbers like cellulose triacetate, citric acid, activated carbon, etc., have applications in poultry and fish.

## INTELLIGENT PACKAGING

Intelligent packaging systems are those that contain an external or internal indicator or sensor to provide information regarding aspects of history of package and/or quality of packaged food. Intelligent packaging has been defined as packaging systems which monitor the condition of packaged foods to give information about the quality of the packaged food during transport and storage. Smart packaging devices, which may be an integral component or inherent property of a foodstuff's packaging, can be used to monitor a plethora of food pack attributes. It refers to packaging that senses and signals or informs. The headspace of food packages undergoes changes in their composition over time. Devices capable for identifying, quantifying, and/or reporting changes in the atmosphere within the package, the temperatures during transfer and storage and the microbiological quality of food provide valuable information both to the final consumer and producer and/or marketer about the effectiveness of the conservation strategies used in the marketing chain.

Basically, there are two types of intelligent packaging: one based on measuring the condition of the package on the outside, the other measuring directly the quality of the food product, i.e., inside the packaging. In the latter case, there is direct contact with the food or with the headspace and there is always the need for a marker indicative of the quality and/or safety of the packed food. Examples include time-temperature indicators (TTI), gas leakage indicators, ripeness indicators, toxin indicators, biosensors, and radio frequency identification. Although distinctly different from the concept of active packaging, features of intelligent packaging can be used to check the effectiveness and integrity of active packaging systems.

## Indicators

### *Time-Temperature Indicators*

The best-before date printed on food packaging is only an indicative value and does not take into account possible fluctuations in temperature that food may suffer during storage. The best-before date must therefore be within the shelflife of the food to ensure that food is safe to consume. They fall into two types: visual indicators or radio frequency identification (RFID) tags. The basic idea underlying visual indicators is that the quality of food deteriorates more rapidly at higher temperatures because chemical reactions, biochemical reactions, and microbial growth are speeded up. The indicators change color in response to cumulative exposure to temperature to point at probable loss of shelflife. The main mechanisms of action include enzymatic reactions, polymerization, or chemical diffusion. These products are used to monitor exposure to unsuitable temperatures during transport and storage and are an indication of quality for the producer because they ensure that the product reaches the consumer in optimal conditions. It is important that the indication is irreversible.

### *Freshness Indicators*

The information provided by intelligent packaging systems on the quality of meat products may be either indirect (i.e., changes in packaging oxygen concentration may imply quality deterioration through established correlation) or direct. Freshness indicators provide direct product quality information resulting from microbial growth or chemical changes within a food product **(Fig. 36.1)**. Microbiological quality may be determined through reactions between indicators included within the package and microbial growth metabolites. The chemical detection of spoilage of foods and the chemical changes in meat during storage provide the basis for which freshness indicators may be developed based on target metabolites associated with microbiologically induced deterioration.

Changes in the concentration of organic acids such as n-butyrate, L-lactic acid, D-lactate and acetic acid during storage offer potential as indicator metabolites for a number of meat products. Biogenic

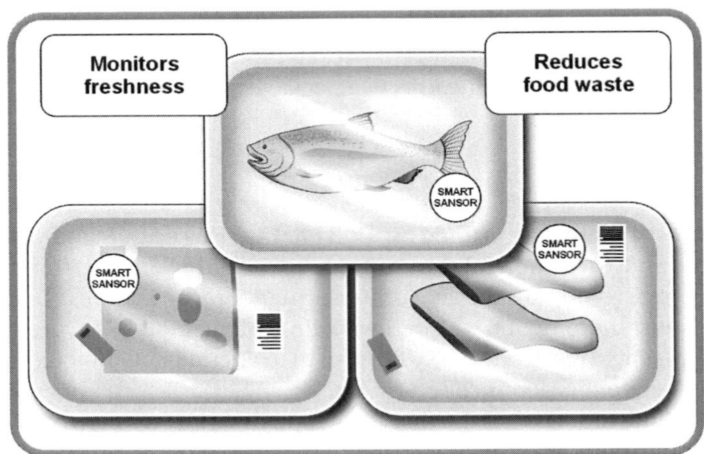


**Fig. 36.1:** Freshness indicators.

amines such as histamine, putrescine, tyramine and cadaverine have been implicated as indicators of meat product decomposition. Carbon dioxide produced during microbial growth can in many instances be indicative of quality deterioration. Hydrogen sulphide, a breakdown product of cysteine, with intense off-flavors and low threshold levels is produced during the spoilage of meat and poultry by a number of bacterial species.

## Sensors

A sensor is defined as a device used to detect, locate or quantify energy or matter, giving a signal for the detection or measurement of a physical or chemical property to which the device responds.

### *Gas Sensors*

Gas sensors are devices that respond reversibly and quantitatively to the presence of a gas by changing the physical parameters of the sensor and are monitored by an external device. Systems presently available for gas detection include amperometric oxygen sensors, potentiometric carbon dioxide sensors, metal oxide semiconductor field effect transistors, organic conducting polymers and piezoelectric crystal sensors. In recent years, a number of instruments and materials for optical oxygen sensing have been described. Such sensors are usually comprised of a solid-state material, which operate on the principle of luminescence quenching or absorbance changes caused by direct contact with the food. These systems provide a noninvasive technique for gas analysis through translucent materials and as such are potentially suitable for intelligent packaging applications.

*Fluorescence-based Oxygen Sensors*

Fluorescence-based oxygen sensors represent the most advanced and promising systems to date for remote measurement of headspace gases in packaged meat products. The active component of a fluorescence-based oxygen sensor normally consists of a long-delay fluorescent or phosphorescent dye encapsulated in a solid polymer matrix. Oxygen is quantified by measuring changes in luminescence parameters from the oxygen-sensing element in contact with the gas or liquid sample, using a predetermined calibration. The process is reversible and clean: neither the dye nor oxygen is consumed in the photochemical reactions involved, nor by-products are generated and the whole cycle can be repeated.

*Biosensors*

Biosensors are compact analytical devices that detect, record and transmit information pertaining to biological reaction. Intelligent packaging systems incorporating biosensors have the potential for extreme specificity and reliability. Market analysis of pathogen detection and safety systems for the food packaging industry suggests that biosensors offer considerable promise for future growth. The majority of available biosensor technology is not yet capable of commercial realization in the food sector.

At present two biosensor systems are commercially available. ToxinGuard® developed by Toxin Alert (Ontario, Canada) is a visual diagnostic system that incorporates antibodies in a polyethylene-based plastic packaging and is capable of detecting *Salmonella* sp., *Campylobacter* sp., *E. coli* 0517 and *Listeria* sp. The Food Sentinel System (SIRA Technologies, California, USA) is a biosensor system capable of continuous detection of contamination through immunological reactions occurring in part of a barcode. The barcode is rendered unreadable by the presence of contaminating bacteria. Such systems give some insight into products likely to become more mainstream in the years to come.

*Radio-frequency Identification Tags*

Radio frequency identification technology does not fall into either sensor or indicator classification but rather represents a separate electronic information-based form of intelligent packaging. RFID uses tags affixed to assets (cattle, containers, pallets, etc.) to transmit accurate, real-time information to a user's information system. In an RFID system, a reader emits radio waves to capture data from an RFID tag, and the data are then passed to a host computer for analysis and decision making. The RFID tag contains a minuscule microchip connected to a tiny antenna.

## BIOBASED AND EDIBLE PACKAGING

In the last decade, there has been a growing interest in the development of thermoplastic materials from biodegradable biopolymers, particularly those derived from renewable resources. The move is directed to produce edible films and coatings capable of protecting the food. Edible Packaging is an edible film or coating and is simply defined as a thin continuous layer of edible material formed on, placed on or between the foods or food components. The edible package is an integral part of the food, which can be eaten as a part of the whole food product. Biopolymers can be an alternative source for packaging development. Many studies have been undertaken for the suitability of various biomolecules mainly includes polysaccharides, lipids and proteins. It is a challenge to incorporate or maintain the functionality of conventional packaging without compromising with intended barrier properties of novel packaging material. These do not generally form coherent standalone films.

**Desirable attributes of package material:** Edible coatings should have an acceptable color, odor, taste, flavor and texture. It must adhere to the food but not stick to the secondary packaging materials. It should melt in mouth, but not in hands. An edible film to be used in food should be generally recognized as safe (GRAS). There should be a declaration about the type of edible materials as some individuals are allergic to certain polymers **(Fig. 36.2)**.

Edible packaging material must meet requirements related to permeability (mainly water vapor, carbon dioxide and oxygen) mechanical properties (especially their resistance to stretching and rupture), optical properties (mainly related with their opacity and color) and optical properties (mainly related with their opacity and

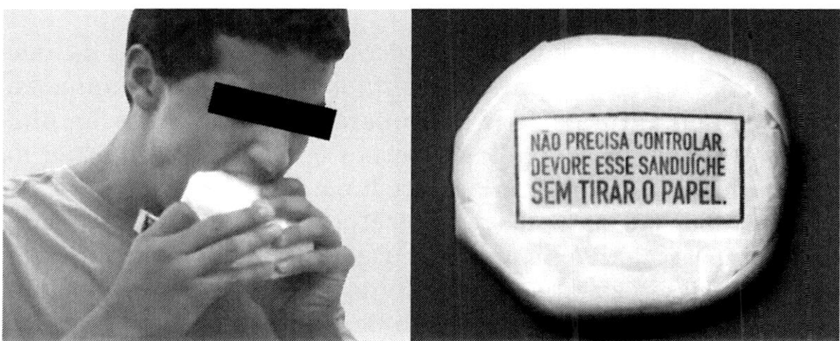


**Fig 36.2:** Burger with edible wrapper.

color) and flavor (in most cases, flavorless coatings are needed). These films/coatings may also serve as carriers of food additives such as anti-browning and antimicrobial agents, colorants, flavors, nutrients and spices. These can be advantageously used on meat and meat products with moisture loss reduction during storage of fresh or frozen meats, retention of juices from fresh meat and poultry, decrease in oxidation of lipids and myoglobin, reduction of spoilage and pathogen microorganisms on the surface of coated meats, and restriction of volatile flavor loss and foreign odor pick up.

Edible coatings should have an acceptable color, odor, taste, flavor and texture. It should be undetectable. It must adhere to the food but not stick to the packaging materials. It should melt in mouth, but not in hands. An edible film to be used in food should be generally recognized as safe (GRAS). There should be a declaration about the type of edible materials as some individuals are allergic to certain polymers.

**Biomolecules of edible packaging:** The use of edible films/coatings based on natural polymers and food grade additives have been constantly increasing in the food industry. The films/coatings can be produced with a great variety of products such as polysaccharides and their derivatives, proteins of animal or vegetable origin, lipids compounds and also from composites consisting of a blend of the previous materials. Normally, plasticizers are added to films/ coatings in order to improve their physical properties. They help to decrease brittleness and improve flexibility by reducing the intermolecular forces and increasing the mobility of polymeric chains.

**Polysaccharides**

Polysaccharides that have been used to form films/coatings include starch and starch derivatives, cellulose derivatives, alginates, carrageenan, various plant and microbial gums, chitosan and pectinates. Their hydrophilic properties provide a good barrier to carbon dioxide and oxygen under certain conditions but a poor barrier to water vapor and deficient mechanical properties. Galactomannans, natural polysaccharides commonly used in food industry, mostly as stabilizer, thickener and emulsifier, are one of the alternative materials that can be used for the production of edible films/coatings based on their edibility and biodegradability. Agar is a gum derived from a variety of red sea weeds and like carrageenan it is a galactose polymer. Agar coatings containing water soluble antibiotics and the bacteriocin nisin have been used on meat and fish.

**Lipids**

Lipids, due to their hydrophobic behavior, are often added to polysaccharide films aiming at decreasing their hydrophilicity and consequently, decreasing the water vapor permeability. The incorporation of active substances such as antibacterial, antifungal and antioxidant is one of the emerging utilizations of edible films/coatings; leading, in some cases, to changes in the physicochemical properties of edible films/coatings. Paraffin wax has been used to give protective coatings on several livestock products.

**Proteins**

A great variety of proteins have been investigated to produce edible films and coatings, such as collagen, common gelatin, corn zein, cotton seed, egg white, wheat gluten, soybean, gelatin, fish myofibrillar protein, pea protein, chitosan, casein, and whey proteins. A process of protein cross linking is necessary to obtain a flexible, easy to handle film. The resulting film properties are affected by the amino acid composition, distribution and polarity; conditions affecting formation of ionic cross linking between amino and carboxyl groups; presence of hydrogen bonding; intra molecular and intermolecular disulfide bonds. Collagen sausage casings are made from regenerated corium layer of animal hides. However, the formation of whey protein-based films has mainly involved heat denaturation in aqueous solution at 75–100°C, which produces intermolecular disulfide bonds, which might be partly responsible for film structure. Heat treatment promotes water insolubility, which may be beneficial to maintain film and food integrity. Whey protein-based films and coatings are generally flavorless, tasteless and flexible materials, water based, and the films varies from transparent to translucent depending on formulation, purity of protein sources and composition.

**Composite film**

Multicomponent and composite films can consist of a lipid layer (moisture barrier) supported by polysaccharide or protein layer (structural matrix). Food-based plasticizers such as glycerol, sorbitol, propylene glycol are generally added to edible films. A potential example of these types of composite packaging materials is gelatinized starch/hydrophobic copolymer/polyethylene. Protein based films appear to be better oxygen barriers than polysaccharides or lipid films. Improved starch and pectin films have been proposed for coating red meat also. Despite considerable research, the use of biobased packaging materials for the packaging of food remains limited.

Thus the package as a simple instrument for the marketing of food is changing to match the needs of consumers and the food industry. Changes in consumer preferences have led to innovations and developments in new packaging technologies. Vacuum packaging and modified/controlled atmosphere packaging maintain the quality of meat and meat products more than 5 weeks at refrigerated temperature. Active packaging is useful for extending the shelf life of fresh, cooked and other meat products. Currently, oxygen scavenger and moisture absorbers are found on the market in increasing numbers. However, antioxidants and antimicrobial active packaging and freshness indicators will be increasingly important and in future demand by the food industry. The potential advantages of intelligent packaging for muscle-based foods are many and varied. Apart from aspects of quality, safety, and distribution already outlined, intelligent packaging offers considerable potential as a marketing tool and the establishment of brand differentiation for meat products. Bio-based materials may find use in short shelflife foods stored at refrigerated temperature due to the fact that the material itself is biodegradable.

37

CHAPTER

# Developments in Sensory Evaluation of Muscle Foods

Sensory evaluation is a scientific testing method that evokes, measures, analyzes and interprets the human responses to those characteristics of food products which can be perceived through the senses of sight, taste, smell, touch and hearing. It is a fairly young science and most of the development and expansion has taken place in the last 25 years. Now, it is being used in the food industry throughout the world. It puts more human element to the overall acceptability of a food product due to multisensory experience. Human physiology and psychology has contributed immensely in evolving the principles of sensory evaluation.

## THE HUMAN SENSES

**Taste:** The four main basic tastes—sweet, salty, sour and bitter were recognized for a long time. However, recently (2002), the existence of a fifth taste called umami (savory or meat like) has been confirmed. The umami receptors detect amino acid glutamate, commonly found in muscle foods.

The classical 'taste map' is an over-simplification. Sensitivity to all tastes is distributed across the whole tongue but some areas are more responsive to certain tastes than others. A human tongue has 2000–10,000 taste buds and each bud has between 50 and 100 taste receptor cells. These are very sensitive and get activated very quickly. So when a food comes in contact with them, they can trigger a neural impulse in less than one tenth of a second.

**Smell:** The inhaled air through the nostrils contain volatile chemical molecules from the food which are detected by 10 million to 20 million olfactory receptor cells (containing protein) embedded in the olfactory membrane of the upper nasal passage. On stimulation of olfactory receptor cells, the membrane sends neural messages to the brain via olfactory nerve.

**Sight:** The eyes perceive general appearance of food such as color, size, shape, texture, consistency, etc. Light entering the lens of the eye is focused on the retina, where the rods and cones convert it to neural impulses that are transmitted to the brain via optic nerve.

**Touch:** The sense of touch delivers the impression of food texture. The tactile feel properties of the texture which are measured as geometric properties (grainy, gritty, crystalline, etc.) or moisture properties (wetness, oiliness, dryness, etc.) are sensed by the tactile nerves in the surface of the skin of the hands, lips or tongue.

**Hearing:** The sense of hearing can perceive sounds like crunching, crackling, popping, etc., can communicate much about a food. Sound is detected as vibrations propagating in the air which are transmitted via middle ear to create hydraulic motion in the fluid of inner ear or cochlea. The agitation in cochlea sends neural impulses to the brain.

## SENSORY TESTING FACILITIES

The sensory evaluation laboratory should have sufficient space with panel booths. It should be quite and odor-free. The temperature and relative humidity in the sensory evaluation area should be 22–24°C and 45–55% respectively. There should be uniform white fluorescent light of 300–500 lux in the evaluation area. Low-intensity red color light can be used to mask visual differences in specific cases **(Fig. 37.1)**.

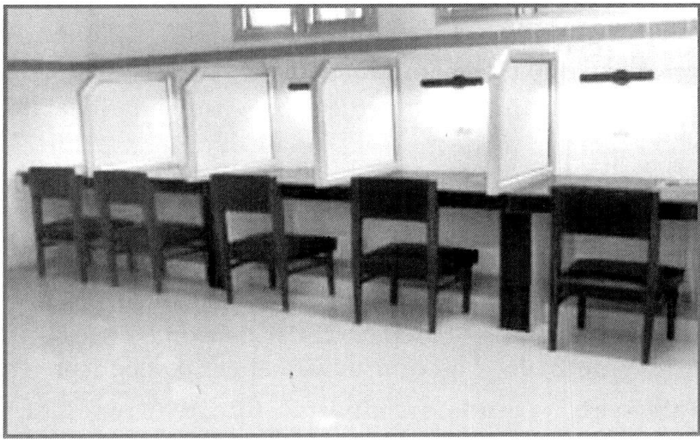

**Fig. 37.1:** Sensory testing facility.

## PANEL SELECTION AND TRAINING

The sensory panelists for analytical tests (discriminative as well as descriptive) have to be properly selected and provided suitable training. They should be healthy persons, preferably drawn from both the sexes and age-groups. People suffering from cold and color blindness do not qualify for the job. Smoking has also been found to dull gustatory and olfactory sensations. The prospective panelists should be subjected to taste recognition and threshold tests. Their threshold can be further improved by conducting training sessions especially difference tests.

## PREPARATION AND PRESENTATION OF SAMPLES

Cooked steaks, chops or roast samples should be cut in 1.25 cm cubes. Cutting of meat patties in pie-shaped or wedge samples is recommended. The minimum serving temperature for meat is 60°C in difference tests because at this temperature most volatile aromatics can be detected.

Samples should be coded with three-digit random numbers and presented in random order. Ideally four samples and maximum six samples can be evaluated per session in order to avoid taste or odor fatigue, lack of interest or concentration amongst the panelists. Palate cleansers such as room temperature distilled water or unsalted crackers can be used to minimize taste fatigue and flavor carryover. In the trained descriptive test, a "first sample bias" can be an issue. So a standardized "warm-up sample" (usually a sample that represents the typical product) should therefore be served to the panelists at the initiation of the sensory session. Ideal time for sensory evaluation is late morning or late afternoon. White-glazed China plates washed in unscented detergent serve best as sample containers.

## TYPES OF SENSORY EVALUATION METHODS

1. **Analytical methods**—based on discernible differences
2. **Affective methods**—based on individual acceptance or preferences

**1. Analytical methods** are divided into two types of tests: (i) Discriminative or difference tests and (ii) descriptive tests.

**(i) Discriminative or difference tests:** These tests are used for finding out the differences between the samples. These are generally employed to check and train the sensitivity of sensory panelists as follows:

A. *Paired comparison test:* It is a comparison test to find out the difference between two samples for a single specific attribute. Two samples are presented at a time to the respondents who are asked to tell whether the samples are same or different. There is 50% chance of the respondent being right in this simple test.

B. *Triangle test:* This is the most widely used difference test. It is employed to check the overall difference between the samples. In the triangle test, three samples are presented simultaneously in which two samples are alike and one is different. Panelists are asked to identify the odd sample. Thus, there is 33.3% chance of getting the right answer.

C. *Duo-trio test:* This test is also an overall difference tests due to multi-attribute evaluation. It is a mix of the earlier two difference tests. In the duo-trio test, the reference sample is presented first; it is then followed by other two samples, one of which is same as the reference. The panelist is asked to identify which of the last two samples is same as/or different from the reference. There is 50% chance of getting the right answer.

**(ii) Descriptive tests:** These are one of the most sophisticated, flexible and widely used tools in the sensory analysis. Descriptive tests have a number of advantages over difference tests and been used to describe and quantify the differences between the meat products and their sensory attributes.

A. *Flavor profile test:* In this test, potential panelists are screened according to their abilities to discriminate aroma and flavor differences. The test uses descriptive terms to characterize the flavor of a product as well as provide the intensities and order of appearance of the various aromas, flavors, and aftertastes detected. After the four to six members of a panel individually evaluate a sample, the results are submitted to the panel leader, who leads a discussion to arrive at a general consensus of the sample **(Fig. 37.2)**. Reference samples can be used to present flavor attributes. Data can be presented in tabular or verbal format. With this method, panelist effects are not accounted for.

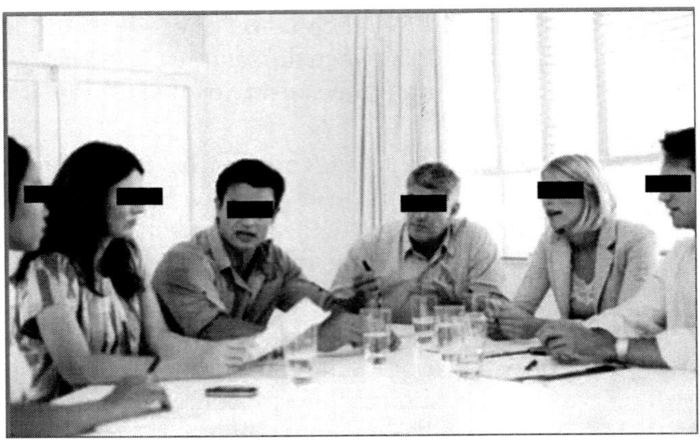

**Fig. 37.2:** Flavor profile test in progress.

B. *Texture profile test:* This test is based on the same concept as flavor profiling in that overall texture of a product is comprised of a number of different texture attributes. Panelists define the procedures and terminology to use in the textural evaluation.

Texture attributes in the texture profile test can be classified as to the following:

- Mechanical
- Geometrical
- Those related to moisture and fat content

Mechanical characteristics are revealed as the meat samples react to stress, such as chewing. Geometrical characteristics relate to size, shape, and orientation of the product before and during breakdown. The contributions of moisture and fat are determined through mouth feel. Texture references have been developed and can be used for training.

C. *Meat descriptive attributes test:* This is a unified method of evaluating several quality attributes of meat product samples at the same time. The test is widely used in the product development as well as shelf-life studies of processed meat products. It uses 8-point or 9-point descriptive scale for each attribute. The test requires training on each attribute and use of uniform cooking as well as product sampling. In the trained meat descriptive attributes test, 'first sample bias' can be an issue. Hence, a standardized 'warm-up sample', usually a sample that represents the typical product, should be served to the panelists at the initiation of sensory session.

D. *Sensory spectrum:* This technique is an expansion of descriptive sensory analysis where instead of panel specific descriptive scale, the panelist use a standardized word list called lexicon. The training of panelists is more extensive and they are provided with the lexicons that are used to describe perceived sensations associated with the samples. The panelists use a numerical intensity scale—usually a 15-point scale and they are supplied with reference standards.

E. *Spider chart (also called Web diagram/Radar chart):* It is a visual tool to organize data in a logical way. It is a graphical method of displaying multivariate data (attributes) in the form of two-dimensional chart of three or more variables (scores) represented on axis starting from the same point. This gives the plot a star-like appearance. The main advantage of spider chart is its capablity of creating more focus and comprehension resulting in quick comparisons **(Fig. 37.3)**.

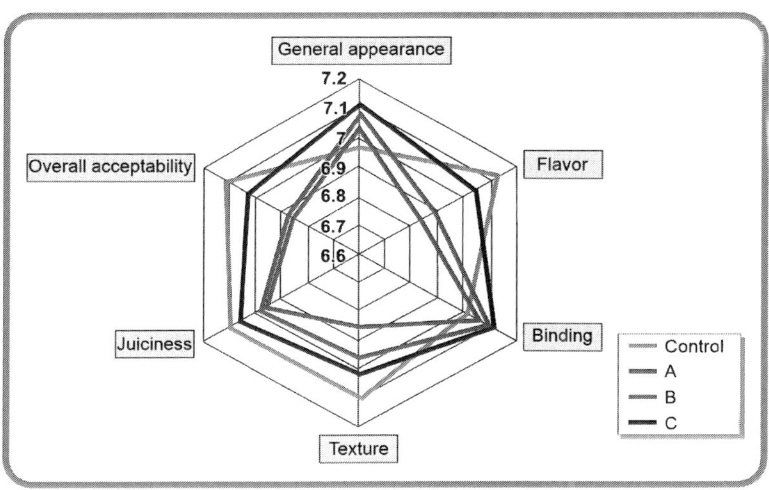


**Fig. 37.3:** Spider chart—sensory attributes.

**2. Affective methods:** These are commonly referred as consumer panel evaluation and usually performed towards the end of product development. The tests are consumer oriented who are not trained but they are potential consumers of the meat product irrespective of their gender, age, social or economic level. In consumer assessment of meat products, the serving size should be standardized in such a way as to get actual consumer eating experience. The serving temperature of meat products for consumer evaluation should be 40°C. The test can be conducted at the market place, grocery store, restaurants, factory premises, fairs, etc. The number of participating consumers should be 100 or more.

A. *Acceptance test:* In this test, the product is rated by the potential consumers on a scale of absolute liking/acceptability. Degree of liking is structured in the short ballot. The option of 'did not like' should also be there. Just About Right (JAR) scale can be used if the product is being tested for specific attribute. In another test form, there may be a paired comparison between the developed product and the existing competitive product in the market. In yet another form of this test, the developed product with minor variations is subjected to acceptance test by potential consumers on a hedonic or eating pleasure scale. The pro forma should be as short as possible in order to avoid 'halo effect'. It is a type of cognitive bias where impression of one attribute influences the acceptance of other attributes of the product. In some western countries, they use Emoji as a simplified version for recording consumer evaluation **(Fig. 37.4)**.

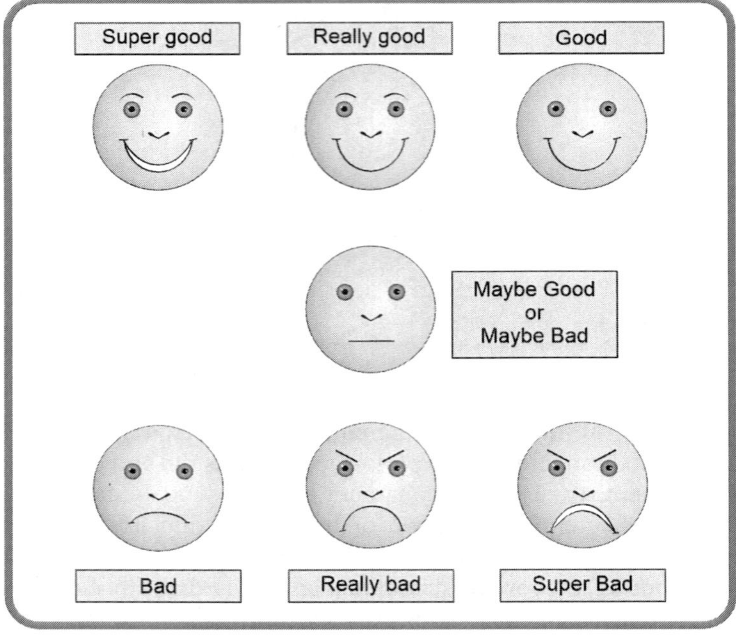


**Fig. 37.4:** Emoji in consumer evaluation.

B. *Preference rest:* These are conducted as ranking test where the various samples of a meat product are ranked by the potential consumers for the intensity of a particular attribute in order of their descending or ascending preferences. This simple test uses large number of prospective consumers. The data is subjected to non-parametric analysis.

Sensory evaluation is a unique science which uses human senses as tools. The food technologists have to rely on sensory evaluation as no instruments can substitute for the instantaneous perception of a food by five human senses. There are several variations and alternative methods even in methods and guidelines suggested by AMSA (2015) and ASTM International. Several concepts are being reviewed, reoriented and realigned in order to derive maximum advantages from these tests. So, we need to apply the right sensory evaluation test in a given situation.

# 38 CHAPTER

# Developments in Sustainable Packaging of Muscle Foods

Packaging plays a crucial role in the modern life. Packaging not only contains, protects and enhances shelf-life a food but also provides base for labeling besides acting as a marketing tool. Traditional plastics are widely used for food packaging materials because of several unique properties. These are chemically inert, light weight and cost-effective. They provide wide choices in respect of transparency, heat sealing, color, heat resistance and barrier properties. They are moldable to make film sheets, shapes and structures.

Most of today's synthetic polymers are produced from petrochemicals and are not biodegradable. Their persistent use generates lot of environment pollution. Worldwide, more than 250 million tonnes of such plastics are being produced annually. Nearly 60% of the total plastic is used for food packaging sector while 40% of plastic produced is used only once and then discarded. Packaging industry has now started getting a bad publicity due to lot of single-use plastic, nonrecyclable materials, excessive use of resources, increasing landfills and harm being caused to marine environment. A plastic bag decomposes in decades and plastic water bottle takes 450 years to decompose. Several widely used packaging plastics can take up to 200–1000 years to degrade in landfills that emit greenhouse gases.

Many of us are well aware of Great Pacific Garbage Patch which is bigger in size than the size of Spain and swimming with non-biodegradable plastic waste. The birds, fish and other marine life are dying because they either eat it or get entangled up in the plastics. Ghent University, Belgium scientists have predicted that by 2050, the volume of plastics accumulated in our oceans will be greater than that of fish. Global warming and climate changes are real threats that are happening right now. These are the results of increase in greenhouse gases in the atmosphere. So, we are required to reduce our individual carbon footprints. It should also be noted that synthetic plastics are manufactured from fossil fuel which is a limited, non-renewable resource and bound to be run out. These conditions call for urgent need to explore, design and use sustainable packaging from renewable resources in order to maintain ecological balance.

Sustainable packaging refers to the development and use of packaging that is reusable, renewable, recyclable and biodegradable/ compostable while being designed to reduce environmental impact and ecological footprint. It takes the holistic view and is always an environmental-friendly packaging. It is also referred as green packaging. Sustainable packaging offers many benefits like (i) reduction in waste (ii) recycling of used product packaging (iii) cleaner production process and (iv) most importantly, reducing threat to the environment.

**3-R Principle:** Sustainable packaging follows the highly popular 3-R principle of waste minimization—reduce, reuse, recycle in the context of both production and consumption.

1. **Reduce:** Reducing the amount of waste at source is the best way to conserve the environment. Only required minimum packaging has to be used.
2. **Reuse:** The packaging can be reusable either for the same purpose or for a different use. Reuse is preferred over recycling because it saves the cost of reprocessing and managing the generated waste.
3. **Recycle:** Recycling is the process of converting the waste of one product which can again be used for creating new product. It reduces the environmental footprint.

The term biodegradable is used to describe those materials which can be degraded by enzymatic action of organisms like bacteria, yeast, fungi, etc. This biodegradation results in the formation of carbon dioxide, water and biomass which are returned to the nature by way of biocycle. Biodegradation occurs in the presence of moisture and microorganisms typically found in the environment. This process is triggered by heat and mechanical stress. Biodegradable materials are made from renewable sources, so they completely breakdown and decompose into natural elements within a short time after disposal—typically in a year or less. Compostable materials are also similar to biodegradable materials but they can degrade at a faster rate in designated sites under specific conditions of sunlight, temperature, wind, etc. They provide rich nutrients once the material is completely broken down.

Ecofriendly packaging can be biodegradable, but it is mostly compostable because of its origin from 100% recyclable plant-based materials. Ecofriendly packaging from biodegradable materials like corn starch, sugarcane bagasse, cassava, etc., contribute to environmental sustainability because (i) they make use of renewable materials (ii) their manufacturing process consumes less energy (iii) they do not release harmful carbon (iv) they decompose in significantly less time and do not pile up in landfills (v) these materials do not pollute our planet.

## SOURCES OF BIODEGRADABLE POLYMERS

1. **Polysaccharides:** Starches, wheat, potatoes, maize, cassava, etc.
2. **Lignocellulose products:** Wood, straw, etc.
3. **Others:** Pectin, chitosan, gums, etc.

Biopolymers are divided into three main categories according to their method of production:

1. Biopolymers obtained from chemically modified natural products
   - Starches (wheat, potato, maize, cassava), cellulose, chitin and chitosan, soy-based plastics, etc.
2. Biopolymers produced through fermentation of microorganisms
   - Polyesters, natural polysaccharide, etc.
3. Biopolymers obtained from chemical synthesis
   - Polylactic acid (PLA), polyglycolic acid (PGA), polycaprolactone, polyvinyl alcohol, etc.

The packaging has to be either recyclable or biodegradable or compostable so that it does not end up in landfill. The use of biodegradable polymer reduces the environmental impact of non-biodegradable plastics.

## SOME RECENT COMMERCIAL DEVELOPMENTS

Bio4Pack, Netherland (2017) has succeeded in producing a sustainable packaging solution for fresh meat that meets the requirements pertaining to renewability as well as compostability. The dish is made out of PLA (polylactic acid), which is made from sugarcane, providing renewable and compostable packaging for fresh meat. The impact additive gives the dish the required strength. A pigment gives the dish its characteristic green color **(Fig. 38.1)**.

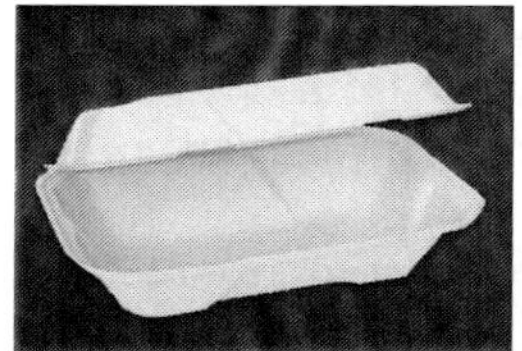 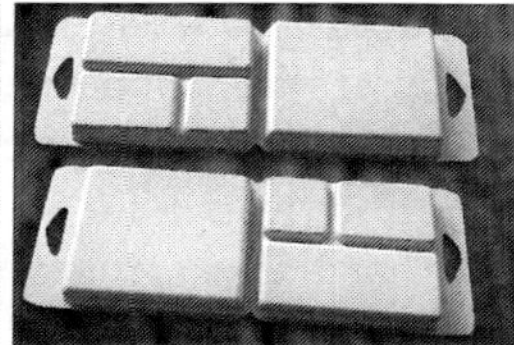 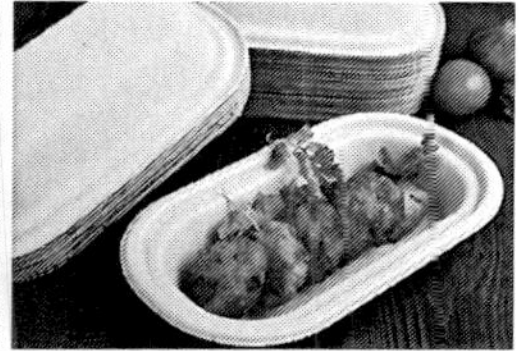

**Fig. 38.1:** Bagasse trays.

Justine Muller (2017) extensively studied the polylactic acid (PLA) and starch as potential replacements for non-degradable petrochemical polymers on the basis of their availability, adequate food contact properties and competitive cost. Their combination as blend or multilayer films could provide properties that are more adequate for packaging purposes on the basis of their complementary characteristics.

CP Foods, Thailand (2018) launched green packaging for meat range. It is also using plant-based polylactic acid (PLA) trays, which is a compostable bioplastic made from natural renewable resources, as a replacement for plastic tray in chilled raw chicken and pork products. The company has redesigned its food packages, for example, packages for fresh chicken, and pork products, to optimize all resources used in food production, reducing waste, especially plastic waste, and promote the use of environmental-friendly materials in accordance with the concept of Circular Economy. As a part of the initiative, CP Foods has redesigned many of its packages such as replacing raw chicken products' multilayer plastic package with a single layer package that is smaller and 100% recyclable, resulting in 24% cost saving.

Plantic Technologies, Australia, is using a combination of plant-based and recycled materials to create meat packaging. This type of packaging is unique when compared to commonly used oil-based packaging. The material is proven to give substantial environmental benefits through a reduction in $CO_2$ emissions Plantic Technologies (2015) primary raw material is a naturally high amylose starch, derived from corn which has been hybridized over a number generations whose special chemical properties allow for a wide range of applications, including thermoforming, injection molding, film extrusion and blow molding, as well as rigid and flexible packaging. PLANTIC™ HP is 100% biodegradable sheet and can be used in a number of packaging applications. It provides outstanding gas barrier properties and is the high performance environmental material. Plantic Eco Plastic is high barrier multilayer rigid and semirigid sheet used for packaging refrigerated goods such as meats and fish. The core layer of the structure is predominately made from corn starch and constitutes about 80% of the total structure. The skin layers are primarily polyethylene and polypropylene.

Sirane's, Iceland launched Earth Packaging range of compostable food packaging solutions in January, 2019. The Earthpouch is made from a paper with a 100% plastic-free heat-sealable coating which is then formed into a preformed stand-up pouch which provides total food security for dry and moist food products. It reduces both packaging waste and food waste. Other compostable food packaging from Sirane includes breathable bags and films for extending the life of fresh produce. Sira-Flex Resolve is a natural biopolymer which can be made into bags or films, can extend shelf-life by many days. Sirane's Sira-Flex™ Resolve® is a unique plant-based breathable film developed to have the optimum balance between humidity control and $O_2$ and $CO_2$ permeability to prevent degradation. Other compostable products include absorbent pads for meat, poultry and seafood. Integrating antimicrobial or antibacterial technology, for example, can help extend the shelf-life even further, helping to achieve 20% reduction in food waste.

Accredo, USA, has come up with recyclable stand-up pouch which provides the consumer a more sustainable proposition of recyclability: Using renewable-sourced resin from sugarcane feedstock (as opposed to hydrocarbon-based feedstock), Accredo has successfully pioneered sustainably produced packaging with a highly renewable content. It has end use market applications for frozen animal protein-based products (chicken, fish and shellfish). It reduces carbon footprint and impact of global warming and climate change. Accredo was the first company globally to manufacture a zippered stand-up pouch made from certified compostable component as per standards for compostability in industrial composting facilities. New developments in compostable film technology enable us to produce compostable packaging that achieves the highest moisture and gas barriers.

Clyser (USA) has made promising advances in commercially viable plastics made from organic materials that can be replenished, such as polylactic acid (PLA) derived from corn. PLAnet™ shrink film from Clysar (USA) for example, is an ideal candidate for packages where renewable, bio-based content is desired. The industry's first 100% renewable, compostable PLA shrink film, 90% this film will biodegrade in 12 weeks in home or industrial composting facilities. It does not sacrifice packaging performance or appearance and display film offers balanced shrink in all directions **(Fig. 38.2)**.

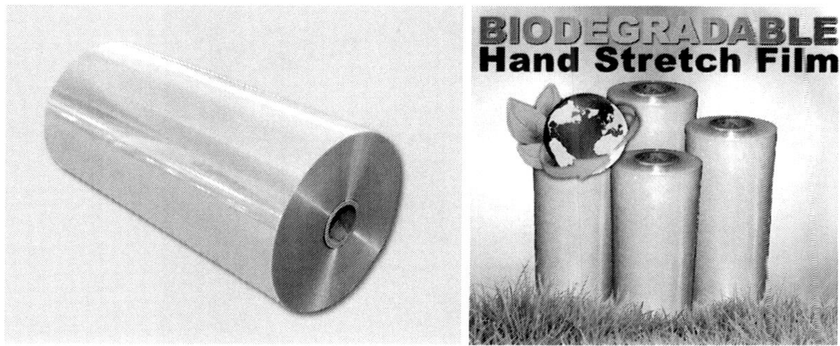


**Fig. 38.2:** PLA shrink film.

Total Packaging Solutions (TPS), USA, provides expert ecofriendly packaging services across the food industry. TPS is source for 'green' ecofriendly solutions—certified disposable containers, tableware, and compostable packaging—made from renewable and sustainable bamboo products. Total Packaging Solutions supplies high quality MAP supplies to leading companies serving the food industry. Total Packaging Solution compostable products include hot soup cups as well as bamboo and bagasse trays. Their barrier products include vacuum bags and vacuum as well as MAP pouches. Biodegradable vacuum pouches have been introduced in the United Kingdom as Eco-pouches **(Fig. 38.3)**. These are made up of corn starch, cassava and eucalyptus fiber. These pouches are 100% decomposable. They are ocean friendly and dissolve in marine environment within 26 weeks and in commercial composting conditions in 12 weeks. The pouches are a natural barrier to aroma, oil and grease. These are suitable for meat cuts, dressed poultry and cooked meat as well as poultry products.

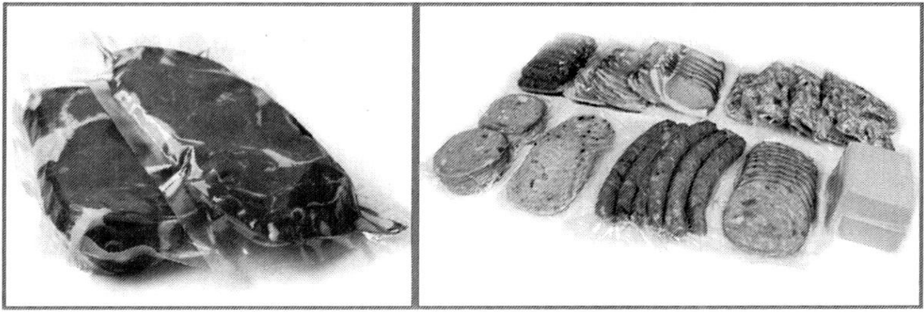

**Fig. 38.3:** Eco-vacuum pouches.

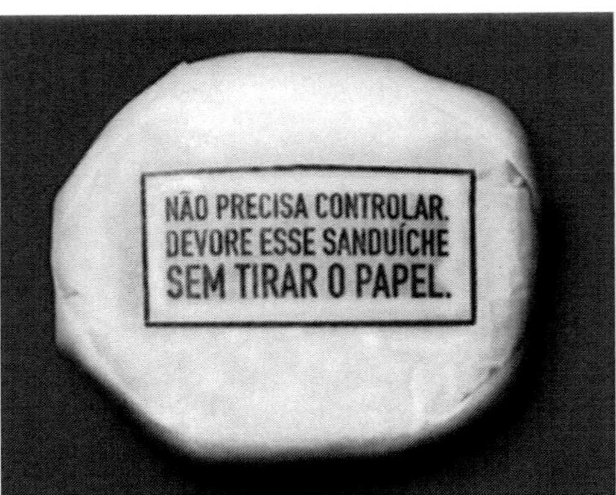


**Fig. 38.4:** Burger with edible wrapper.

Edible packaging is also environment friendly and reduces the waste and solid disposal problem. It is a thin continuous layer of edible material formed on or placed on the food. Thus package is an integral part of food and can be eaten along with food **(Fig. 38.4)**. Edible packaging retards moisture migration as well as gas permeability retains volatile flavor compounds and may improve mechanical handling. Edible collagen casings for salami and smoke house snacks are quite popular in this category. These casings are required to be kept in refrigerator when not in use and soaked in water for 2–3 minutes before putting on the stuffer.

## NANOCOMPOSITES

A newer development in this field addresses the issues of poor barrier properties and weak mechanical properties generally encountered in biopolymers.

The application of nanocomposites could bring about modification in the properties of biomaterials. It can make them lighter and improve the strength as well. This technique promises to expand the use of biopolymers in processed muscle foods by supporting preservation and extending shelf-life. Antimicrobials such as nanoparticles of silver or titanium can be used for this purpose. Whey protein isolate (WPI) film embedded with titanium nano-particles have great potential for extending shelf-life of packaged meat products.

Plant-based sustainable packages made from renewable, low carbon or recycled materials are emerging as good alternative to plastic packaging. Their use is bound to increase and ultimately replace the fossil fuel-based packages in future.

# Bibliography


- Agricultural and Processed Food Products Export Development Agency (APEDA) Report, 2020-21.
- Animal Welfare Board of India,1962.
- APEDA National Programme for Organic Production (NPOP), 2001 to 2014.
- Bartholonew DT, Osualo CI. Acceptability of flavour, texture and appearance in processed meat products. Journal of Food Science. (1986):51(6):1560-62.
- Centre for Science and Environment (CSE), 2004.
- Chander M. Organic Animal Husbandry Standards – Proceeding of National Workshop. IVRI: Izatnagar; 2002.
- Codex Alimentarious Commission. Report of the 26th Session of the Codex Alimentarious Commission. Rome, FAO, 2003.
- Cole DJA, Lawrie RA. *Meat.* The Butterworth and Company (Publishers) Ltd., London; 1975.
- FAO/WHO (2003). Expert consultations on the safety assessment of foods derived from genetically modified animals, including fish. Rome, FAO; 2003.
- Food Safety and Standard Act, 2006.
- Frazier WC, Westhoff DC. *Food Microbiology,* 3rd edn. Tata McGraw Hill Publishing Company, New Delhi; 1978.
- FSSAI Food Safety and Standards (Food Products Standards and Food Additives) Amendment Regulations, 2018 on various types of meat.
- Golomski WA. ISO 9000: The global perspective. Food Technology. 1994;48(12):57-59.

- Gopakumar K. Textbook of Fish Processing Technology. Indian Council of Agricultural Research. New Delhi; 2006.
- Hofstad MS, Calnek BW, Helmboldt CF, Reid WM, Yader, Jr HW. Diseases of Poultry. Oxford and IBH Publishing Co., New Delhi; 1975.
- http://www.monsanto.com/monsanto/gurt/default.htm
- http://www.csa.com/discoveryguides/gmfood/overview.php
- Japson A. Danish Standards in Meat Hygiene. WHO/FAO, Geneva; 1957.
- Jay JM. Modern Food Microbiology, 3rd edn. CBS Publishers and Distributors, Delhi; 1986.
- Komark LS, Tressler DK and Long L. Food Products Formulatory, Vol. I. The AVI Publishing Company Inc., Westport, Connecticut; 1974.
- Kondaiah N. Export potential of meat and meat products. National symposium on meat and milk industry: Trends and Developmental Strategies. Hisar; 1994.
- Kumar S, Sharma BD. Prospects of processing meat from spent animals in 21st century. In: Prospects of Livestock and Poultry Development in 21st Century (ed. Rishendra Verma *et. al.*), IAAVR Publication, Bareilly, 1996.
- Lawrie RA. Meat (eds DJA Cole and RA Lawrie). Butterworth and Company (Publishers) Ltd., London,1975; p. 249.
- Lawrie RA. Meat Science, 3rd edn. Pergamon Press, Oxford. 1979.
- Leistner L, Rodel W. The stability of intermediate moisture food with respect of microorganisms. In "Intermediate Moisture Foods", (eds Davies R, Birch GG, Parker KJ), Applied Science Publishers, London. 1976.
- Levie A. The Meat Handbook. The AVI Publishing Company, Inc.,Westport, Connecticut. 1970.
- Mendiratta SK, Kumar S, Keshri RC, Sharma BD. Comparative efficiency of microwave oven for cooking of chicken meat. Fleischwirtschaft. 1998;78(7):827-28.
- Mountney GT. Poultry Products Technology, 2nd edn. The AVI Publishing Company, Westport, Connecticut. 1976.
- Nag S, Sharma BD, Kumar S. Quality attributes and shelf life of chicken nuggets extended with rice flour. Indian Journal of Poultry Science. 1998;32(2):182-6.

- Padda GS, Sharma BD, Sharma N. Oxidative discolouration and rancidity in meat - a review. Indian Food Packer. 1987;41(6):31-45.
- Padda GS, Sharma BD. Massaging and tumbling (M&T): Recent development in meat technology. Livestock Advisor. 1985;10(8):13-15.
- Padda GS, Sharma BD, Keshri RC. Research priorities for meat in India. Indian Food Industry. 1986;7(2):1-8.
- Padda GS, Sharma N, Sharma BD. Profiles of some processed meat products developed at IVRI. Beverage and Food World. 1988;15(1):31-34.
- Panda B, Mahapatra SC. Poultry Production, ICAR Publication, New Delhi. 1989.
- Panda PC. Textbook on Egg and Poultry Technology. Vikas Publishing House Pvt. Ltd., New Delhi. 1976.
- Pearson AM, Tauber FW. Processed Meats. The AVI Publishing Company, Inc., Westport, Connecticut. 1973.
- Press Information Bureau, Govt. of India 2oth Livestock Census, 2019.
- Prevention of Cruelty to Animals Act, 1960.
- Price JF, Schweigert BS. The Science of Meat and Meat Products, 2nd edn. WH Feeman and Company, USA. 1971.
- Sen AR, Sharma BD, Yadav, PL. Effect of milk-co-precipitate incorporation on physico-chemical and sensory quality of chicken loaf. Indian Journal of Poultry Science. 1994;29(2):201-203.
- Sharma BD. Meat and Meat Products Technology, 2nd Edition. Jaypee Brothers Medical Publishers, New Delhi. 2020.
- Sharma BD, Bachhil VN, Bisht GS. Effect of hot and chilled boning and subsequent processing on the quality characteristics of pork. Indian J. Meat Sci. 1990;3(1):1-9.
- Sharma BD. Meat and Meat Products Technology, 2nd edition. Jaypee Brothers Medical Publishers, New Delhi. 2020.
- Sharma BD, Padda GS, Joshi HB. Use of milk proteins in meat products: A review. Indian Dairyman. 1985;37(11):48-491.
- Sharma BD, Padda GS, Yadav PL. Development of gravy bases for meat curry. Beverage and Food World. 1994;21(4):7-8, 12.
- Sharma BD, Padda GS, Sharma N. Off flavors in meat. Livestock Advisor. 1986;11(9):5-8.

- Sharma BD, Rao VK, Sanyal MK, Yadav PL. Effect of colostrum incorporation on the physico-chemical and palatability properties of mutton loaf. Beverage and Food World. 1992;19(1):37-38.
- Sharma BD, Sharma N, Chatterjee AK, Padda GS. Packaging of meat and meat products. Indian Food Packer. 1985;39(6):40-44.
- Sharma BD, Singh SP, Singh P. Processed meat products–emerging scenario and potential in India. Livestock Advisor. 1995;20(3)28-30.
- Sharma BD, Wani SA, Sharma N. Sensory Evaluation Manual for Meat and Meat Products. Publication No. 36, IVRI, Izatnagar, 1997.
- Sharma N, Keshri RC, Sharma BD, Padda GS, Kondaiah N. Studies on processing and palatability properties of pork tikka. In: Advances in Meat Research. R and B Cross Publishers, Bombay. 1987;96-102.
- Sohrab. ISO-9000 through HACCP. Indian Food Industries, 1977.
- Singh SP, Singh P, Prakash R, Sharma BD. Estimation of yield of livestock byproducts at state and national level in India. Agricultural situation in India. 1987;159-63.
- Singh SP, Singh P, Sharma BD, Prakash R. Perspectives on meat production and marketing. The Economic Times, Bombay. 1987.
- Singh YP, Sharma BD. Consumer attitude towards poultry meat. Processed Food Industry. 1998;1(11):17-18.
- Suzuki T. Fish and krill protein processing technology. Applied Science Publishers, London. 1981.
- Thatcher FS. Meat and Meat Products Technology Including Poultry Products Technology. Journal of Applied Bacteriology. 1963; 16:226.
- Watt BK, Merril AL. Composition of Foods: Raw, Processed, Prepared. USDA Handbook No. 8. 1963.
- Winton LA, Winton KB. Fish and fish products. Allied Scientific Publishers, Bikaner. 1999.

# Index

Page numbers followed by *f* refer to figure, *fc* refer to flowchart, and *t* refer to table.

## B

# D

# F

# I



# J

## K



## L

## N

## S